MECHANISMS IN RECOMBINATION

MECHANISMS IN RECOMBINATION

Edited by

Rhoda F. Grell

Biology Division
Oak Ridge National Laboratory
Oak Ridge, Tennessee

PLENUM PRESS • NEW YORK AND LONDON

Library of Congress Cataloging in Publication Data

Main entry under title:

Mechanisms in recombination.

"Proceedings of the twenty-seventh Biology Division research conference held
in Gatlinburg, Tennessee, March 31-April 4, 1974."
Includes bibliographies and index.
1. Genetic recombination. I. Grell, Rhoda Frank,   ed. II. United
States. National Laboratory, Oak Ridge, Tenn. Biology Division. [DNLM: 1.
Recombination, Genetic—Congresses. QH443 011m 1974]
QH443.M42   575.2'1   74-20987
ISBN 0-306-30823-1

Proceedings of the Twenty-Seventh Biology Division Research Conference
held in Gatlinburg, Tennessee, March 31-April 4, 1974

© 1974 Plenum Press, New York
A Division of Plenum Publishing Corporation
227 West 17th Street, New York, N. Y. 10011

United Kingdom edition published by Plenum Press, London
A Division of Plenum Publishing Company, Ltd.
4a Lower John Street, London, W1R 3PD, England

This volume is dedicated to three pioneers in the study of recombination

CARL C. LINDEGREN

MARY B. MITCHELL

ALEXANDER WEINSTEIN

Foreword

This book contains the papers presented at the Twenty-Seventh
Annual Biology Division Research Conference which was held April
1-4, 1974 in Gatlinburg, Tennessee. The topic of the symposium
was Mechanisms in Recombination and it follows by exactly twenty
years the previous Gatlinburg Symposium on Genetic Recombination.
During this interval, and the preceding years as well, the process
of recombination has remained a central and tantalizing problem
for geneticists. The subject assumes added significance with the
recent appeal by a committee of leading scientists for a moratorium
on the construction of certain types of recombinant molecules.
That autonomously replicating molecules linking portions of prokaryotic and eukaryotic DNA can now be produced *in vitro* attests
to the technical advances that have taken place in this field.
Nevertheless, the details underlying the process *in vivo* continue
to be elusive.

This symposium brought together individuals studying recombination in organisms as widely separated as bacteriophage and mammals
and using disciplinary approaches of comparable diversity. Consequently the present volume summarizes much of current strategies
and concepts concerning the subject.

The meeting was sponsored by the Biology Division of the Oak
Ridge National Laboratory (operated by the Union Carbide Corporation
for the U. S. Atomic Energy Commission) with the support and encour-
agement of its director, H. I. Adler. The organizing committee was
chaired by J. K. Setlow and included R. F. Grell, R. D. Hotchkiss
and E. Volkin. Special thanks are due to the speakers, to I. R.
Lehman, G. Mosig, S. H. Goodgal, R. K. Mortimer, C. W. Hinton, and
R. D. Hotchkiss who acted as chairmen of the sessions, and to M. J.
Loop for arranging many of the details. I am happy to acknowledge
the invaluable assistance of C. L. Smith and the generous help of
W. E. Cohn in the editing of this volume.

Rhoda F. Grell
Editor

September, 1974

Contents

RECOMBINATION IN FUNGI

RECOMBINATION IN HIGHER EUKARYOTES

MODELS OF RECOMBINATION

RECOMBINATION IN BACTERIA AND THEIR PHAGES

EXCHANGE OF PARENTAL DNA DURING GENETIC RECOMBINATION IN

BACTERIOPHAGE φX174

Robert M. Benbow*, Anthony J. Zuccarelli[†], Alma J.

Shafer and Robert L. Sinsheimer

Division of Biology, California Institute of Technology,

Pasadena, California 91109

SUMMARY

Two-factor crosses were performed between *am* mutants of φX174 in which one or both of the single-stranded parental bacteriophages were labeled with heavy isotopes. Recombinants were formed that contained DNA from each of the two parental phages and were composed almost entirely of parental RF DNA. A small amount of the parental-strand DNA (less than 700 nucleotides on the average) was removed and replaced during the formation of a recombinant molecule.

INTRODUCTION

Genetic recombination often involves breakage and reunion of preexisting parental chromosomes (Meselson, 1967). This was first established by examining the density of recombinants of bacteriophage λ formed in two-factor crosses in which one parental chromosome was labeled with heavy isotopes, and one with light isotopes (Meselson and Weigle, 1961; Kellenberger *et al.*, 1961). That such

---

* Present address: MRC Laboratory of Molecular Biology, Hills Road, Cambridge, England CB2-2QH.

[†] Present address: Fachbereich Biologie, Universität Konstanz, D-775 Konstanz, West Germany.

3

recombinants were formed almost entirely of parental DNA was established by examining the density of recombinants formed in two-factor crosses carried out in an unlabeled host between bacteriophages both labeled with heavy isotopes (Meselson, 1962). Furthermore, since the recombinants formed in these heavy-heavy crosses were found to contain small amounts of light isotopes, Meselson suggested that a small amount of DNA was removed and resynthesized during the formation of recombinant molecules (Meselson, 1964).

RECOMBINANT FORMATION BETWEEN ϕX174 PARENTAL RF DNA MOLECULES

The density exchange experiments described below involved the use of heavy isotopes incorporated into one or both of the original single-stranded parental ϕX DNA molecules. As reported previously (Sinsheimer *et al.*, 1962) infection of the host cell with heavy bacteriophage resulted in the formation of parental RF DNA molecules of hybrid (heavy-light) density. The heavy isotopes, when employed, were always found in the (+) or parental strand; the (-) or complementary strand always contained only light isotopes. Because of this inherent symmetry in our experimental design, we found it desirable to reexamine the key evidence establishing the major pathway of ϕX174 recombinant formation (Benbow *et al.*, 1974b), paying particular attention to the parental (+) DNA strand. As we shall show, interpretation of our density exchange experiments involves several assumptions about the recombinational equivalence of the two strands of an RF molecule.

FATE OF THE PARENTAL STRAND DURING RECOMBINANT FORMATION

The major pathway for ϕX174 recombinant formation is summarized in Fig. 1 (Benbow *et al.*, 1974b). Two single-stranded parental phages of different genotype (Fig. 1a) attach to a single host cell and undergo eclipse, and their DNA [*i.e.* the parental (+) strand, which may or may not be density labeled] penetrates into the cell (Newbold and Sinsheimer, 1970). Double-stranded parental RF DNA is formed immediately (Sinsheimer *et al.*, 1962; Zuccarelli *et al.*, 1974), at an essential bacterial site (Yarus and Sinsheimer, 1967) (Fig. 1b).

Recombinant formation is initiated (Fig. 1c) by the occurrence of a single-strand "break" in either strand (see below) of one of

---

Figure 1. The major pathway for ϕX174 recombinant formation. The original parental (+) DNA strands and genetic markers are represented by solid heavy lines (━━). All subsequently synthesized DNA strands and genetic markers are represented by solid thin lines

φX174 RECOMBINANT FORMATION

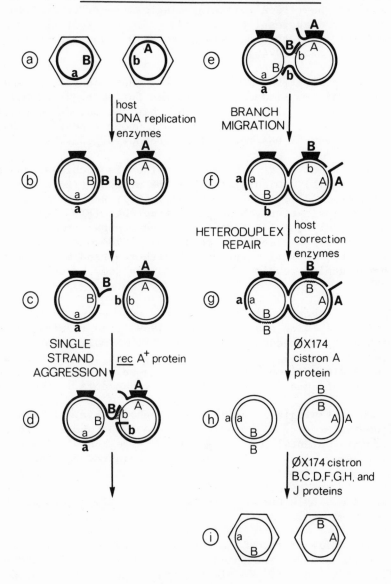

(———). Heteroduplex mismatch repair synthesis is indicated by a
jagged thin line (⋀⋀⋀). To minimize confusion, the actions of ligase, polymerase I, and repair of nucleolytic enzymes usually are
not indicated. Enzymes or proteins known to be involved in specific
steps are indicated in lower-case type. Branch migration definitely
does not require any enzyme.

the two parental RF DNA molecules (Benbow *et al.*, 1974c).   In the
presence of the host *recA*[+] protein, single-strand "breaks" in
either strand are aggressive (Fig. 1d).   Figure-eight DNA molecules
are formed (Fig. 1e) that contain parental DNA and can be recombinant (Benbow *et al.*, 1974b).

Only parental RF DNA molecules [*i.e.* those containing the infecting parental (+) strand] are utilized for most ϕX recombinant
formation (Benbow *et al.*, 1974a).   For this reason, our density
exchange experiments could be carried out under conditions that
restricted progeny RF DNA replication (Benbow *et al.*, 1972a).

The next event in recombinant formation is double-strand branch
migration (Fig. 1f), which stabilizes the nascent figure-eight DNA
molecules (Lee *et al.*, 1970; Kim *et al.*, 1972; Benbow *et al.*, 1974b).
Heteroduplex repair of any base-pair mismatches (Fig. 1g) then may
take place rapidly [at least repair has been shown in *artificial*
heteroduplexes by Weisbeek and van de Pol (1970) and by Baas and
Jansz (1972a,b)].   Short stretches of either strand may be removed
during heteroduplex repair (Fig. 1g) and replaced by unlabeled nucleotides.

In normal recombinant formation, the subsequent formation of
progeny RF DNA (Levine and Sinsheimer, 1969) then results in a high
yield of homozygous recombinant progeny RF DNA molecules (Fig. 1h).
However, since most of our density exchange experiments were designed to examine only parental RF DNA, these progeny RF molecules
usually were not detected in representative amounts.

Recombinant single-stranded bacteriophage (Fig. 1i) are replicated from the progeny RF, and these recombinant phage in general
do not contain parental DNA.   None of the nine known ϕX174 cistron
products (Benbow *et al.*, 1971, 1972b) are required for recombinant
formation.   Recombinants are produced in about 1% of all multiply
infected cells and can be recovered from single cells in nonreciprocal asymmetric single bursts (Benbow *et al.*, 1974a; Doniger *et al.*,
1973).

If this model of recombinant formation is correct, it is cru-
cial to decide whether the three key processes — single-strand
aggression (Fig. 1d), figure-eight formation (Fig. 1e), and double-
strand branch migration (Fig. 1f) — exhibit any strand preferences.
Any strand bias will be reflected in the results of our density
exchange experiments.

ARE BOTH STRANDS AGGRESSIVE?

Evidence that ϕX174 recombinant formation is stimulated (in
recA[+] cells) by introduction of single-strand "breaks" into one of

the two parental RF DNA molecules is summarized in Fig. 2. The
clearest evidence was obtained by ultraviolet irradiation of the
single-stranded parental bacteriophage prior to infection; this resulted in the formation of damaged replicative-form structures
after infection that were recombination proficient. Unfortunately,
however, the ultraviolet lesions were necessarily in the parental
or (+) strand only, and synthesis of the complementary (-) strand
was halted at most lesions (Benbow *et al.*, 1974c). The net result
was that most parental (+) strands remained intact and circular,
while most complementary (-) strands contained a "break."   Therefore, this experiment provided solid evidence only for complementary
strand aggression*.

    In contrast, recombination-proficient single-strand "breaks"
were introduced into *both* strands of parental RF DNA molecules by
thymine starvation (Benbow *et al.*, 1974c). Since these "breaks"
were not visible in electron micrographs (Fig. 2), no more than 50
nucleotides could have been missing at each "break" (Davis *et al.*,
1971). In addition, since both strands contained "breaks" with
similar frequencies, it was likely (though not rigorously proven)
that parental (+) as well as complementary (-) strand aggression
occurred during recombinant formation.

    Our third line of evidence for single-strand aggression corre-
lated the presence of specific single-strand "breaks" within cistron A with a recombination "hot spot" observed in that cistron
(Fig. 2) (Benbow *et al.*, 1971; Benbow *et al.*, 1974c). Thus, nascent
parental RF DNA molecules were expected to contain a "break" in
cistron A as a result of the initiation of the first complementary
strand near or in that cistron (Zuccarelli *et al.*, 1974a). These
"breaks" would be available early in infection when most φX174 recombinant formation occurs. Therefore, we have attributed the high
recombination region within cistron A to complementary (-) strand
aggression arising from these "breaks." We wish to point out, however, that a parental (+) strand "break" in cistron A also is observed (Fig. 2) later in infection (Johnson and Sinsheimer, 1974).
Therefore, parental (+) strand aggression may occur, depending on

---

    * In principle we cannot decide whether the incomplete comple-
mentary (-) strand was aggressive against the intact duplex, or
alternatively whether a random "nick" in the complementary (-)
strand of the *other* duplex allowed its complementary (-) strand to
pair with the extensive single-stranded region of the parental (+)
strand of the damaged molecule. However, we favor the former interpretation because ultraviolet irradiated episomes transferred
during conjugation are recombination proficient (Benbow *et al.*,
1973).

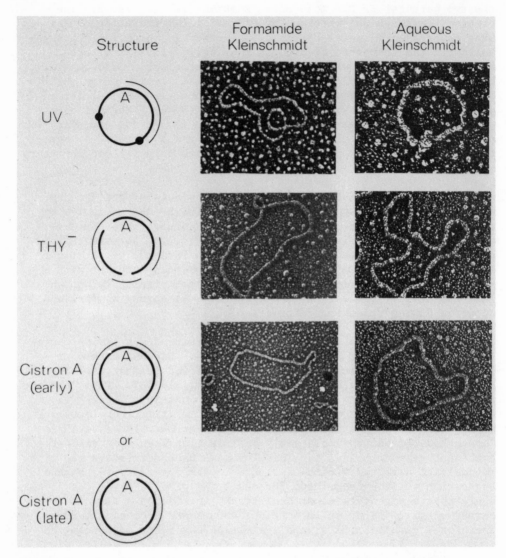

Figure 2. Recombination-proficient structures. Electron micrographs of ultraviolet-damaged and thymine-starvation-damaged RF DNA
molecules (Benbow *et al.*, 1974c) spread by aqueous and formamide
Kleinschmidt procedures (Davis *et al.*, 1971). The putative structure of these molecules also is indicated; the parental strand is
represented by the solid thick line, the newly synthesized complementary strand by the solid thin line. In addition we have drawn
hypothetical structures initiating recombination preferentially
within cistron A. The corresponding electron micrographs are of
RFII molecules isolated late in infection, which presumably are
specifically gapped in the parental strand in the cistron A region
(Johnson and Sinsheimer, 1974).

how early the "break" is introduced into the parental (+) strand, but again this is not proven.

We conclude that complementary strand aggression *does* occur, and that parental strand aggression *may* occur during φX174 recombinant formation. A strand bias could exist (but see below).

CAN BOTH STRANDS BRANCH MIGRATE?

Formation of a stable recombinant figure-eight molecule (Fig. 1f) requires double-strand branch migration (Benbow *et al.*, 1972a). A proof (of sorts) that double-strand branch migration can and does occur in φX174 DNA molecules is offered in Fig. 3. Artificial heteroduplexes were formed from *del*E (Zuccarelli *et al.*, 1972) dimeric complementary (−) strands and two *wt* parental (+) strand monomers (Kim *et al.*, 1972). In almost every case, the two deletion loops were rapidly juxtaposed as a result of branch migration, and structures containing separated (*i.e.* partially migrated or unmigrated) deletion loops were exceedingly rare. A very elegant study of the kinetics of branch migration was carried out by Kim *et al.* (1972), using our φX174 multimeric DNA preparations; and further examples of branch migration in φX174 DNA molecules were given by Benbow *et al.* (1972a).

To interpret our density exchange experiments it is important to note that branch migration is a symmetric process: both strands participate equally in branch migration. Furthermore, the presence of heavy isotopes in one or more strands is unlikely to alter significantly the rate of, or distance traversed during, migration.

WHERE ARE THE PARENTAL DNA STRANDS IN FIGURE-EIGHT DNA MOLECULES?

Two classes of recombinant figure-eight DNA molecules are likely to arise, depending on whether the parental(+) or the complementary (−) strand receives the initial single-strand "break." These are diagrammed in Fig. 4 next to an electron micrograph of a typical φX174 figure-eight DNA molecules. We now describe density exchange experiments which show that *both* of these recombinant structures are likely to be formed *in vivo*, though not necessarily with equal probability. Furthermore, these experiments apparently exclude the breakage and copy mechanism of Boon and Zinder (1969, 1971), which requires extensive DNA replication.

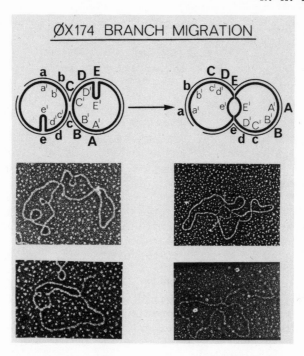

Figure 3.   Branch migration in bacteriophage φX174.   Artificial
heteroduplexes of two *wt* monomer (+) strands with one double length
*del*E(-) strand (Benbow *et al.*, 1972a) were formed as described by
Kim *et al.* (1972).   In most molecules, the two deletion loops
branch migrated to juxtaposition as diagrammed on the right.   Two
additional examples of branch migration in φX174 are shown: a
Cairns structure with a whisker (single-strand branch migration)
and an H-branched structure analogous to those described by Broker
and Lehman (1971).   (We thank Mrs. J. S. Kim for the rare electron
micrograph showing two deletion loops that had not branch migrated
to juxtaposition.)

RECOMBINANT FORMATION BETWEEN TWO HEAVY PARENTAL GENOMES

[3]H-Labeled heavy *am*3(E) phage and cold heavy *am*86(A) phage were
used to infect the host strand HF4704 in the presence of 0.003 M KCN
and [^{14}C]thymidine.   Parental RF DNA molecules of hybrid density
were formed as shown in Fig. 5, but the presence of KCN inhibited
the formation of progeny RF DNA molecules (Benbow, 1972).   The
initial events in recombinant formation are known to occur under
these conditions (Benbow, 1972).   After removal of the KCN, RF DNA
was extracted either early (4 min) or late (20 min) in the infection
process.   After purification by velocity sedimentation in neutral

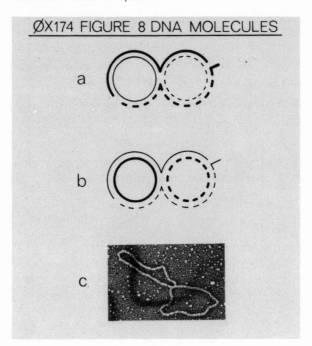

ØX174 FIGURE 8 DNA MOLECULES

Figure 4. Figure-eight DNA molecules. Two classes of figure-eight
DNA molecules are formed, depending on whether the parental (+) or
the complementary (-) strand receives the initial single-strand
break. Parental (+) strands are represented by thick lines, complementary (-) strands by thin lines. One genotype is represented by
solid lines, and the other by interrupted lines. Only the parental
(+) strands were labeled with heavy isotope in our experimental design.

sucrose gradients, the RF DNA molecules were examined by banding in
CsCl, and *wt* recombinants were assayed across the gradient with a
spheroplast assay in which further recombination was unable to take
place (Benbow *et al.*, 1974b).

Early in infection, a peak of *wt* recombinants was observed one
fraction lighter than "heavy" (*i.e.* heavy-light hybrid) DNA molecules (Fig. 5a). A small number of fully light *wt* recombinants
were also seen, presumably representing homozygous *wt* progeny RF
DNA molecules. Later in infection (Fig. 5b), after progeny RF DNA
replication had occurred, the vast majority (>99%) of *wt* recombinants were detected at densities corresponding to fully light RF
DNA molecules.

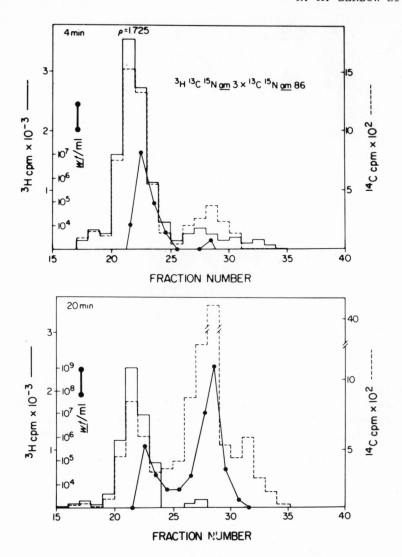

Figure 5. A two-factor cross between two heavy bacteriophage φX174. ³H,¹³C,¹⁵N-labeled *am*3(E) and ¹³C,¹⁵N-labeled *am*86(A) phage were grown in heavy minimal medium (Kelly and Sinsheimer, 1967) as described by Levine and Sinsheimer (1969), using host strains HF4704 (Lindqvist and Sinsheimer, 1970) and Su2$_{am}$ (Funk and Sinsheimer, 1970), respectively. [³H]Thymidine (Schwarz/Mann, 10 Ci/mmole), if employed, was added during the last generation only. Auxotrophic supplements, if necessary, were present at all times. Heavy phage were purified by banding and rebanding in CsCl as described by Sinsheimer *et al.* (1962).

HF4704, a *thy* host, was grown at 37°C with aeration to a con-

RECOMBINANT FORMATION BETWEEN ONE HEAVY AND ONE
LIGHT PARENTAL GENOME

[3]H-Labeled heavy $am3$(E) phage and ^{14}C-labeled light $am9$(G)
phage were used to infect the host strain HF4704 in the presence
of 0.003 M KCN. Parental RF DNA molecules of hybrid ($\rho \cong 1.725$)
and of light ($\rho \cong 1.705$) density were formed. KCN was removed
after 15 min and RF DNA was extracted 4 min later. The purified
RF molecules were examined by banding in CsCl, and wt recombinants
were detected in peaks one or two fractions lighter than "heavy"
($i.e.$ heavy-light hybrid) RF, in the fully light RF molecules, and
midway between the two peaks (Fig. 6).

EXCHANGE OF PARENTAL DNA DURING RECOMBINANT FORMATION

Interpretation of these density exchange experiments is particularly complex because of an unfortunate circumstance: relaxed
figure-eight DNA molecules containing a "break" sediment in neutral
sucrose gradients with nearly the same S value as RFI DNA molecules
(Benbow, Eisenberg, and Sinsheimer, to be published). Therefore,
although less than 1% of the purified replicative-form DNA molecules
banded in these experiments were figure-eight structures, it was
often impossible to decide whether the observed wt recombinants in
a particular region of the CsCl gradient arose from monomeric RF
molecules or from figure-eight molecules. With this qualification,
we offer the following interpretation of our results.

Recombinants formed from two "heavy" parental genomes were of
slightly less than hybrid density early in infection (Fig. 5a).
This suggests that only a small amount (less than 1 fraction in 8,

---

centration of 2×10^8 cells per ml in TPG-AA + 2 μg/ml thymine
(Lindqvist and Sinsheimer, 1970). The culture was made 0.003 M in
KCN and aerated for 10 min.   [3]H,[13]C,[15]N-labeled $am3$(E) and ^{13}C,[15]N-
labeled $am86$(A) were added at a multiplicity of infection of 10,
along with 2 μCi/ml [^{14}C]thymidine (Schwarz/Mann, 50 Ci/mmole).
After 15 min at 37°C (without aeration) for adsorpotion, the culture
was pelleted, washed three times in 0.05 M borate-0.005 M EDTA, and
resuspended in fresh medium. At 4 min (a) and at 20 min (b), half
of the culture was pelleted; RF DNA was extracted as described by
Benbow et $al.$ (1974c), and was purified by repeated sedimentation
through 5-20% sucrose (1.0 M NaCl, 0.05 M Tris, pH 7.5, 0.005 M
EDTA) in an SW41 rotor at 40,000 rpm for 8 hr. The region from 16
to 22S was pooled, dialyzed against 0.05 M Tris, pH 8.0, and banded
in CsCl as described by Sinsheimer et $al.$ (1962) in a Type 50 rotor
at 36,000 rpm for 36-48 hr, and wt recombinants were assayed across
each gradient as described by Benbow et $al.$ (1974b).

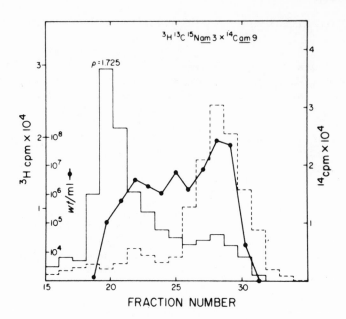

Figure 6. A two-factor cross between one heavy and one light bacteriophage ϕX174. ^{3}H,^{13}C,^{15}N-labeled *am*3(E) was prepared as described in the legend to Fig. 5. ^{14}C-labeled *am*9 was prepared as
described by Benbow *et al.* (1974c). Infection, RF DNA extraction,
and banding were carried out as described in the legend to Fig. 5,
except that 0.003 M KCN was again added 4 min after dilution of the
infected cells into fresh medium.

or 12%) of parental (+) strand DNA was removed and resynthesized
during recombinant formation. However, recombinants formed from
one heavy and one light parental genome were found throughout the
gradient (Fig. 6). Furthermore, a majority of the recombinants
formed in these crosses were found at positions only slightly removed from hybrid or fully light densities.

Several additional conclusions can be drawn from the heavy-
light experiments: (i) most recombination events ($\sim$80%) involved
exchange of only small lengths ($\sim$700-1400 nucleotides) of parental-
strand DNA. (ii) A significant but minor fraction of recombinant
events involved exchange of longer lengths of parental-strand DNA
(>2000 nucleotides). (iii) Parental (+) strand aggression did occur.

We were unable to identify with certainty the peak of intermediate density (Fig. 6), although it is perhaps of interest that
an intact figure-eight DNA molecule containing one "heavy" and one
light RF DNA molecule would be of this density.

The results obtained late in infection (Fig. 5b) demonstrate that homozygous recombinant progeny RF DNA is produced in large quantities. This confirms our indirect evidence (Benbow, 1972; Benbow *et al.*, 1974a), which showed that large single bursts of recombinants were obtained.

In addition, the observations of extensive losses of recombinants from the "heavy" (*i.e.* heavy-light hybrid) DNA region, and of the increased numbers at intermediate densities later in infection (Fig. 5b) suggest that considerable *in vivo* heteroduplex repair occurred. The cumulative sum of repaired regions often extended for over 1000 bases.

We thus argue that the density exchange experiments presented in this paper support our model of the major pathway of φX174 recombinant formation and are exceedingly difficult to reconcile with the extensive DNA replication required by the breakage and copy model of Boon and Zinder (1969, 1971). In addition, our density exchange experiments suggest that both of the recombinant figure-eight structures diagrammed in Fig. 4 can be formed (*i.e.* that both parental and complementary strand aggression can occur), but not necessarily with equal probability. Finally, the data suggest that extensive *in vivo* repair of natural heteroduplexes occurs during the first 20 min after infection.

REFERENCES

Baas, P. D. and H. S. Jansz. 1972a. Asymmetric information transfer during φX174 DNA replication. J. Mol. Biol. 63: 557.

Baas, P. D. and H. S. Jansz. 1972b. φX174 replicative form DNA. Replication, origin and direction. J. Mol. Biol. 63: 569.

Benbow, R. M. 1972. On the genetic recombination of bacteriophage φX174 DNA molecules. Ph.D. Thesis, California Institute of Technology.

Benbow, R. M., R. Devoret and P. Howard-Flanders. 1973. Indirect ultraviolet induction and curing in *E. coli* cells lysogenic for bacteriophage λ. Molec. Gen. Genet. 120: 355.

Benbow, R. M., M. Eisenberg and R. L. Sinsheimer. 1972a. Multiple lenth DNA molecules of bacteriophage φX174. Nature New Biol. 237: 141.

Benbow, R. M., C. A. Hutchison, J. D. Fabricant and R. L. Sinsheimer. 1971. Genetic map of bacteriophage φX174. J. Virol. 7: 549.

Benbow, R. M., R. F. Mayol, J. C. Picchi and R. L. Sinsheimer. 1972b. Direction of translation and size of bacteriophage φX174 cistrons. J. Virol. 10: 99.

Benbow, R. M., A. J. Zuccarelli, G. C. Davis and R. L. Sinsheimer. 1974a. Genetic recombination in bacteriophage φX174. J. Virol. in press.

Benbow, R. M., A. J. Zuccarelli and R. L. Sinsheimer. 1974b. Recombinant DNA molecules of bacteriophage φX174. Proc. Nat. Acad. Sci. U.S.A. in press.

Benbow, R.M., A. J. Zuccarelli and R. L. Sinsheimer. 1974c. An aggressive role for single-strand "breaks" in bacteriophage φX174 genetic recombination. J. Mol. Biol. in press.

Boon, T. and N. D. Zinder. 1969. A mechanism for genetic recombination generating one parent and one recombinant. Proc. Nat. Acad. Sci. U.S.A. 64: 573.

Boon, T. and N. D. Zinder. 1971. Genotypes produced by individual recombination events involving bacteriophage f1. J. Mol. Biol. 58: 133.

Broker, T. R. and I. R. Lehman. 1971. Branched DNA molecules: Intermediates in T4 recombination. J. Mol. Biol. 60: 131.

Davis, R. W., M. N. Simon and N. Davidson. 1971. Electron microscope heteroduplex methods for mapping regions of base sequence homology in nucleic acids. In (L. Grossman and K. Moldave, eds.) Methods in Enzymology, Vol. XXI, part D, pp. 413-428. Academic Press, New York.

Doniger, J., R. C. Warner and I. Tessman. 1973. Role of circular dimer DNA in the primary recombination mechanism of bacteriophage S13. Nature New Biol. 242: 9.

Funk, F. and R. L. Sinsheimer. 1970. Process of infection with bacteriophage φX174. XXXV. Cistron VIII. J. Virol. 6: 12.

Johnson, P. H., and R. L. Sinsheimer. 1974. Structure of an intermediate in the replication of bacteriophage φX174 deoxyribonucleic acid: the initiation site for DNA replication. J. Mol. Biol. 83: 47.

Kellenberger, G., M. L. Zichichi and J. Weigle. 1961. Exchange of DNA in the recombination of bacteriophage lambda. Proc. Nat. Acad. Sci. U.S.A. 47: 869.

Kelly, R. B. and R. L. Sinsheimer. 1967. The replication of bacteriophage MS2. VII. Non-conservative replication of double-stranded RNA. J. Mol. Biol. 26: 169.

Kim, J. S., P. A. Sharp and N. Davidson. 1972. Electron microscope
studies of heteroduplex DNA from a deletion mutant of bacteriophage
φX174. Proc. Nat. Acad. Sci. U.S.A. 69: 1948.

Lee, C. S., R. W. Davis and N. Davidson. 1970. A physical study
by electron microscopy of the terminally repetitious, circularly
permuted DNA from the coliphage particles of Escherichia coli 15.
J. Mol. Biol. 48: 1.

Levine, A. J. and R. L. Sinsheimer. 1969. The process of infection
with bacteriophage φX174. XXV. Studies with bacteriophage φX174
mutants blocked in progeny replicative form DNA synthesis. J. Mol.
Biol. 39: 619.

Lindqvist, B. and R. L. Sinsheimer. 1970. The process of infection
with bacteriophage φX174. XIV. Studies on macromolecule synthesis
during infection with a lysis defective mutant. J. Mol. Biol. 28:
87.

Meselson, M. 1962. Genetic recombination at the molecular level.
Pontif. Acad. Sci. Scr. Varia 22: 173.

Meselson, M. 1964. On the mechanism of genetic recombination
between DNA molecules. J. Mol. Biol. 9: 734.

Meselson, M. 1967. The molecular basis of genetic recombination.
In (R. A. Brink, ed.) Heritage from Mendel, pp. 81-104. Univ. of
Wisconsin Press, Madison.

Meselson, M. and J. J. Weigle. 1961. Chromosome breakage accompanying genetic recombination in bacteriophage. Proc. Nat. Acad. Sci.
U.S.A. 47: 857.

Newbold, J. E. and R. L. Sinsheimer. 1970. The process of infection with bacteriophage φX174. XXXII. Early steps in the infection
process: attachment, eclipse and DNA penetration. J. Mol. Biol.
49:49.

Sinsheimer, R. L., B. Starman, C. Nagler and S. Guthrie. 1962. The
process of infection with bacteriophage φX174. I. Evidence for a
"replicative form." J. Mol. Biol. 4: 142.

Weisbeek, P. J. and J. H. van de Pol. 1970. Biological activity
of φX174 replicative form DNA fragments. Biochim. Biophys. Acta
224: 328.

Yarus, M. J. and R. L. Sinsheimer. 1967. The process of infection with bacteriophage φX174. XIII. Evidence for an essential bacterial 'site'. J. Virol. <u>1</u>: 135.

Zuccarelli, A. J., R. M. Benbow and R. L. Sinsheimer. 1972. Deletion mutants of bacteriophage φX174. Proc. Nat. Acad. Sci. U.S.A. <u>69</u>: 1905.

Zuccarelli, A. J., R. M. Benbow and R. L. Sinsheimer. 1974. Synthesis of the first complementary strand of φX174. J. Mol. Biol. in press.

RECOMBINATION IN BACTERIOPHAGE f1

Norton D. Zinder

The Rockefeller University, New York, New York 10021

The bacteriophage f1 is a small, single-stranded DNA-containing phage. The DNA is in a ring form containing about 6000 nucleotides. The phage particle itself is filamentous, does not kill its host cells, and is continuously extruded from the cell surface while the cells continue to grow (Marvin and Hohn, 1969).

Complementation analysis of a set of amber mutants indicates that the phage has eight genes. On the basis of the sizes of the proteins these genes specify, they should just about saturate the genome (Model and Zinder, 1974). The order of the genes around the circular map is II, IV, I, VI, III, VIII, V, VII with some ambiguity about the relative order of genes V and VII (Lyons and Zinder, 1972) (Fig. 1).

Under non-permissive conditions, gene II mutants block phage replication beyond the conversion of input single-strands to the double-stranded form (Pratt and Erdahl, 1968). Therefore the experimental design we used was to infect nonpermissive cells with two different amber mutants in gene II and determine the genotypes of the progeny phage by plating samples on bacterial hosts which can differentiate all of the possible combinations of genetic markers present in any particular cross. Barring leakage and freeloading, the only progeny emerging from these infected cells should be wild-type recombinants and all other phage genotypes that were generated in the recombination event.

The first experiments were designed to test the system: Was recombination occurring between input DNA molecules? The approach was based on a preconception about genetic recombination, that is,

19

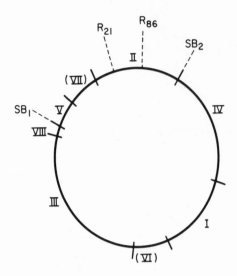

Figure 1.   Genetic map of phage f1.   The map as drawn is more or
less proportional to gene product sizes (Model and Zinder, 1974),
with the location of specific reference points determined from
fragments produced by a restriction endonuclease from *Haemophilus
aegyptius* (Horiuchi and Vovis, unpublished).   The genes in parentheses have not as yet been associated with a protein product and
hence can not be given a size.

that recombination involved some kind of breakage and joining of
DNA molecules (Meselson and Weigle, 1961).   Arber and Kuhnlein
(1967) had shown that f1 phage could transfer input DNA from parent
to the progeny in relatively intact form.   Thus we attempted to
show that a reasonable fraction of the recombinants obtained under
these conditions contained parental atoms.   Isotopic labeling experiments were difficult because of the low frequency of recombination (only one in a thousand of mixedly infected cells yield
progeny), so in order to reduce infection by more than two parental phage (freeloading) we infected only a small fraction of the
cells.   We therefore chose to use the biological system of Ihler
and Meselson (1963) to mark DNA molecules (Boon and Zinder, 1970).

We digress for a moment to describe some properties of f1 and
anticipate their subsequent use.   Phage f1 undergoes a restriction
modification cycle during growth on *Escherichia coli* K versus *E.
coli* B (Arber, 1966).   This system has been used extensively in
these studies.   Phage grown on *E. coli* K plate with an efficiency
of 7 X 10^{-3} on *E. coli* B, while phage grown on *E. coli* B grow as
well on *E. coli* K as on *E. coli* B.   The resistance of "B grown"
phage to restriction is attributable to the methylation of two

specific adenine residues in the DNA. This methylation renders the
DNA molecule resistant to action of the B restriction endonuclease.
Progeny of methylated phage are not resistant to the enzyme unless
they too are methylated, or unless they inherit a methylated strand
from a parent. Hybrid double-stranded molecules which have one
methylated and one unmethylated strand are resistant to the enzyme.
Mutants can be selected which have lost one or both sites responsible for sensitivity to the B restriction endonuclease. There is
both genetic (Boon and Zinder, 1971) and biochemical evidence
(Horiuchi and Vovis, unpublished results) that these mutations are
located at specific points on the phage chromosome. Mutant phage
are not modified; they do not accept methyl groups. Hybrids in
which one strand of a double-stranded molecule is mutant and the
other is wild type are resistant to the restriction endonuclease,
as is the case with hybrids in which only one strand is methylated
(Vovis *et al.*, 1973). Preliminary results suggest, however, that
mutant-wild type hybrids differ from methylated-unmethylated hybrids in that the mutant hybrid cannot be methylated. Segregation
of the strands of such a hybrid would lead, therefore, to the
generation of one restriction-sensitive molecule and one restriction-
resistant molecule. Both genetic (Hartman and Zinder, 1974a) and
biochemical evidence shows that the sites of mutation and/or methylation are not necessarily the sites of endonucleolytic cleavage
(Horiuchi and Zinder, 1972). This cleavage can apparently occur
at many sites, possibly at random. Thus the specific sites of
methylation and mutation probably serve as recognition elements for
binding of the enzyme.

These properties of the restriction-modification system and
the mutants to it have been used in the following ways: (1) To
inquire into parent-to-progeny transfer of DNA, *E. coli* K are infected with methylated phage grown on *E. coli* B. Progeny which
have received the DNA containing the methyl groups will plate on
E. coli B, while those containing newly synthesized (unmethylated)
DNA can do so only at much reduced efficiency. (2) The mutants
are used as unselected markers for crosses done in *E. coli* K. The
progeny can be assayed for the SB markers on *E. coli* B. (3) They
are used as a means of introducing breaks into one of the two
parents in a cross. The parent to be protected may be either mutant,
or may be methylated by having been grown in *E. coli* B. The other
parent will have at least one unmethylated, wild-type site and will
be attacked by the restriction endonuclease if the cross is done in
E. coli B.

We now return to the experiments that have been done to date.
E. coli K was infected with phage grown on *E. coli* B to determine
whether some of the progeny remember their prior growth on *E. coli*
B. Of the cells infected with a low multiplicity of wild-type phage,
about 0.2 put out a phage particle that could grow on *E. coli* B.

When crosses between two different gene II mutants were done,
among the cells that yielded recombinant progeny about 0.2 released
a recombinant that grew on *E. coli* B (Boon and Zinder, 1970).

This result supports two points: (1) some recombination
occurs between input molecules without their prior replication,
other than becoming double-stranded, and (2) that recombination
involves some kind of breakage and joining of these molecules. We
had hoped that generalized recombination in f1, which is recA dependent, would turn out to be simple reciprocal breakage and joining.
Single-strand exchange in recombination would pose for us the
following problem: F1 is a single-stranded DNA phage and the messenger RNA strand is equivalent to the DNA strand in the phage (Sugiura
et al., 1969). Since some atoms of parental phage were in the recombinant phage strand and gene function is necessary for progeny
to be produced, a heteroduplex DNA molecule with a parental genome
in the complementary strand and a wild-type recombinant gene in the
viral equivalent strand should be nonviable unless some kind of base
correction occurred.

Crosses were done between phage containing two different gene
II amber mutants in nonpermissive hosts. The phage stocks also
contained some non-selective markers. Although the crosses were
done in several different symmetries and different markers, we will
illustrate the results with one type of cross in which the same nonselective marker was segregating. The two counter-selected amber
mutants in gene II are called 21 and 86. The nonselective marker
segregating is always the mutant SB_2^0 and its wild-type allele SB_2^+.
This mutant is partially resistant to the B restriction endonuclease.
When grown on *E. coli* K it has an efficiency of plating on *E. coli*
B of about 0.03 instead of 7×10^{-3}. The order of these genes on
the circular f1 map is 21, 86, and SB_2^0; with 21 and 86 being about
300 nucleotides apart and SB_2^0 closely linked to the 86 marker but
probably at least 500 nucleotides away (Fig. 1). In some of the
crosses shown the marker SB_1^0 was also present. It is close to the
21 marker but was not segregating in these particular crosses as
both of the parental phages carry this marker. Phage containing
this marker also plate on *E. coli* B with an efficiency of 0.03.
Phage containing both SB_1^0 and SB_2^0 are completely resistant to B
restriction. The phage progeny from single cells were analyzed.
The yields from these cells contained for the most part only two
types of phage, and these were not the reciprocal recombinants.
The majority of bursts contained one intact parental phage genome
and one recombinant genome with a particular combination of the
nonselective markers. The bursts were therefore tabulated with regard to the parental genome and the kind of recombinant with which
it emerged (Boon and Zinder, 1971).

Table 1 contains the data from one such cross. The bias in
association of the nonselective marker of the wild-type recombinants

Table 1. Tabulation of single bursts with regard to the parental phage and recombinant phage which emerged together. From Boon and Zinder (1971).

$$R21 \quad SB_1^o \quad SB_2^o \quad \text{by} \quad R86 \quad SB_1^o \quad SB_2^+$$

Parent	Am+ Recombinants	
	SB_2^+	SB_2^o
R86 SB_1^o SB_2^+	19	80
R21 SB_1^o SB_2^o	28	34

with the two different parental genomes indicated that these parental phage were indeed the result of the recombination event and not "freeloaders" or the result of leakage. The crosses were done with a variety of markers, and all lead to the general conclusion that the majority of recombination events generate one wild-type recombinant and one single amber mutant. In general the single amber phage that emerges has retained all of its genes--genetic conservation of one parent. Although many of the recombinants differed from the parent for the nonselective markers, a significant fraction did carry the same marker--a kind of coconversion. This resembles the asymmetric coconversion found by Fogel and Mortimer (1969) in yeast. Since these crosses were done under selective conditions (all of the products might not be recovered) and all that was ascertained was the segregation of the markers, and since replicating DNA itself is double-stranded, we could not be sure whether a single double helix or two double helixes were segregating.

There were a number of ways to explain these data by mechanisms other than reciprocal breakage and reunion--particularly asymmetric heteroduplex formation, the transfer of a single strand from one DNA molecule to the other. However, at that time we could not see how such a mechanism for genetic recombination could ever generate a reciprocal recombinant (but see Radding, this volume). Therefore, in an attempt to be more general, we developed a breakage-copy model for genetic recombination which could explain these data and could still give rise to reciprocal recombinants (Boon and Zinder, 1971).

The second set of crosses was designed to test the effect of a known lesion introduced into a parental DNA molecule at a specific point. We would use the B restriction endonuclease to introduce such a lesion. Our rationale was (1) our model for genetic recombination had a double-strand break at the initiation site for recom-

Table 2. Tabulation of single bursts with regard to parental
phage and recombinant phage which emerged together. Above the
diagonal, data from crosses performed in *E. coli* K; below the
diagonal crosses performed in *E. coli* B.

$$R21 \quad SB_2^+(B) \quad by \quad R86 \quad SB_2^o(K)$$

Parent	Am+ Recombinants	
	SB_2^o	SB_2^+
R86 SB_2^o	9 / 1	29 / 4
R21 SB_2^+	34 / 45	44 / 50

bination, and (2) more generally the effect of site-specific breaks
could well be revealing of mechanism. Thus all simple notions
predicted that such lesions would alter linkage values and might
give us a clue as to what was happening. The experiments were pre-
dicated on the hypothesis that the SB sites were the sites of
cleavage by restriction enzymes. Therefore, one parent was protected by being B-modified phage, while the other parent had one of
the SB sites available for restriction. The same crosses were done
in B and K hosts. The crosses in *E. coli* K gave the familiar one
parent and one recombinant pattern, while the crosses in B also
gave one parent and one recombinant but only the class with the non-
restricted parent. The major effect of restriction was to reduce
the proportion of bursts emerging with the sensitive parent and
those recombinants associated with it (Table 2). The missing class
of recombinants was not found among the bursts that did not yield
parental phage (Hartman and Zinder, 1974a). During these experiments
our fundamental assumption that the SB sites were the sites of cleavage came into question. *In vitro* experiments with the B restriction
endonuclease indicated that the SB sites were not the sites of
cleavage but rather recognition sites on the DNA and that cleavage
could take place at many different points on the molecules (Horiuchi
and Zinder, 1972), although generally only one break per molecule
was found.

Given this fact and the fact that we obtained in the "restriction" crosses something resembling half of the usual data, we obviously could say little more about genetic recombination in f1,
other than that since this recombination was also recA dependent,
these data supported donor-recipient models of genetic recombination
(Hartman and Zinder, 1974a). Perhaps at this point we should have
left well enough alone.

Table 3. Tabulation of single bursts with regard to parental phage and recombinant phage which emerged together. Above the diagonal crosses in *E. coli* K; below the diagonal crosses in *E. coli* B.

$$R21 \quad SB_1^0 SB_2^0 \quad \times \quad R86\, SB_1^0 SB_2^+\,(K)$$

Parent		Am+ Recombinants	
		SB_2^+	SB_2^0
R86	$SB_0^1 SB_2^+$	8 / 0	26 / 1
R21	$SB_0^1 SB_2^0$	10 / 1	12 / 16

However, there are two ways to protect a parental DNA molecule from restriction: (1) by B modification as described above, or (2) by mutation of the SB sites. We therefore performed a similar set of crosses with the protected parent now protected by mutation at one or both of the SB sites. Without a significant change in the recombination frequency, the results markedly changed. The recombinant progeny tended to emerge with the same set of nonselective markers as those of the protected parent (Hartman and Zinder, 1974b). Table 3 shows one of many such crosses. The SB_2^0 marker no longer segregates.

Let us try to put this all into a single picture. All models of recombination involving double-strand transfers, breakage, or copying or transfer of short single strands should give primarily homoduplex DNA. It is hard to envision how the B restriction system could discriminate between two pairs of homoduplexes, one pair in which one homoduplex is B modified and the other normal, versus the pair in which one is mutant and the other is normal. However, given the formation of long heteroduplex DNA, a heteroduplex between a DNA molecule with a modified site and a normal site might well be discriminated from a heteroduplex between a mutant and a normal site. Threfore we suggest that in genetic recombination in f1 there is a tendency to insert as long a DNA strand as possible making heteroduplex DNA. This would explain the one parent one recombinant yields, with the different nonselective alleles. This occurs by the simple segregation of such heteroduplexes during the next round of replication. When one strand is protected by B modification there is no restriction, and the complementary strand can be modified and hence is protected. In the absence of site-specific breakage, and with restriction determining which is the donated strand, we thus obtain in these restriction crosses half of the usual data. When the heteroduplex is between a mutant site and a normal site it could either be directly restricted or not modifiable and cleaved following replication. Therefore the only recombinant progeny that can be obtained are those from which heteroduplex DNA did not cover an SB site, and therefore they must resemble the protected SB mutant parent.

In vitro experiments show that heteroduplexes between mutant and normal DNA cannot be restricted (Vovis *et al.*, 1973), although preliminary results suggest they *cannot* be modified. *In vivo*, such heteroduplexes are operationally restricted in transfection experiments; that is, they are less efficient in infecting B versus K hosts, but here we can't distinguish a failure to modify progeny from restriction of the parents (Enea and Zinder, unpublished).

The model of recombination for phage f1, now proposed, still leaves us with the problem of how parental atoms are transferred to the progeny viral strands. However, we cannot say that all recombination events involve the viral strand (Boon and Zinder, 1970). In addition, some of the bursts (30-50%) yield only recombinant progeny (Boon and Zinder, 1971; Hartman and Zinder, 1974a, b). It is possible that these pure bursts are the result of transfer of the viral strand and base correction of the complementary strand. Hence gene II could function to yield the progeny which are the source of recombinants with parental atoms. Alternatively, the temporary nick that must be present in a transferred viral strand could mimic the gene II function for the first round of replication and thus give recombinant progeny with parental atoms.

Another problem posed by the single-strand exchange model of genetic recombination for f1 described above is the fate of the residual strand of the donor parent and the displaced strand of the recipient parent. Most of the possible answers were touched upon by Boon and Zinder (1971). Others come to mind, but since we still have only segregation data and no physical data, further comment at this time would only be gratuitous.

In summary, we believe we have shown that, in phage f1, recA-dependent recombination involves breakage and joining of DNA molecules with the formation of long segments of heteroduplex DNA. This latter finding contradicts a prediction of the breakage-copying model of Boon and Zinder (1971) for genetic recombination in f1, although I still find the model aesthetically pleasing in that it couples two of the fundamental attributes of DNA, replication and recombination (see Stahl and Stahl, this volume).

REFERENCES

Arber, W. 1966. Host specificity of DNA produced by *Escherichia coli*. J. Mol. Biol. <u>20</u>: 483.

Arber, W. and U. Kuhnlein. 1967. Mutationeller Verlust B-spezifischer Restiktion des Bakteriophagen fd. Pathol. Microbiol. <u>30</u>: 946.

Boon, T. and N. D. Zinder. 1970. Genetic recombination in bacteriophage f1: Transfer of parental DNA to the recombinant. Virology <u>41</u>: 444.

Boon, T. and N. D. Zinder. 1971. Genotypes produced by individual recombination events involving bacteriophage f1. J. Mol. Biol. <u>58</u>: 133.

Fogel, S. and R. K. Mortimer. 1969. Informational transfer in meiotic gene conversion. Proc. Nat. Acad. Sci. U.S.A. <u>62</u>: 96.

Hartman, N. and N. D. Zinder. 1974a. The effect of B specific restriction and modification of DNA on linkage relationships in f1 bacteriophage: Studies on the mechanism of B restriction *in vivo*. J. Mol. Biol. in press.

Hartman, N. and N. D. Zinder. 1974b. The effect of B restriction and modification on linkage relationships in f1 bacteriophage: Evidence for a heteroduplex intermediate. J. Mol. Biol. in press.

Horiuchi, K. and N. D. Zinder. 1972. Cleavage of f1 DNA by the restriction enzyme of *Escherichia coli* B. Proc. Nat. Acad. Sci. U.S.A. <u>69</u>: 3220.

Ihler, G. and M. Meselson. 1963. Genetic recombination in bacteriophage λ by breakage and joining of DNA molecules. Virology <u>21</u>: 7.

Lyons, L. and N. D. Zinder. 1972. The genetic map of the filamentous bacteriophage f1. Virology <u>49</u>: 45.

Marvin, D. A. and B. Hohn. 1969. Filamentous bacterial viruses. Bacteriol. Rev. <u>33</u>: 172.

Meselson, M. and J. Weigle. 1961. Chromosome breakage accompanying genetic recombination in bacteriophage. Proc. Nat. Acad. Sci. U.S.A. <u>47</u>: 857.

Model, P. and N. D. Zinder. 1974. *In vitro* synthesis of bacteriophage f1 proteins. J. Mol. Biol. <u>83</u>: 231.

Pratt, D. and W. S. Erhdahl. 1968. Genetic control of bacteriophage M13 DNA synthesis. J. Mol. Biol. <u>37</u>: 181.

Sugiura, M., T. Okanoto and M. Takanami. 1969. Studying nucleotide sequences of RNA synthesized on the replicative form DNA of
coliphage fd. J. Mol. Biol. <u>43</u>: 299.

Vovis, G., K. Horiuchi, N. Hartman and N. D. Zinder. 1973. Restriction endonuclease B and f1 heteroduplex DNA. Nature New
Biol. <u>246</u>: 13.

ON THE ROLE OF *ESCHERICHIA COLI* DNA POLYMERASE I AND OF T4

GENE 32 PROTEIN IN RECOMBINATION OF PHAGE T4

Gisela Mosig

Vanderbilt University, Nashville, Tennessee 37203

As discussed repeatedly during this symposium, recombination between DNA molecules proceeds in several steps (see Fig. 1): (A) Breakage or nicking of parental molecules (Meselson and Weigle, 1961), (B) formation of "joint" intermediates (Anraku and Tomizawa, 1965), some of them branched (Broker and Lehman, 1971; Benbow *et al.*, this symposium), (C) conversion of "joint" into covalently linked "recombinant" molecules, which may still contain mismatched base pairs in the heteroduplex regions (Tomizawa, 1967; Kozinski *et al.*, 1967), (D) repair of mismatches in heteroduplex regions (Spatz and Trautner, 1970; Fox, Meselson, this symposium), and (E) replication of "recombinant" DNA molecules, which resolves unrepaired mismatches in heteroduplex regions. The temporal sequence of some of these steps is not well defined; *i.e.*, breakage may precede or follow the formation of "joint" molecules and repair may precede or follow the conversion of "joint" into "recombinant" molecules. Holliday (1964) and Whitehouse (1963) pointed out that two kinds of heteroduplex structures could be derived from intermediate branched structures: (I) "insertion" heteroduplexes, in which outside markers retain parental configurations, and (II) "recombinant" heteroduplexes, in which outside markers are exchanged (see Fig. 1, step B). The different modes to form and resolve branched intermediates are sterically equivalent and, therefore, considered equally likely (Sigal and Alberts, 1972; Meselson, 1972; Radding, this symposium; Meselson, this symposium; Sobell, this symposium). All of the present models imply that a DNA-binding protein, *e.g.* the gene 32 protein of T4 (Alberts and Frey, 1970), facilitates formation of heteroduplex regions and their extension by branch migration (Lee *et al.*, 1970), because T4 gene 32 *am* mutants do not even form "joint" molecules (Tomizawa, 1967; Kozinski and Felgen-

29

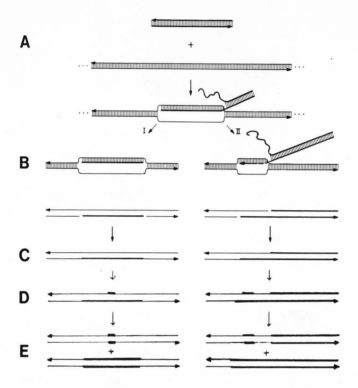

Figure 1. A model for recombination near ends of DNA fragments,
modified from Fox (1966). Steps A through E are described in the
text. This model most readily accounts for recombination patterns
near ends of incomplete T4 chromosomes (Mosig *et al.*, 1971).

hauer, 1967; Broker, 1973). Some of the models postulate a role
of DNA polymerases and/or nucleases for the conversion of branched
into nonbranched, "joint" or "recombinant" molecules (Hotchkiss,
1971; Radding, this symposium). Tomizawa (1967) has shown that T4
DNA polymerase is involved in the conversion of "joint" into "recombinant" T4 molecules. In subsequent studies (Anraku *et al.*,
1969) T4 DNA polymerase appeared to be required *in vitro*, but not
in vivo for this conversion. This apparent difference could be
explained by the finding that *Escherichia coli* DNA polymerase I is
involved in T4 recombination (Mosig *et al.*, 1972a). This enzyme
may be involved in covalent linkage *in vivo*.

Our first set of experiments suggests that the lack of polymerase I in the *pol*Al mutants of *E. coli* specifically inhibits
formation of "recombinant" heteroduplexes (Fig. 1, step BII), but
not of "insertion" heteroduplexes (Fig. 1, set BI). Our second

set of experiments shows that the gene 32 protein of T4 is involved both in the formation of "joint" molecules *and* in their conversion to "recombinant" molecules. The latter step requires the interaction of the gene 32 protein with the *r*II proteins of T4 or with equivalent host protein(s). These results imply that covalent linkage occurs at the membrane.

THE EFFECT OF *E. COLI pol*A MUTATIONS ON T4 RECOMBINATION

T4 produces, in addition to normal particles, some small morphological variants containing incomplete chromosomes (for summary see Mosig *et al.*, 1972b). These small particles produce progeny only after coinfection of a bacterium with other particles which provide the missing genes. The incomplete chromosomes of these small particles represent random segments of the genetic map (Mosig, 1968; Parma, 1969; Childs, 1971), and two or more incomplete chromosomes cooperate in wild-type hosts with an efficiency equal to the probability that the incomplete chromosomes contain between them a complete set of T4 genes. In *pol*Al hosts, however, at 42°C the efficiency of cooperation of incomplete wild-type chromosomes is reduced to approximately 30% of the expected probability (Mosig *et al.*, 1972a). We have now asked whether the *pol*Al mutation affects all T4 recombination or whether it specifically affects the resolution of branched intermediates into (I) "insertion" or (II) "recombinant" heteroduplexes (Fig. 1, step B). (The former eventually yield double-exchange recombinants in short intervals, associated with negative interference. The latter eventually yield singleexchange recombinants in large intervals, associated with positive interference.) The rationale of our experiments is based on the results of previous 19-factor single-burst crosses involving incomplete T4 chromosomes (Mosig *et al.*, 1971). In such crosses, the ends of the infecting incomplete chromosomes are recombinogenic (Mosig, 1963; Doermann and Parma, 1967). Contrary to the interpretation of Doermann and Parma, we find that recombination in some terminal regions of the incomplete chromosomes is associated with negative interference [coefficient of coincidence (c.o.c.)>1, *within the single burst*], while other terminal regions show positive interference (c.o.c. <1). After an incomplete chromosome coinfects a bacterium together with a complete chromosome (for a representative example see Fig. 2, left), terminal regions showing positive or negative interference occur, on the average, with approximately equal frequencies. There are bursts in which both ends show positive or both ends show negative interference, there are also bursts in which both patterns occur together. These patterns are best explained by the model in Fig. 1; the ends of the incomplete chromosome invade the complete chromosome and the resulting branched intermediates are resolved into "insertion" or "recombinant" heteroduplexes with equal probability. (Note that this is analogous to

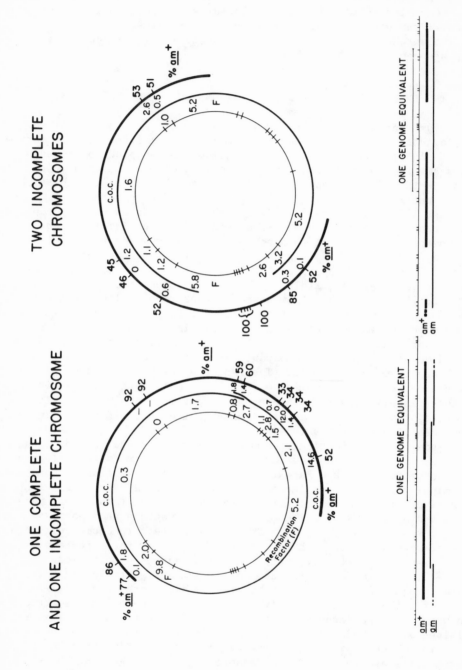

the situation in eukaryotes, where intragenic recombination is
equally likely associated with exchange or nonexchange of outside
markers (Chovnick, this symposium; Fogel, this symposium).

We find, on the other hand, that when two incomplete chromosomes coinfect a bacterium (Fig. 2, right) most terminal regions
show positive interference. We assume that for successful cooperation of two incomplete chromosomes "recombinant" heteroduplexes
(Fig. 1, step BII) are required and selected because only they will
join the incomplete chromosomes to a packageable structure that is
longer than genome length. Thus, we consider the possibility that
the poor cooperation of incomplete T4 chromosomes in *polA*1 hosts
could result from the inability of branched intermediates to become
"recombinant" heteroduplexes in these hosts. To test this possibility, we crossed, in *polA*1 and in *polA*$^+$ hosts, phage strains with
the marker combinations shown in Table 1 and Fig. 3, and measured
the percentage of wild-type recombinants in the progeny. We assume
that many of the wild-type recombinants in the large interval are
formed via "recombinant" heteroduplexes, while most wild-type recombinants in the three-factor cross are formed via "insertion"
heteroduplexes. The results are summarized in Table 1 and in Fig.
3. The *polA*1 mutation specifically reduces single-exchange recombination in the large interval but does not significantly affect
the double-exchange recombination in the short intervals. Single-
exchange recombination, like cooperation of incomplete chromosomes,
is more affected at 42°C than at 30°C. Note that the reduction of
recombinants in the large interval is an underestimate of the reduction in "recombinant" heteroduplexes because some recombinants
for the large interval must be formed via "insertion" heteroduplexes
for one of the markers.

Double-exchange recombination is not significantly affected in
*polA*1 hosts. This suggests that the lack of polymerase I in *polA*1
strains does not shift the equilibrium between "insertion" and
"recombinant" heteroduplexes, but that it specifically inactivates
the potential "recombinant" heteroduplexes. We assume that the

---

Figure 2. Frequencies of wild-type alleles (% *am*$^+$), recombination
factors (F), and coefficients of coincidence (c.o.c.) in two representative single bursts from 19-factor crosses involving incomplete
chromosomes. The inner circle gives the map positions of the 19
markers. The recombination factor F =

$$F = \frac{\text{percentage of recombinants in given interval in given burst}}{\text{mean percentage of recombinants in given interval}}$$

The bursts shown are #14 from Table 4 (left) and #7 from Table 5
(right) of Mosig *et al.* (1971). The lower part of the figure indicates the equivalence of linear and circular arrangements of the
markers.

Table 1. Percentage of wild-type recombinants in different T4 crosses in *E. coli* $polA^+$ (B, or nonlysogenic K) and $polA1$ (p3478 or H560) hosts. Data are the averages of 5 or 6 crosses ± standard deviation, except for rb_{41} X rb_{42}.

Cross	$polA^+$		$polA1$	
	30°C	42°C	30°C	42°C
rb_{41} X E1 ($rIIB_1$ X 36)	16.5 ± 1.0	12.9 ± 1.3	10.8 ± 0.5	5.2 ± 2.2
rb_{41} X $r220rb_{42}$ $rIIB_1$ X $rIIA$ $rIIB_2$	0.08 ± 0.01	0.06 ± 0.01	0.09 ± 0.06	0.07 ± 0.02
rb_{41} X $r220$ $rIIB_1$ X $rIIA$	0.62 ± 0.11	0.64 ± 0.13	0.57 ± 0.03	0.44 ± 0.09
rb_{41} X rb_{42} $rIIB_1$ X $rIIB_2$	1.55 ± 0.34	1.25	1.17 ± 0.13	1.12 ± 0.19

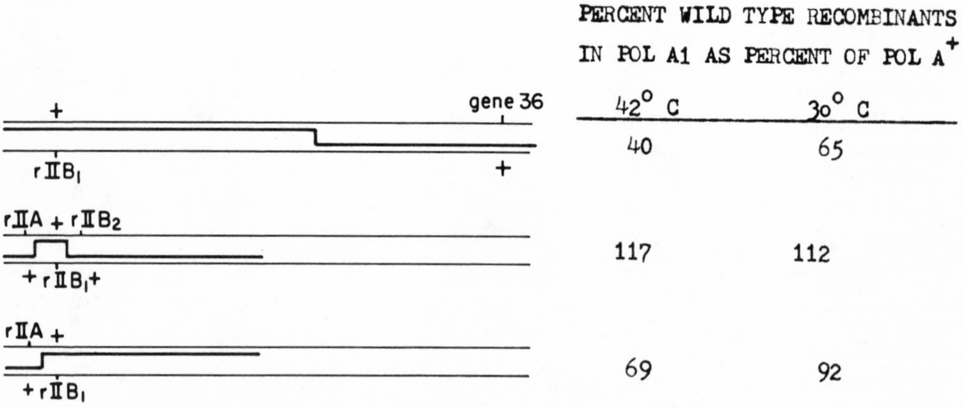

	PERCENT WILD TYPE RECOMBINANTS IN POL A1 AS PERCENT OF POL A^+	
	42° C	30° C
(gene 36 / rIIB₁)	40	65
(rIIA + rIIB₂ / +rIIB₁+)	117	112
(rIIA + / +rIIB₁)	69	92

Figure 3. Comparison of T4 recombination in $polA1$ hosts with $polA^+$ hosts.

recombination deficiency of the *pol*A1 mutants results predominantly from the imbalance of nucleolytic and polymerizing activity (Lehman and Chien, 1973). Possibly, the DNA polymerase I binds to the branch points of the recombinational intermediates to perform "nick-translation" or strand assimilation, a requirement for the formation of "recombinant" heteroduplexes (Fig. 1B). In the absence of compensating polymerase activity the enzyme may specifically destroy potential "recombinant" heteroduplexes. It is also possible that the nuclease activity of the defective polymerase I generally destoys branched intermediates and that most of the insertion heteroduplexes are not derived from branched intermediates. It appears that the nucleolytic activity of DNA polymerase I is not required for T4 recombination (it could possibly be substituted for by a phage function). In a *pol*A mutant 107 (Heijneker *et al.*, 1973), which is defective in the 5'→3' nucleolytic activity of polymerase I, cooperation of incomplete T4 chromosomes is as high as in wild-type hosts. [Experiments with the temperature-sensitive *pol*A 12 mutant (Monk and Kinross, 1972) give ambiguous results, since this mutant adsorbs T4 very poorly.]

THE ROLE OF GENE 32 IN T4 RECOMBINATION

Our second conclusion, that gene 32 protein is involved in at least two different steps of recombination, comes from experiments with one of the gene 32 *ts* mutants (L171), which does not produce phage progeny but shows considerable (although limited) DNA replication after infection at the restrictive temperature of 42°C. The complete details of these experiments will be published elsewhere (Mosig, Breschkin and Berquist, in preparation). Some *r*II mutations (both in the *r*II A and in the *r*II B cistron) partially suppress the L171 defect; *i.e.*, the double mutants produce some progeny at the restrictive temperature. Other *r*II mutations have no effect or even enhance the sensitivity of the L171 mutant to high temperatures. When the parental DNA is labeled with ^{13}C, ^{15}N, and ^{32}P and the progeny DNA is labeled with ^{3}H, it can be seen in sedimentation and density analyses that the gene 32 mutant L171 produces considerable amounts of light-light progeny DNA and that DNA molecules of hybrid and of light-light density form base-paired "joint" molecules. Clearly, L171 differs from the gene 32 *am* mutant A453. Since L171 does form "joint" molecules very efficiently, we can ask whether the gene 32 protein is also involved in covalent linkage during recombination by asking whether L171 can complete this step. Fig. 4A shows that in the intracellular L171 DNA dense ^{32}P-labeled parental and light ^{3}H-labeled progeny strands do not become covalently linked; *i.e.*, they are well separated in alkaline Cs_2SO_4 density gradients. A suppressing *r*II mutation permits some covalent linkage between parental and progeny DNA strands (Fig. 4B). It does not, however, increase the amount of progeny DNA that is produced per

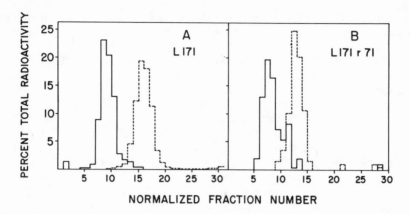

Figure 4. Separation of replicated phage DNA into ^{13}C, ^{15}N, ^{32}P-
labeled parental and ^{3}H, ^{12}C, ^{14}N-labeled progeny strands in alkaline
Cs_2SO_4 gradients. *E. coli* B bacteria were multiply infected with
labeled L171 (A) or L171 *r*71 (B) particles, incubated at 42°C for
16 min, and lysed. The unsheared lysates were fractionated in
neutral Cs_2SO_4 density gradients. Replicated phage DNA was pooled
and recentrifuged in denaturing alkaline Cs_2SO_4 gradients.

replicated template; *i.e.*, the double mutant produces the same
limited amount of progeny DNA per replicated chromosomes as the
single L171 mutant. The inability of the single L171 mutant to
convert "joint" into covalently linked "recombinant" molecules can
completely account for the lack of viable progeny production in
spite of the considerable DNA synthesis, and suppression of this
defect by an *r*II mutant is correlated with measurable progeny production.

Thus, we conclude that gene 32 protein is required not only to
form "joint" molecules but also to convert "joint" into "recombinant"
molecules. In the latter process (but not in the former) it must
interact with the *r*II proteins (or with equivalent host proteins).
Since the *r*II proteins are found almost quantitatively in membrane
preparations (Weintraub and Frankel, 1972; Ennis and Kievitt, 1973),
this implies that covalent linkage occurs at the membrane. In this
respect it is noteworthy that *E. coli* DNA polymerase I transiently
associates with the membrane after T4 infection (Majumdar *et al.*,
1972). Our first set of experiments indicates that *E. coli* polymerase I is involved in the processing of branched recombinational
intermediates. It is presently not clear whether polymerase I and
the gene 32 protein interact in this step of recombination. Huberman *et al.* (1971) have reported that *in vitro* the gene 32 protein
does not interact with *E. coli* DNA polymerase I. Its *in vivo* in-

teraction may, however, have been inaccessible because it involves more cellular components than were present in the assays.

ACKNOWLEDGMENTS

I thank Susan Bock for excellent technical assistance and Alan Breschkin and Richard Dannenberg for stimulating discussions. Supported by NIH grant GM 13221.

REFERENCES

Alberts, B. M. and L. Frey. 1970. T4 bacteriophage gene 32: a structural protein in the replication and recombination of DNA. Nature 227: 1313.

Anraku, N., Y. Anraku and I. R. Lehman. 1969. Enzymic joining of polynucleotides VIII. Structure of hybrids of parental T4 DNA molecules. J. Mol. Biol. 46: 481.

Anraku, N. and J. Tomizawa. 1965. Molecular mechanisms of genetic recombination of bacteriophage V. Two kinds of joining of parental DNA molecules. J. Mol. Biol. 12: 805.

Broker, T. R. 1973. An electron microscopic analysis of pathways for bacteriophage T4 DNA recombination. J. Mol. Biol. 81: 1.

Broker, T. R. and I. R. Lehman. 1971. Branched DNA molecules: Intermediates in T4 recombination. J. Mol. Biol. 60: 131.

Childs, J. D. 1971. A map of molecular distances between mutations of bacteriophge T4D. Genetics 67: 455.

Doermann, A. H. and D. H. Parma. 1967. Recombination in bacterio-phage T4. J. Cell. Physiol. 70 (Suppl. 1): 147.

Ennis, H. L. and K. D. Kievitt. 1973. Association of the *r*IIA protein with the bacterial membrane. Proc. Nat. Acad. Sci. U.S.A. 70: 1468.

Fox, M. S. 1966. On the mechanism of integration of transforming deoxyribonucleate. J. Gen. Physiology 49: 183.

Heijneker, H. L., D. J. Ellens, R. H. Tjeerde, B. W. Glickman, B. van Dorp and P. H. Pouwels. 1973. A mutant of *Escherichia coli* K12 deficient in the 5'-3' exonucleolytic activity of DNA polymerase I. II. Purification and properties of the mutant enzyme. Molec. Gen. Genet. 124: 83.

Holliday, R.   1964.   A mechanism for gene conversion in fungi.
Genet. Res. 5: 282.

Hotchkiss, R. D.   1971.   Toward a general theory of genetic recombination in DNA.   Advan. Genet. 16: 325.

Huberman, J. A., A. Kornberg and B. M. Alberts.   1971.   Stimulation
of T4 bacteriophage DNA polymerase by the protein product of T4
gene 32.   J. Mol. Biol. 62: 39.

Kozinski, A. and Z. Felgenhauer.   1967.   Molecular recombination in
T4 bacteriophage deoxyribonucleic acid   II. Single-strand breaks
and exposure of uncomplemented areas as a prerequisite for recombination.   J. Virol. 1: 1193.

Kozinski, A. W., P. B. Kozinski and R. James.   1967.   Molecular recombination in T4 bacteriophage deoxyribonucleic acid   I. Tertiary
structure of early replicative and recombining deoxyribonucleic
acid.   J. Virol. 1: 758.

Lee, C. S., R. W. Davis and N. Davidson.   1970.   A physical study
by electron microscopy of the terminally repetitious, circularly
permuted DNA from the coliphage particles of *Escherichia coli* 15.
J. Mol. Biol. 48: 1.

Lehman, I. R. and J. R. Chien.   1973.   DNA polymerase I activity in
polymerase I mutants of *Escherichia coli*.   In (R. D. Wells and R.
B. Inman, eds.) DNA Synthesis In Vitro. p. 3-12.   University Park
Press, Baltimore.

Majumdar, C., M. Dewey and F. R. Frankel.   1972.   Bacteriophage-
directed association of DNA polymerase I with host membrane: A
dispensable function.   Virology 49: 134.

Meselson, M.   1972.   Formation of hybrid DNA by rotary diffusion
during genetic recombination.   J. Mol. Biol. 71: 795.

Meselson, M. and J. J. Weigle.   1961.   Chromosome breakage accompanying genetic recombination in bacteriophage.   Proc. Nat. Acad.
Sci. U.S.A. 47: 857.

Monk, M. and J. Kinross.   1972.   Conditional lethality of *rec* A and
*rec*B derivatives of a strain of *Escherichia coli* K-12 with a temperature-sensitive deoxyribonucleic acid polymerase I.   J. Bacteriology
109: 971.

Mosig, G.   1963.   Genetic recombination in bacteriophage T4 during
replication of DNA fragments.   Cold Spring Harbor Symp. Quant.
Biol. 28: 35.

Mosig, G. 1968. A map of distances along the DNA molecule of phage T4. Genetics 59: 137.

Mosig, G., D. W. Bowden and S. Bock. 1972a. *E. coli* DNA polymerase I and other host functions participate in T4 DNA replication and recombination. Nature New Biol. 240: 12.

Mosig, G., J. R. Carnighan, J. B. Bibring, R. Cole, H-G. O. Bock and S. Bock. 1972b. Coordinate variation in lengths of deoxyribonucleic acid molecules and head lengths in morphological variants of bacteriophage T4. J. Virol. 9: 857.

Mosig, G., R. Ehring, W. Schliewen and S. Bock. 1971. The patterns of recombination and segregation in terminal regions of T4 DNA molecules. Molec. Gen. Genet. 113: 51.

Parma, D. H. 1969. The structure of genomes of individual petit particles of the bacteriophage T4D mutant E920/96/41. Genetics 63: 247.

Sigal, N. and B. Alberts. 1972. Genetic recombination: the nature of a crossed strand-exchange between two homologous DNA molecules. J. Mol. Biol. 71: 789.

Spatz, H. C. and T. A. Trautner. 1970. One way to do experiments on gene conversion? Transfection with heteroduplex SPP1 DNA. Molec. Gen. Genet. 109: 84.

Tomizawa, J-I. 1967. Molecular mechanisms of genetic recombination in bacteriophage: Joint molecules and their conversion to recombinant molecules. J. Cell Physiol. 70: 201.

Weintraub, S. B. and F. R. Frankel. 1972. Identification of the T4 rIIB gene product as a membrane protein. J. Mol Biol. 70: 589.

Whitehouse, H. L. K. 1963. A theory of crossing-over by means of hybrid deoxyribonucleic acid. Nature 199: 1034.

HETEROZYGOTES AS INTERMEDIATES OF BACTERIOPHAGE RECOMBINATION

Maurice S. Fox and Raymond L. White*

Department of Biology, Massachusetts Institute of

Technology, Cambridge, Massachusetts 02139

The specificity of the interaction between the complementary strands of DNA molecules provides an attractive way of thinking about the structure of the joint between the two parental contributions of a recombinant DNA molecule. Several lines of evidence demonstrate that heteroduplex regions, in which one strand of DNA is contributed by one of the parental molecules and its complementary strand by the other, are a prominent feature of the primary products of genetic recombination.

Investigations of bacteriophage recombination provide evidence for genetic exchange by a double-strand breakage and joining mechanism in which a region of heteroduplex overlap constitutes the joint between the parental components of the recombinant molecule (Meselson, 1967). The primary recombinant product of bacterial transformation contains a single-stranded fragment of donor DNA that has been inserted into the continuity of the recipient chromosome to form a heteroduplex structure (Fox, 1966). Genetic exchanges involving such single-strand insertions may also occur in bacteriophage recombination but may have escaped detection in the case of λ, since a double-strand exchange appears to be an essential prerequisite for maturation of unduplicated phage (Stahl *et al.*, 1973).

When the two complementary parental strands present in a heteroduplex structure differ in genetic composition, the recombinant molecule is heterozygous.

---

* Present address: Department of Biochemistry, Stanford University School of Medicine, Stanford, California 94304.

Aberrant meiotic segregation or gene conversion has been interpreted in terms of reduction to homozygosity of heterozygous recombinant molecules (Meselson, 1965; Holliday, 1964; Whitehouse and Hastings, 1965). Transfection with heteroduplex bacteriophage DNA has provided evidence for such reduction events (Doerfler and Hogness, 1968; Spätz and Trautner, 1970; Wildenberg, personal communication).

Some features of the structure and fate of heterozygous recombinant molecules have been revealed by investigation of undulplicated bacteriophage λ heterozygotes issuing from crosses carried out under conditions severely restricting DNA synthesis. In addition, transfection experiments with artificially prepared heteroduplex heterozygotes serve to confirm our interpretation of the genetic results. In particular, the observations suggest an explanation for the clustering of recombination events often observed on selection for genetic exchanges within small intervals--high negative interference (Amati and Meselson, 1965; Chovnick *et al*, 1971; Fogel *et al.*, 1971). They also suggest a singularity with regard to the chemical orientation of the heteroduplexes that occur in recombinant molecules of λ (White and Fox, 1974).

The results suggest that double-strand recombinant molecules contain long heteroduplex overlap regions that are initially non-recombinant for closely linked markers but perhaps recombinant for markers that are more widely separated. Markers that are heterozygous within the overlap region are often reduced to homozygosity, and many, perhaps most, of the products exhibiting recombination between closely linked markers arise by this route. The mechanism giving rise to recombination between closely linked markers would therefore depend on, but differ qualitatively from, the mechanism giving rise to recombination between distant markers.

Three suppressible point mutations, O*am*29, P*am*3, and P*am*80, were used as selected genetic markers in these experiments. Their location on an abbreviated physical map of λ are shown in Fig. 1 (Davidson and Szybalski, 1971). Three-factor crosses with these

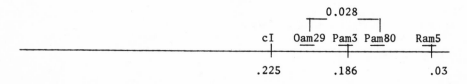

Figure 1. Abbreviated map of phage λ showing physical locations of markers used. Numbers shown are distances from the right end, as fractions of the total λ length.

markers exhibit high negative interference (Amati and Meselson, 1965). Employing the strategy of McMilan and Russo (1972), crosses were performed in the bacterial strain FA77, which is temperature sensitive for DNA synthesis of phage λ (dnaB) and *suppressor negative*, between a λ 0am29 Pam80 parent and a λ Pam3 parent at high temperature. Since neither parent can make active P gene product, DNA synthesis is doubly blocked in this cross (Ogawa and Tomizawa, 1968). The recombinant phage that mature under this stringent limitation of DNA synthesis contain, to a first approximation, only parental DNA. If the two parental genotypes carry different isotopic density labels, then the density of progeny phage in a cesium formate equilibrium gradient will be a measure of the DNA contribution of each of the parents.

To show that DNA synthesis is minimal for 0^+P^+ recombinant, as well as for overall phage progeny, a cross was performed between phage of the two parental genotypes both containing heavy density label (D, ^{15}N) under DNA$^-$ conditions in light medium. Any excess DNA synthesis by the P^+ recombinants should cause them to be density-shifted away from the conserved progeny peak.

The density gradient profile of the progeny of a cross of heavy λcI60 Pam3 by heavy λcI^+ 0am29 Pam80 is shown in Fig. 2. The phage appear at a density position in the gradient expected of particles containing unduplicated DNA with the isotopic composition of the parental phage. The 0^+P^+ recombinants appear at very nearly the same density, demonstrating that their DNA has also been conserved and to very nearly the same extent as the DNA of the total phage progeny. The recombinant peak is density-shifted about 1 fraction (about 3%) to the light side of the peak of total phage.

In order to determine the parental DNA contribution to the double recombinants, a DNA$^-$ cross of heavy λcI60 Pam3 by light λcI^+ 0am29 Pam80 was performed. Since the physical distance between the markers 0am29 and Pam80 is only 2.8% the length of the λ genome, single-strand or double-strand insertion double recombinants should appear as a discrete band, slightly lighter in density than conserved heavy progeny in a density gradient. The appearance of the density-gradient profile of the double recombinants from such a cross (Fig. 3) is contrary to this expectation. The double recombinants are distributed in a broad band from a density position representing substitution of about 15% light DNA into heavy molecules to a position representing substitution of about 15% heavy DNA into light molecules. This result excludes the possibility that the double recombinants observed are the result of a simple insertion event both of whose termini reside between the outside markers.

The results of a cross between cI60 Pam3 as the heavy parent and cI^+ Pam80 as the light parent (Fig. 4) show that single recom-

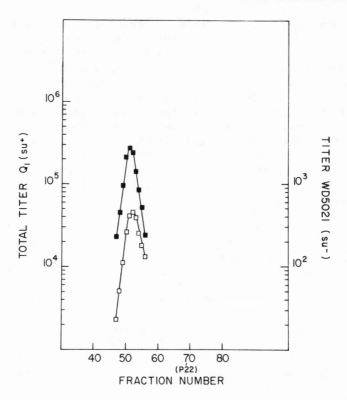

Figure 2.   Cesium formate density-gradient profile of progeny from
cross of heavy c160 Pam3 by heavy cI857 Oam29 Pam80 in FA77 (su⁻,
tsDNA) at 41.5°C.   Bacteria were grown at room temperature in supplemented λ broth to a density of 4×10^8/ml, shifted to 41.5°C
for 15 min, and infected with prewarmed parent phage at 4×10^9/ml,
incubated for 60–70 min at 41.5°C, and terminated by addition of
3 volumes of $CHCl_3$ saturated D_2O buffer.   Lysates were centrifuged
to remove bacterial debris, light Salmonella phage P22 was added,
and cesium formate was added to a refractive index of 1.3710–1.3715.
Centrifugation was for 40–48 hr at 27,000 rpm at 20°C in a Beckman
swinging-bucket rotor (SW39, SW50L, or SW50.1).   One-drop fractions
were collected (130–150 per tube), 1 ml SM was buffer added, and
tubes were titered on Q_1 (su⁺) [■] and WD5021 (su⁻) [□].   P22
position markers were titered on Salmonella strain DB21.   The unadsorbed phage, fully heavy in density (not shown), constitute a
heavy position marker in these gradients.

binants are distributed in a manner very similar to the distribution of double recombinants.   It would appear here too that many of
these recombinants are not likely to arise from simple events involving breakage and joining events that occur in the interval between
Pam3 and Pam80.

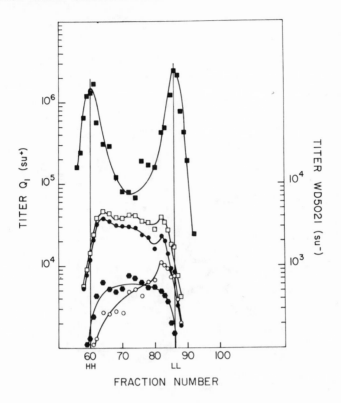

Figure 3. Cesium formate density-gradient profile of progeny from cross of heavy cI60 Pam3 by light cI$^+$ Oam29 Pam80 in FA77 (su$^-$, tsDNA) at 41.5°C (see legend to Fig. 2). ■ , Total phage titer Q$_1$ (su$^+$); □ , total phage titer WD5021 (su$^-$); ● , titer of clear plaques on WD5021 (su$^-$); O, titer of turbid plaques on WD5021 (su$^-$); ⬢ , titer of mottled plaques on WD5021 (su$^-$).

A further analysis of the structure of unduplicated double re-combinants was made by examining the genotypes represented among their progeny. If both alleles of a genetic locus are represented in the progeny of a single infection, then the infecting phage must have been heterozygous at that locus. If only one allele is found there is less certainty, since both alleles may have been present in the infecting phage particles but only one allele transmitted to progeny phage.

The progeny of a cross between heavy λcI60 Pam3 Ram5 and light λcI$^+$ Oam29 Pam80 were distributed in the density gradient shown in Fig. 5. Phage from three regions of the gradient--heavy recombinant, central recombinant, and light recombinant--were adsorbed at low

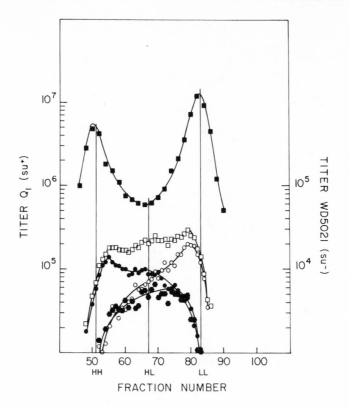

Figure 4. Cesium formate density-gradient profile of progeny from cross of heavy cI60 P*am*3 by light cI⁺ P*am*80 in FA77 (su⁻, *ts*DNA) at 41.5°C. ■, Total phage titer Q_1 (su⁺); □, total phage titer WD5021 (su⁻); ●, titer of clear plaques on WD5021 (su⁻); O, titer of turbid plaques on WD5021 (su⁻); ◉, titer of mottled plaques on WD5021 (su⁻).

multiplicity to su⁻ cells and distributed into tubes for single-burst analysis. After incubation, the cells were lysed with chloroform and lysozyme to release λR*am*5 (lysis deficient) phage, allowing us to use the R*am*5 mutation as an unselected outside marker.

The progeny genotypes found for the selected markers O*am*29⁺, P*am*3⁺, P*am*80⁺ for the three regions of the gradient are displayed in Table 1. The pattern of heterozygous bursts among heavy and light recombinants are distinctly different. Bursts heterozygous for P*am*3, the central allele, occur among double recombinants from heavy fractions but are relatively infrequent among recombinant bursts from light fractions. Light recombinant bursts are *frequently heterozygous* for only the O*am*29 allele. The recombinant bursts from

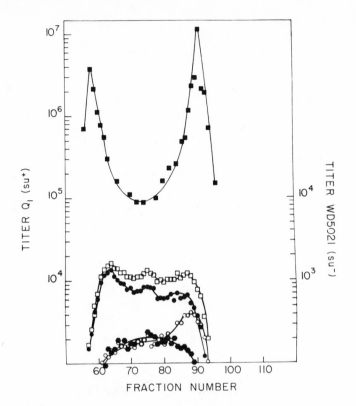

Figure 5. Cesium formate density-gradient profile of progeny from
cross of heavy cI60 Pam3 Ram5 by light cI$^+$ Oam29 Pam80 in FA77
(su$^-$, tsDNA) at 41.5°C. ■ , Total phage titer Q$_1$ (su$^+$); □ , total
phage titer WD5021 (su$^-$); ● , titer of clear plques on WD5021 (su$^-$);
0, titer of turbid plaques on WD5021 (su$^-$); ◆ , titer of mottled
plaques on WD5021 (su$^-$).

the central fractions include both Oam29/+ and Pam3/+ heterozygous
bursts. Bursts heterozygous for the third locus, Pam80, are rarely
found in any region of the gradient. Heterozygosity at the unselected cI60 and Ram5 loci was ubiquitous among all classes of bursts
whether heterozygous or homozygous for the selected alleles. About
40% of the selected recombinant bursts were heterozygous at the cI
locus and about 15% were also heterozygous at the Ram5 locus.

    In a similar analysis of a cross in which the heavy phage
carried the markers cI857 Oam29 Pam80 by light phage cI60 Pam3 Qam73
Ram5, a similar asymmetry is prominent, with Oam29/+ as the major
heterozygote class (60%) among heavy recombinants and Pam3/+ the
major heterozygote class (40%) among light recombinants. Among

Table 1.   Progeny genotypes from three gradient regions

Majority progeny genotypes	Gradient fraction		
	Heavy recombinant	Central recombinant	Light recombinant
+ + +	0.75	0.63	0.43
+ + + and + Pam3 +	0.22	0.13	0.08
+ + + and Oam29 + Pam80	0.02	0.02	0.08
+ + + and + + Pam80	0	0	0
+ + + and Oam29 + +	0.02	0.21	0.41
Total number of wild type containing bursts examined	51[a]	97	51[a]

Phage were absorbed to WD5021 (2-4 X 10^8/ml) at a total multiplicity of 10^{-3} for 10 min at 37°C, anti-λ serum (k=1) for 10 min. Infective centers were diluted in supplemented λ broth, 0.1-ml volumes were distributed in tubes containing 0.1 infective centers/tube and incubated for 60 min at 37°C, and 0.3 ml of iced $CHCl_3$-saturated λ broth containing 20 μg/ml lysozyme was added and incubated at 37°C an additional 45 min. Q_1 plating bacteria were added to each tube, the total contents were plated, and about 20 plaques were picked to identify genotypes.

[a] In addition to the above bursts, among the 538 tubes from the heavy fraction, 21 contained only + Pam3 + phage (setting an upper limit on the extent of leakage of parental phage through the su⁻ host), and among the 549 tubes from the light fraction, four contained only Oam29 + +, six contained only Oam29 + Pam3, and one contained + Pam3 + phage.

the selected recombinants about 40% were heterozygous for cI and about 30% were simultaneously heterozygous for markers on either side of the O,P region.

Some of the features of the density distribution of recombinants as well as the differences in marker content of heterozygous bursts found among heavy and light recombinant phage could be accounted for in the following way.

The products of a double-strand exchange between DNA molecules include a heteroduplex region that is long compared to the intervals between the selected markers. Selected markers present in such heteroduplex regions are usually present as nonrecombinant heterozygotes in the progeny of DNA⁻ crosses. Reduction to homozygosity of some loci within the heterozygous overlap region occurs in the selective indicator, constituting the primary route for formation of the close double recombinants observed in DNA⁻ crosses. Since the termini of the heteroduplex region are not specified, variable parental material contributions to the recombinants may be accomodated.

We further propose that the heterozygous overlaps that give rise to the O,P recombinants occur with only one of the two possible chemical polarities. If both chemical polarities were formed, the set of heterozygous molecules from which recombinants derive would appear as in Fig. 6. Structure a differs from structure b in that both the base-pair mismatches and the genetic composition of the l and r strands are nonidentical in the overlap region. However, in both these respects structure a is identical to structure d, and b is identical to c. The presence of structures a and b, yielding phage that appears at a relatively heavy density, and c and d, yielding phage of a lighter density, would yield a set of similar nonrecombinant heterozygous intermediates among both heavy and light recombinants. In fact, the single-burst data presented show that the genetic content of heterozygous bursts from heavy recombinants differs markedly from that of the light recombinants.

If only one of the two overlap polarities were formed, the heterozygous bursts of heavy and light recombinants might be expected to differ since they would result from heterozygous intermediates a and c or b and d, both pairs consisting of distinguishable structures.

Confidence in this argument would be gained if infections with nonrecombinant, artificially constructed heterozygotes of known structure were to yield recombinant bursts qualitatively similar to those described for recombinant phage from DNA⁻ crosses. The r and l strands of DNA from purified λ stocks of cI⁺ Oam29 Pam80 and cI60 Pam3 genotypes were separated on poly(U,G)-CsCl gradients and heteroannealed (Szybalski et al., 1971). These molecules were used to form infective centers by transfection of su⁻ cells (Mandel and Higa, 1970). The infective centers were plated on a permissive lawn, and the genotypes present in the resulting plaques were examined. The genotypes found are presented in Table 2. By comparison with su⁺ bacteria and with DNA from wild-type phage, we estimate that between 1% and 5% of the su⁻ bacteria transfected with heteroannealed molecules yielded bursts containing O⁺P⁺ phage.

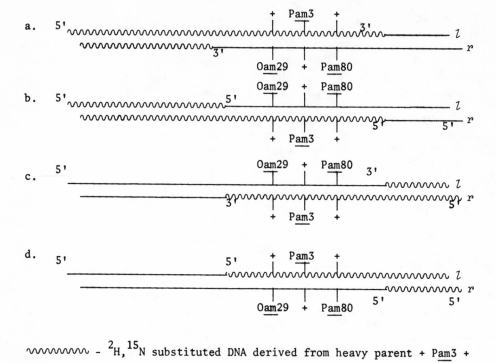

wwwww - ^{2}H,^{15}N substituted DNA derived from heavy parent + P$\underline{am}$3 +

————— - light DNA derived from light parent O$\underline{am}$29 + P$\underline{am}$80

Figure 6. Possible heterozygous molecules giving rise to O,P recombinants. wwww, ^{2}H,^{15}N-substituted DNA derived from the heavy
parent, + Pam3 +; ————, light DNA derived from the light parent,
Oam29 + Pam80.

It is apparent that recombinants can be formed from these
heteroduplex substrates. Furthermore, the heterozygous recombinant
bursts are very similar in frequency and type to the heterozygous
bursts found among the phage progeny of the DNA$^-$ crosses. Infec-
tion with $\dfrac{\text{O}am29 + \text{P}am80 \ (1)}{+ \ \text{P}am3 + \ (r)}$ molecules yields both wild-type recombinants and Oam29 recombinants, as was found for phage particles from
a light region of the density gradient. The $\dfrac{+ \ \text{P}am3 + \ (1)}{\text{O}am29 + \text{P}am80 \ (r)}$ input
molecules yield wild-type homozygous bursts and heterozygous recom-
binant bursts containing wild type and + Pam3 +, as was found for
phage particles from the heavy region of the density gradient. This
result supports the proposal that close double recombinants arise
from nonrecombinant heterozygous intermediates and identifies a

Table 2. Progeny genotypes from transfected su⁻ cells

Progeny genotype found in burst	Genotype of transfecting DNA	
	cI60 + Pam3 + ‒‒‒‒‒ l / ‒‒‒‒‒ r + Oam29 + Pam80	+ Oam29 + Pam80 ‒‒‒‒‒ l / ‒‒‒‒‒ r cI60 + Pam3 +
	Frequency	Frequency
+ + +	0.70	0.25
+ + + and + Pam3 +	0.21	0.02
+ + + and Oam29 + Pam80	0.05	0.07
+ + + and + + Pam80	0.05	0
+ + + and Oam29 + +	0	0.67
Total number of bursts	66	57

Strands of phage DNA were separated by the method of Szybalski (1971), and l strands of each genotype were annealed with r strands of the other genotype by the method of Davis *et al.* (1971). Transfection was carried out by the method of Mandel and Higa (1970). Two volumes of competent MR93/λ were added to one volume of DNA at 0°C for 15 min and 30°C for 3 min, then 1/10 volume of 10X λ broth was added, incubation was continued for an additional 12 min, and infected bacteria were plated with LS446a (su⁺) indicator bacteria. Plaques were picked, and those containing wild-type phage were tested for genotypes present.

unique heteroduplex overlap polarity of 3'-3' as shown in Fig. 6a, c. This result further suggests that many or all of the phage progeny from the DNA⁻ crosses that form plaques on nonpermissive indicators are actually nonrecombinant heterozygotes that generate recombinants after infection of the su⁻ indicator.

DISCUSSION

Evidence has been provided to support the idea that closely
linked multiple recombination events are the result of operations
on long, heterozygous, heteroduplex overlaps that cause some or all
of the heterozygous sites to become homozygous. These operations
would account for high negative interference, since both single
and multiple recombination products would be derived from the nonrecombinant heterozygous overlaps that result from single physical
exchange events.

Support for the existence of extensive heteroduplex overlaps
comes from the observations reported by Russo (1973) as well as
those reported here, that many phage that give rise to double recombinants in the O,P region exhibit associated heterozygosity extending from cI to gene R, a distance of about 1/5 of the λ chromosome length. Since reduction to homozygosity of heterozygotes has
been shown to occur, this value must represent an underestimate of
the actual length distribution of heterozygotes. Although not
easily predictable, the density-gradient profile of double recombinants issuing from heavy by light DNA⁻ crosses is probably consistent with the notion that recombinants arise from molecules containing overlap regions of variable length, sometimes including a substantial fraction of the phage genome. If the overlap is long, the
break points could be very far from the region of selected recombination. The resulting population of recombinant molecules would be
heterogeneous in density, limited by the requirement that the $Oam29^+$,
$Pam3^+$, and $Pam80^+$ alleles of the two parents be present.

If close double recombinants arise in the manner we have suggested, then the single recombinant products of a cross between
closely linked markers should occur by the same mechanism. The results of the cross between $Pam3$ and $Pam80$ substantiate this view.

It would appear that among the progeny of a λ cross the frequency of products exhibiting recombination between closely linked
markers will ultimately be influenced by the following variables:
the frequency with which markers appear within heteroduplex overlaps,
the specificity of the function responsible for the reduction to
homozygosity of the individual base-pair mismatches, and the polynucleotide extent of the region rectified by the reduction mechanism.
Markers that are very closely linked would be expected to exhibit
reduced recombination frequencies by virtue of simultaneous reduction of adjacent heterozygous sites giving rise to one or the other
parental genotype. It seems likely that the specificity with which
base-pair mismatches are recognized and reduced to homozygosity
could readily account for difficulties that have been reported in
using recombinational analysis to determine the linear arrangement
of closely linked markers (Norkin, 1970).

We estimate that only a few percent of the su⁻ bacteria transfected with heteroannealed heteroduplex molecules yield double-
recombinant progeny. It would appear therefore that the recombinants
detected in the progeny of a DNA⁻ cross represent only a small fraction of those phage particles that mature with a heteroduplex overlap
that includes the O,P region. In fact many of the particles of
intermediate density (Fig. 5) exhibit evidence of heterozygosity in
the O,P region. About 12% of the plaques plated permissively contain
either phage with both $Oam29^+$ and $Pam3^+$ alleles or phage with both
$Pam3^+$ and $Pam80^+$ alleles. About 75% of the plaques derived from
plating infective centers, resulting from transfection of permissive
bacteria with heteroannealed heteroduplex DNA, contain phage of one
parental type or the other. It could be, therefore, that as many as
half of the phage of intermediate density derived from the phage
cross contain DNA molecules whose heteroduplex region is sufficiently
extensive to include heterozygosity in the O,P region of the genome
(White and Fox, in preparation).

The events required for the transition of nonrecombinant heterozygotes to recombinants remain unclear. Possibilities include specific editing or repair of base-pair mismatches, random excision and
repair followed by selection for recombinant messenger-producing
strands, elimination of one of the products of aborted synthesis
initiating at the normal origin of replication, or even localized
duplication of the heterozygous region followed by additional recombination events. Extensive duplication does not seem to be required,
however, since $\dfrac{Oam29 + Pam80}{+ Pam3 +}$ artificial heterozygotes form recombinants in su⁻ cells even though neither infecting strand can produce
the functional P gene product required for DNA synthesis.

Although neither of the mechanisms are, as yet, clear, the
processes giving rise to recombination between closely linked markers
seems to be qualitatively different from the process giving rise
to recombination between distant markers.

ACKNOWLEDGMENTS

This work was supported by grant #AI 05388 from the National
Institutes of Health and by grant #B33622 from the National Science
Foundation.

REFERENCES

Amati, P. and M. Meselson. 1965. Localized negative interference
in bacteriophage λ. Genetics 51: 369.

Chovnick, A., G. H. Ballantyne and D. G. Holm. 1971. Studies on gene conversion and its relationship to linked exchange in *Drosophila melanogaster*. Genetics 69: 179.

Davidson, N. and W. Szybalski. 1971. Physical and chemical characteristics of lambda DNA. In (A. D. Hershey, ed.) The Bacteriophage Lambda. p. 45. Cold Spring Harbor Laboratory, New York.

Davis, R. W., M. Simon and N. Davidson. 1971. Electron microscope heteroduplex methods for mapping regions of base sequence homology in nucleic acids. Methods Enzymol. 21 (part D): 413.

Doerfler, W. and D. S. Hogness. 1968. Gene orientation in bacteriophage lambda as determined from the genetic activities of heteroduplex DNA formed *in vitro*. J. Mol. Biol. 33: 661.

Fogel, S., D. D. Hurst and R. K. Mortimer. 1971. Gene conversion in unselected tetrads from multipoint crosses. In (G. Kimber and G. P. Redei, eds.) Stadler Genetics Symposia, Vols. 1 and 2, p. 89. University of Missouri Agricultural Experiment Station, Columbia, Mo.

Fox, M. S. 1966. On the mechanism of integration of transforming deoxyribonucleate. J. Gen. Physiol. 49: 183.

Holliday, R. 1964. A mechanism for gene conversion in fungi. Genet. Res. 5: 282.

Mandel, M. and A. Higa. 1970. Calcium-dependent bacteriophage DNA infection. J. Mol. Biol. 53: 159.

McMilan, K. D. and V. E. A. Russo. 1972. Maturation and recombination of bacteriophage lambda DNA molecules in the absence of DNA duplication. J. Mol. Biol. 68: 49.

Meselson, M. 1965. The duplication and recombination of genes. In (J. A. Moore, ed.) Ideas in Modern Biology, p. 3. The Natural History Press, Garden City, N. Y.

Meselson, M. 1967. The molecular basis of recombination. In (R. A. Brink, ed.) Heritage from Mendel, p. 81. University of Wisconsin Press, Madison.

Norkin, L. C. 1970. Marker-specific effects in genetic recombination. J. Mol. Biol. 51: 633.

Ogawa, T. and J. Tomizawa. 1968. Replication of bacteriophage DNA. I. Replication of DNA of lambda phage defective in early functions. J. Mol. Biol. 38: 217.

Russo, V. E. A. 1973. On the physical structure of λ recombinant DNA. Molec. Gen. Genet. 122: 353.

Spätz, H. Ch. and T. A. Trautner. 1970. One way to do experiments on gene conversion? Transfection with heteroduplex *SPP1* DNA. Molec. Gen. Genet. 109: 84.

Stahl, F., S. Chung, J. Crasemann, D. Fualds, J. Haemer, S. Lam, R. Malone, K. McMilan, Y. Nozu, J. Siegel, J. Strathern and M. Stahl. 1973. Recombination, replication, and maturation in phage lambda. In (C. F. Fox and W. S. Robinson, eds.) Virus Research, p. 487. Academic Press, New York.

Szybalski, H., H. Kubinski, Z. Hradecna and W. C. Summers. 1971. Analytical and preparative separation of the complemenatry DNA strands. Methods Enzymol. 21 (part D): 383.

White, R. L. and M. S. Fox. 1974. On the molecular basis of high negative interference. Proc. Nat. Acad. Sci. U.S.A. in press.

Whitehouse, H. L. K. and P. J. Hastings. 1965. The analysis of genetic recombination on the polaron hybrid DNA model. Genet. Res. 6: 27.

MAPPING OF POINT MUTATIONS ON THE PHYSICAL MAP OF COLIPHAGE LAMBDA: ABSENCE OF CLUSTERING FOR ODD-NUMBERED EXCHANGES

F. R. Blattner, J. D. Borel, T. M. Shinnick and W. Szybalski

McArdle Laboratory for Cancer Research, University of Wisconsin, Madison, Wisconsin 53706

One of the classic problems of genetics concerns the relationship between the genetic map, measured in recombination frequency units, and the physical map, measured in nucleotide pairs along a DNA molecule. For *Escherichia coli* bacteriophage λ the gross correlation between the genetic and physical maps was discussed by Campbell (1971), Davidson and Szybalski (1971) and Signer (1971). In the present study we undertook to analyze recombination very precisely and quantitatively within a short segment of the λ genome in the so-called immunity region. The advantage of this region is the availability of many point mutations and deletions, studied intensively by earlier authors (see *e.g.*, Kaiser, 1957; Kayajanian, 1968, 1970; Lieb, 1966; Gussin *et al.*, 1973), and of a precise physical map (Fiandt and Szybalski, 1973; Blattner *et al.*, 1972, 1974). The position of mutations can be established by several methods, including calculations based on recombination frequency between point mutations, the techniques of deletion mapping, and the present method of extrapolation mapping. This work is an extension of our earlier and current mapping of the p_L mutant *sex*1 (Blattner *et al.*, 1972, 1974), and was summarized by Blattner and Borel (1973).

MAPPING OF "CLEAR" MUTATIONS

For this study we developed the technique shown in Fig. 1. Each cross was performed in a rec^+su host between a λbio phage, which cannot form plaques on the recA bacteria because of its Fec$^-$ phenotype (Signer, 1971; Blattner *et al.*, 1972, 1974), and a

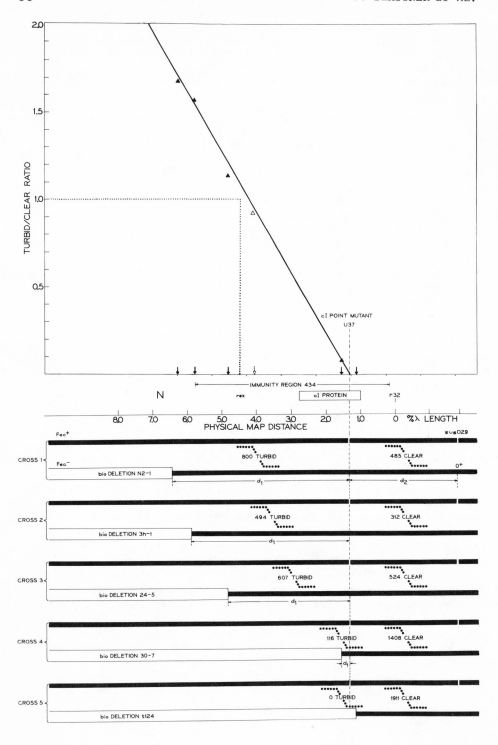

Figure 1. Graphic representation of a typical recombination experiment. The five crosses are shown schematically. Recombinants in the variable d_1 interval give rise to turbid recombinants, whereas those in the constant d_2 region produce clear plaques. The tu/cl ratios for the Fec^+O^+ recombinants are plotted (solid triangles) against the physical positions of the *bio* endpoints measured from the site of the *r*32 insertion. The result of the cross between λ*bio*t75 and λ*c*IU37*sus*029 (open triangle; see Fig. 2) is included. The use of the tu/cl ratios automatically normalizes all results in relation to the constant d_2 interval. The tu/cl value equals 1 when interval d_1 equals d_2 (dotted lines).

λ*c*I⁻*sus*0, which cannot plate on a *su*° host. The products of these crosses were plated on the N100(*recA*⁻*su*°) indicator lawn, which selected only for Fec^+O^+ recombinants. The endpoints of the *bio* substitutions have been precisely determined by electron micrographic mapping (Fiandt and Szybalski, 1973; Blattner *et al.*, 1974). Recombinants occurring in the constant d_2 interval between the *c*I⁻ and *O*⁻ mutation formed clear (cl) plaques and recombinants in the variable *bio*-to-*c*I interval formed turbid (tu) plaques. Plotting the tu/cl ratio as a function of the physical position of the *bio* endpoints permitted us to extrapolate the least-squares line to the position for the *c*I⁻ mutation on the physical map of the λ immunity region, as the point of intersection on the abscissa. Several such extrapolations for a series of *c*I⁻ mutations and for other "clear" mutants (*sex*1, *v1v*3, *c*17) are shown in Fig. 2.

The following properties of such plots can be noted in Figs. 1 and 2. (1) The extrapolation plots are straight lines. (2) They intersect with the abscissa between those two *bio* endpoints which bracket the clear mutation, as determined by deletion mapping. This result lends credence to this method of mapping. Indeed, in the case of the *sex*1 mutation, the position of which is known from nucleotide sequence analysis, the intercept is within 15 nucleotides of the correct position (Blattner *et al.*, 1974). Such high accuracy might be fortuitous, especially since for some other *c*I mutations -- *e.g.*, *ts*2 where long extrapolations were made -- the margin of error is large (Fig. 2). (3) As expected, most of the plotted lines pass through the point equal to 1 (or near it) on the tu/cl axis when the variable distance d_1 equals the constant interval d_2 (see dotted line on Fig. 1). Some exceptions to this result, for instance caused by the *v*2 marker, which differentially affects the growth of the clear and turbid recombinants, are discussed in more detail by Blattner and Borel (1974). It will suffice to state here that although such markers change the slope of the plotted line, they do not affect the position of the intercept.

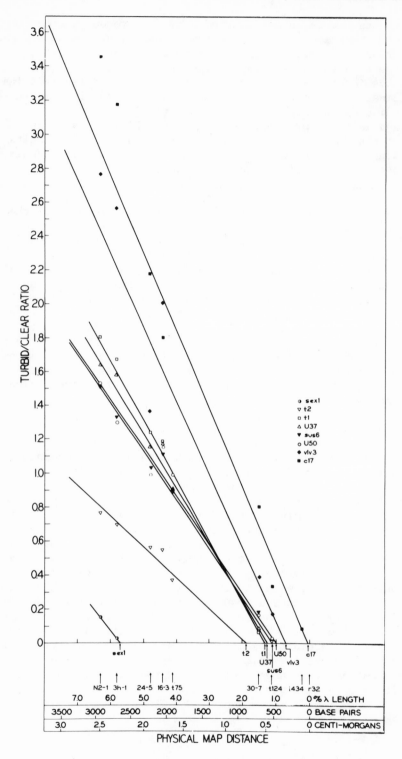

Figure 2. Extrapolation mapping of point mutations on the physical
map. Eight experiments analogous to the one illustrated in Fig. 1
were performed, using the following "clear" markers: the p_L promoter mutation $sex1$; cI mutants $ts2$, $ts1$, $tsU37$, $tsU50$, and $sus6$;
the o_L operator mutations $v1v3$; and a new promoter mutation $cl7$
(see Blattner $et\ al.$, 1974; Lieb, 1966; Szybalski, 1972). The scale
on the abscissa is in %λ units, with 1% of the λpapa length corresponding to 0.66 centimorgans and 465 nucleotide pairs (Davidson
and Szybalski, 1971). The straight lines are fitted by the least-
squares method, and the position of the "clear" marker corresponds
to the intercept on the abscissa.

THE NATURE OF RECOMBINATIONAL CLUSTERING

The phenomenon of localized high negative interference has
been observed in a number of genetic systems, including phage T4
(Chase and Doermann, 1958; Doermann and Parma, 1967), the lac operon
(Sadler and Smith, 1971) and phage λ (Amati and Meselson, 1965).
Its principal experimental manifestation is the occurrence of
closely spaced multiple crossovers at unexpectedly high frequency
in a population of recombinants selected for a single exchange.
This has been interpreted to mean that a single recombination event
is likely to produce a cluster of crossovers near the selected region. A mathematical model was described that postulates a recombinationally active region, the "switch area," with many crossovers
distributed at random within it (Chase and Doermann, 1958; Barricelli and Doermann, 1960). Models of this type were applied by
Sadler and Smith (1971) and Amati and Meselson (1965) to data derived
mostly from double crossovers, and they concluded that a typical
cluster would measure 1500 to 3000 nucleotide pairs, with crossovers
distributed at random at about one crossover per 500 nucleotide
pairs within the recombinationally active cluster. These parameters,
when applied to the present data, predict an extreme downward curva-
ture for the plots shown in Figs. 1 and 2. The theoretically derived curves (Fig. 3) bend downward as the variable region d_1
increases, basically for the same reason that markers very far apart
on a "classical" chromosome appear to be unlinked; $i.e.$, the frequency of recombination ceases to depend on distance and the plot
becomes horizontal in the extreme case. It should be stressed that
in the experiments shown in Figs. 1 and 2 the departure from linearity is a very sensitive measure of the recombinational clustering
or high negative interference phenomenon. For example, the p = 1.0
curve in Fig. 3 corresponds to one crossover per one %λ unit (465
nucleotide pairs), which, as discussed above, is a typical density
of crossovers in an assumed recombinational cluster.

Our present results appear to be incompatible with the concept
of "switch areas" because of the strict linearity of the plots shown
in Figs. 1 and 2. What could be the reason for this disagreement?

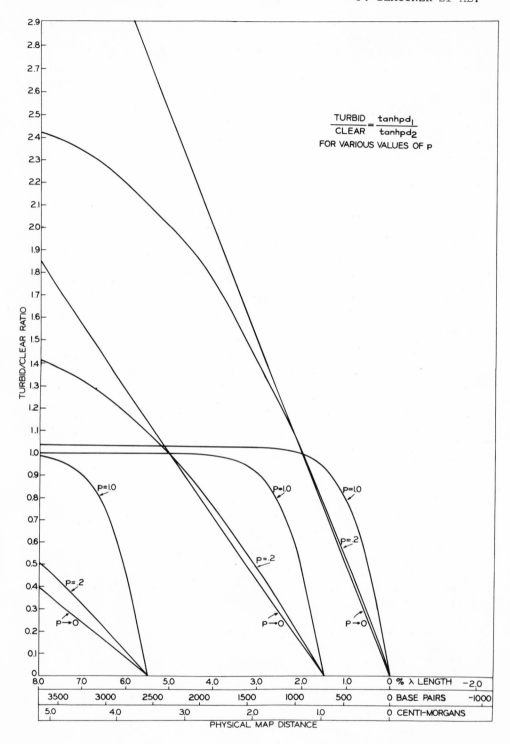

Figure 3. Calculated effects of recombinational clustering on the extrapolation mapping. Three imaginary clear point mutants were analyzed according to a simple cluster model (Blattner and Borel, 1974). The parameter p specifies the average spacing of crossovers (Poisson distribution) within a cluster (p = 1 corresponds to one crossover per 1 %λ; p = 0.2 corresponds to one crossover per 5 %λ). The length of a cluster is assumed to be on the order of 1500 to 3000 base pairs. These predictions (especially for p = 1; Amati and Meselson, 1965) are clearly different from the experimental data shown in Figs. 1 and 2.

The peculiar design of our experiment is that it scores only for the odd-numbered genetic exchanges, since all the double and higher even-numbered crossovers are removed from consideration by our selective procedure. On the other hand, in most of the Amati and Meselson (1965) experiments, the recombinational clustering and high negative interference were observed for double exchanges. Formally, this would indicate that the basic premise of the switch area hypothesis, namely that crossovers are distributed at random, may not be true. Instead, it could be that double exchanges can occur as a single event (Fig. 4, D_1 and E_1), so that the localized high negative interference is observed for the double crossovers and not for the odd-numbered exchanges. Is there any recombinational model that would predict such a recombinational behavior? Indeed, the chiasma migration model of Holliday (1964) predicts that double exchanges should be as frequent as single exchanges over distances traveled by the DNA strand chiasma (Fig. 4), but that triple exchanges should occur only by multiple chiasma migration events.

THE CHIASMA MIGRATION MODEL

The chiasma migration model, which has been extensively discussed during this conference, is shown in Fig. 4. It postulates the formation of an exchange between two DNA strands of the same orientation (DNA strand chiasma) derived from two parental DNA molecules. This chiasma can migrate up or down the DNA, driven by "speedometer cable" rotation of the parental duplexes, and can be cut in two different ways to separate the two recombinant DNA molecules. One type of cut produces a single recombinant (Fig. 4, D_2 and E_2) and the other results in a double recombinational event in a single step (Fig. 4, D_1 and E_1). As a first approximation, this model would explain the high negative interference due to the excess of double crossovers and the absence of recombinational clustering for triple and higher-numbered odd exchanges observed in our experiments.

There are three basic models for explaining high negative interference: (1) the switch area hypothesis, (2) the mismatch

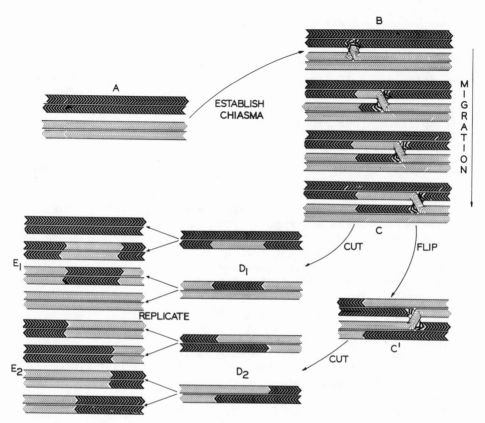

Figure 4. Chiasma migration model (Holliday, 1964; Sigal and
Alberts, 1972). The polarity of the DNA strands in the DNA duplexes
is indicated. Two parental duplexes (A) give rise by an unspecified
mechanism to a crossed-strand chiasma (B). Chiasma migration leads
to formation of heteroduplex regions (C). The chiasma may be cut
and resolved to produce strand-insertion heteroduplex molecules
(D_1), or it might "flip" ("strand equivalence"; Sigal and Alberts,
1972) to produce an equivalent isomeric form of the chiasma (C')
and then be cut to yield strand-overlap heteroduplex molecules (D_2).
Replication of these molecules yields eight homoduplex types (E_1
and E_2). By this mechanism the double (E_1) and single (E_2) crossovers occur at comparable frequencies over the distance of chiasma
migration, whereas apparent triple and higher crossover events can
only occur by repeated exchanges or by mismatch repair events in
the heteroduplex regions (C and D) before establishment of the
homoduplex structures (E).

correction (or repair) hypothesis, and (3) the chiasma migration
hypothesis. As already discussed, the third hypothesis would
explain both the absence of high negative interference observed in

our experiments and the seemingly opposite results of Amati and Meselson (1965). However, the second mechanism might play an important role when DNA replication is severely inhibited and the DNA heteroduplexes, formed by DNA strand chiasma migration, persist for a long time. In our case λ DNA replication was not inhibited and, thus, the mismatch corrections must have played a very minor role. Indeed, if any substantial fraction of recombinants in our experiment were due to mismatch correction, the tu/cl ratio would hardly depend on the d_1 (*bio*-clear) distance (Fig. 1). There is no evidence for the first (switch area) hypothesis on the basis of our data.

CONCLUSIONS AND SUMMARY

1. The extrapolation mapping of point mutations on the physical map of phage λ is a very accurate and reasonably simple technique. It is quite useful whenever accurate physical maps for clustered deletions are available.

2. The extrapolation plots were all linear, indicating that no localized high negative interference was encountered in this system, which was designed to select only for single and odd-numbered crossovers.

3. The absence of high negative interference for odd-numbered exchanges and the presence of frequent clusters of double crossovers can be predicted by the chiasma migration model (Fig. 4). This would be especially true for áctively replicating phages, in which repair replication is minimized. When DNA synthesis is blocked during the recombinational process, mismatch repair of nonreplicated heteroduplexes formed during the chiasma migration (Fig. 4; stages C and D) might lead to more complex phenomena.

ACKNOWLEDGMENT

These studies were supported by grants from the National Cancer Institute (CA-07175) and the National Science Foundation (GB-2096). We are indebted to Mr. M. Fiandt and Dr. E. H. Szybalski for unpublished electron micrographic mapping data and to Drs. M. Lieb, H. O. Smith, and W. F. Dove for helpful suggestions and phage strains.

REFERENCES

Amati, P. and Meselson. 1965. Localized negative interference in bacteriophage λ. Genetics **51**: 369.

Barricelli, N. A. and A. H. Doermann. 1960. An analytical approach to the problem of phage recombination and reproduction. II. High negative interference. Virology 11: 136.

Blattner, F. and J. Borel. 1973. High negative interference in bacteriophage λ: absence of multiple odd exchanges. Abstract for Symposium on Genetic Recombination, p. 44. Roche Institute of Molecular Biology, Nutley, New Jersey.

Blattner, F. R. and J. D. Borel. 1974. Recombination in bacteriophage lambda -- absence of correlated triple exchanges; a method for mapping point mutations on the physical map. J. Mol. Biol., submitted for publication.

Blattner, F. R., J. E. Dahlberg, J. K. Boettiger, M. Fiandt and W. Szybalski. 1972. Distance from a promoter mutation to an RNA synthesis startpoint on bacteriophage λ DNA. Nature New Biol. 237: 232.

Blattner, F. R., M. Fiandt, K. K. Hass, P. A. Twose and W. Szybalski. 1974. Deletions and insertions in the immunity region of coliphage lambda: revised measurements of the promoter-startpoint distance. Virology, in press.

Campbell, A. 1971. Genetic structure. In (A. D. Hershey, ed.) The Bacteriophage Lambda. p. 13. Cold Spring Harbor Laboratory, Cold Spring Harbor, New York.

Chase, M. and A. H. Doermann. 1958. High negative interference over short segments of the genetic structure of bacteriophage T4. Genetics 43: 332.

Davidson, N. and W. Szybalski. 1971. Physical and chemical characteristics of lambda DNA. In (A. D. Hersehy, ed.) The Bacteriophage lambda. p. 45. Cold Spring Harbor Laboratory, Cold Spring Harbor, New York.

Doermann, A. H. and D. H. Parma. 1967. Recombination in bacteriophage T4. J. Cell. Physiol. 70 (Suppl. 1): 147.

Fiandt, M. and W. Szybalski. 1973. Electron microscopy of the immunity region in coliphage lambda. Abst. Ann. Meet. Amer. Soc. Microbiol., p. 218.

Gussin, G. N., V. Peterson and N. Loeb. 1973. Deletion mapping of the λ *rex* gene. Genetics 74: 385.

Holliday, R. 1964. A mechanism for gene conversion in fungi. Genet. Res. 5: 282.

Kaiser, A. D. 1957. Mutations in a temperate bacteriophage affecting its ability to lysogenize *Escherichia coli*. Virology $\underline{3}$: 42.

Kayajanian, G. 1968. Studies on the genetics of biotin-transducing, defective variants of bacteriophage λ. Virology $\underline{36}$: 30.

Kayajanian, G. 1970. Deletion mapping of the c_{III}-c_{II} region of bacteriophage λ. Virology $\underline{41}$: 170.

Lieb, M. 1966. Studies of heat-inducible lambda bacteriophage. I. Order of genetic sites and properties of mutant prophages. J. Mol. Biol. $\underline{16}$: 149.

Sadler, J. R. and T. F. Smith. 1971. Mapping of the lactose operator. J. Mol. Biol. $\underline{62}$: 139.

Sigal, N. and B. Alberts. 1972. Genetic recombination: The nature of a crossed strand-exchange between two homologous DNA molecules. J. Mol. Biol. $\underline{71}$: 789.

Signer, E. 1971. General recombination. In (A. D. Hershey, ed.) The Bacteriophage Lambda. p. 139. Cold Spring Harbor Laboratory, Cold Spring Harbor, New York.

Szybalski, W. 1972. Transcription and replication in *E. coli* bacteriophage lambda. In (L. Ledoux, ed.) Uptake of Informative Molecules by Living Cells. p. 59. North-Holland Publ. Co., Amsterdam.

SITE-SPECIFIC RECOMBINATION: GENES AND REGULATION

Harrison Echols, Stephen Chung and Linda Green

Department of Molecular Biology, University of

California, Berkeley, California 94720

A dozen years have passed since Allan Campbell (1962) suggested that prophages might associate with the host chromosome through an insertion mechanism accomplished by a reciprocal recombination event. We now know that insertion does occur for most temperate phage and that the insertion reaction is typically catalyzed by a phage-specified pathway of recombination, which is notable for its localization to one or a small number of sites on the phage and host DNA (for reviews see Echols, 1971; Gottesman and Weisberg, 1971).

For phage λ, the genetic analysis of site-specific recombination has been particularly extensive (Echols, 1971; Gottesman and Weisberg, 1971). This paper will attempt to summarize this analysis, with emphasis on some recent developments concerning two aspects of site-specific recombination: essential genes and regulation of the direction of the reaction.

RECENT CLASSICAL CONCEPTS (ca. 1971)

The general features of site-specific recombination by phage λ (as of the reviews noted above) are indicated in Fig. 1. The viral DNA circularizes after infection, and a reciprocal recombination event between the phage attachment site (aa') and the bacterial attachment site (bb') leads to a covalent insertion of the viral DNA into that of the host. When the prophage is induced to lytic growth, the process is reversed: a reciprocal recombination event between the prophage attachment sites (ba' and ab') leads to a regeneration of the original viral DNA.

The concept of a phage-specified, site-specific recombination

69

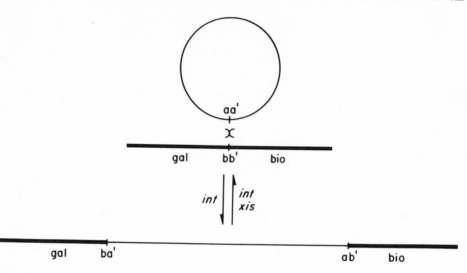

Figure 1. The integration-excision reaction. Phage DNA is indicated by a light line and bacterial DNA by a heavy line. Site-specific recombination between the phage attachment site *aa'* and the host
attachment site *bb'* results in insertion of the viral DNA (integrative recombination). The inserted prophage is flanked by the recombinant prophage attachment sites *ba'* and *ab'*. Site-specific recombination between *ba'* and *ab'* results in detachment of the viral DNA
(excisive recombination).

pathway developed from the isolation of mutants defective in integration (Zissler, 1967; Gingery and Echols, 1967; Gottesman and
Yarmolinsky, 1968a) and from the demonstration that these mutants
affected a recombination event at a single site of λ DNA (Echols
et al., 1968; Weil and Signer, 1968). Further studies showed that
these mutants also affected excision (Gottesman and Yarmolinsky,
1968b; Gingery and Echols, 1968). Thus the product of the *int* gene
(Int protein) is necessary for both integration and excision. However, one can ask whether the Int protein is sufficient in itself.
Because regulatory features of the reaction appeared to require
greater complexity, we sought evidence for an excision-specific
gene through a search for mutants which could integrate but not
excise. These mutants defined the *xis* gene, another component of
the site-specific recombination reaction (Guarneros and Echols,
1970; Echols, 1970). The Xis protein is essential for excision but
not for integration. New information summarized here indicates that
there exists a gene which has a role in integration like that of the
xis gene in excision. We term this gene *hen*, for help to integration.

    The general regulatory concepts for site-specific recombination

by phage λ (as of the reviews noted above) are indicated in Fig. 2.
The genes for site-specific recombination are expressed as part of
an *N*-activated, *c*I-repressed unit of transcription, the recombination region of λDNA (Echols, 1971, 1972; Gottesman and Weisberg,
1971). This view is based on two observations. First, the integrated state is stable in a lysogen, and superinfecting phage integrate poorly (Campbell and Zissler, 1966); thus, site-specific
recombination is subject to repression. Second, *N*⁻ mutants of λ
integrate inefficiently (Signer, 1969). Three additional features
of this regulation are now known from recent experiments (Echols,
1974; Shimada and Campbell, 1974), and the evidence is summarized
briefly here. First, integrative recombination can occur at a low
level in a repressed lysogen. Second, this constitutive integrative recombination is much more effective in the repressed lysogen
than excisive recombination. Third, the synthesis of the proteins
responsible for this constitutive integrative recombination probably
involves transcription from a separate promoter site from that used
for most of the transcription of the recombination region during
normal lytic growth of λ.

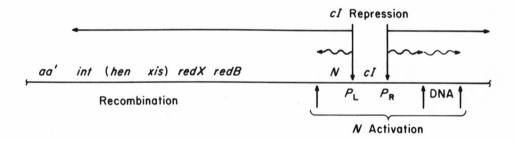

Figure 2. Regulation of the recombination region. Transcription
during the immediate-early stage of λ development (〜〜〜) is
carried out by the host transcription machinery; efficient transcription of the recombination region occurs during the delayed-early
stage of λ development (⇌), activated by the product of gene
N. The probable sites at which *N*-activation occurs are indicated
by the vertical arrows (↑). The virus may then enter the lysogenic
pathway or the late stage of the lytic pathway. Lysogeny is maintained by the cI protein, which acts at operator sites to the left
and right of the *c*I gene [vertical arrows (↓)] to repress immediate-
early RNA synthesis initiated at the promoter sites P_L and P_R. For
a complete review of the lysogenic and lytic pathways see Echols
(1972) or Herskowitz (1973).

CONSTITUTIVE INTEGRATIVE RECOMBINATION

The experimental system we have used to study integrative recombination in a repressed lysogen is indicated in Fig. 3. In this case, a λ*gal* DNA has integrated by excisive recombination. The λ*gal* carries the left-hand prophage attachment site (*ba'*) and integrates into a defective lysogen which carries only the right-hand prophage attachment site (*ab'*). Insertion of the λ*gal* DNA and *gal* transduction derive from an excisive recombination event requiring the Int and Xis proteins; detachment of this λ*gal* DNA requires an integrative recombination event. Thus the normal catalytic features of integration and excision are reversed. The utility of this λ*gal* lysogen for the study of integrative recombination and its stability derive from the fact that the stability of the λ*gal* prophage depends on the frequency of integrative recombination in a repressed state.

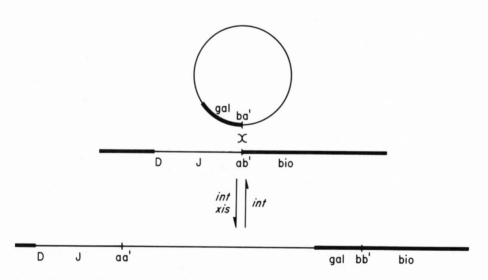

Figure 3. The "reversed" integration-excision reaction used to study integrative recombination in a repressed lysogen and to isolate *hen* mutants. A λ*gal* transducing phage undergoes site-specific recombination in a host that carries the right prophage attachment site but lacks most other λ genes through a prophage deletion (only the genes D to J of the head and tail region remain). In this case, insertion and detachment occur by the *reverse* of the normal recombination reactions: insertion occurs by excisive recombination (*ba'* X *ab'*) and detachment occurs by integrative recombination (*aa'* X *bb'*).

In the absence of all general recombination (through appropriate mutations), the λgal lysogen depicted in the figure is significantly unstable. The frequency with which gal^- segregants are
produced is approximately 5 X 10^{-3}; in contrast, a normal prophage
of the type depicted in Fig. 1 will segregate at a frequency less
than 5 X 10^{-6} (Echols, 1974; R. A. Weisberg, personal communication). Thus integrative recombination not only occurs in a repressed lysogen but is many orders of magnitude more effective than
excisive recombination. The value of this regulatory mechanism for
a virus is presumably to provide an additional mechanism by which
the stability of the prophage state is maintained.

The constitutive features of the integrative recombination
reaction have also been explored by Shimada and Campbell (1974),
utilizing an experimental system in which transcription of an adjacent host gene is used to monitor the presumptive constitutive
expression of the λint gene. They have shown that it is possible
to delete the normal leftward promoter (P_L in Fig. 2) without
altering this capacity for synthesis. Thus the protein synthesis
required for constitutive integrative recombination probably
involves transcription from a promoter site separate from that used
for most of the recombination region during lytic growth. The precise location of this promoter site (P_I) has not been specified;
however, Shimade and Campbell present indirect evidence that it may
be located in the xis gene itself.

EVIDENCE FOR ANOTHER INTEGRATION FUNCTION

Because of some peculiar asymmetries between integrative and
excisive recombination, one of which we have just noted, we decided
to ask whether there might be a gene which played a role in integration analogous to the role played by xis in excision. In order
to look for mutants in such a gene we employed the recombinational
system shown in Fig. 3, in which λgal inserts by excisive recombination and detaches by integrative recombination. In such an experimental system a λgal phage which reaches the prophage state should
have normal int and xis genes, but need not have normal expression
of the hypothetical ancillary function for integrative recombination, because insertion has occurred by an excisive recombination
reaction. Thus one can seek mutants defective in this hypothetical
additional gene by a search for mutants of λgal for which gal transduction can occur but for which loss of prophage does not occur with
the normal frequency. The characterization of these mutants so far
indicates that they involve a previously unidentified λ gene, which
we have termed hen for "help to integration" (Chung et al., 1974).
We have analyzed these mutants by measurements of the normal integration and excision reactions and of site-specific recombination
between phage in lytic crosses. A summary of the results is

Table 1. The Hen phenotype

Phage genotype	% Integration (lysogeny)	% Excision (curing)	% Recombination in lytic crosses	
			aa'/bb'	*ba'/ab'*
int+	58	69	14	4
*int*2	<0.1	<0.1	0.03	0.06
*xis*1	49	<0.1	8	0.02
*hen*1	4	75	0.2	18

Integration frequencies represent the stable inheritance of a prophage following infection of initially nonlysogenic cells; excision frequencies represent the loss of a stable prophage following brief derepression of initially lysogenic cells (for procedures see Guarneros and Echols, 1970). Integrative recombination in lytic crosses was measured between a "normal" λ phage with attachment site *aa'* and a λ*gal bio* phage with attachment site *bb'*; excisive recombination was measured between a λ*gal* phage with attachment site *ba'* and a λ*bio* phage with attachment site *ab'* (for procedures see Echols, 1970).

presented in Table 1. A *hen*⁻ mutant is defective in normal integration, although not as defective as a phage mutant in the *int*
gene itself (Column 1); however, excision is normal (Column 2).
In lytic crosses the *hen*⁻ mutant is defective in integrative recombination but not in excisive recombination (Columns 3 and 4).
A similar phenotype has been found for two other *hen*⁻ mutants.

It is clearly important to establish whether the *hen*⁻ mutations define a gene which is distinct from the *int* and *xis* genes.
As judged by a complementation test, the *hen*⁻ mutations are distinct from previously identified mutations in the *int* gene; a deletion of most of the *int* gene can complement *hen*⁻ mutants to provide
for normal integrative recombination. Thus we believe that the *hen*
gene is distinct from the *int* gene.

Further functional analysis with deletions has indicated that
the *hen* gene is close to the *xis* gene, because the same deletion
eliminates both functions. Therefore we must ask whether the *hen*⁻
mutations define a gene distinct from *xis* or represent a particular
type of *xis*⁻ mutation. We have done two types of experiments which
we believe indicate strongly that the *hen*⁻ mutations define a separate gene. In the first, we constructed a phage which carries a
nonsense mutation in the *xis* gene in addition to a *hen*⁻ mutation.
If the *hen*⁻ mutation provided for an altered Xis protein, the *hen*⁻
phenotype should disappear in the double mutant, because no functional Xis protein should be made at all. However, we find that the
xis nonsense *hen*⁻ double mutant retains the *hen*⁻ phenotype. This
indicates that *xis* and *hen* are not the same gene. We were concerned,
however, that the previous isolation of *xis*⁻ mutants required that
the phage integrate normally and therefore that a rather special
class of mutations may have been selected, which were not indicative
of total absence of activity for the Xis protein. To investigate
this possibility further we isolated 10 new *xis*⁻ mutants by a technique which did not require integration. We selected for *either*
int⁻ or *xis*⁻ mutations by inability of λ*gal* phage to integrate in
the experimental system shown in Fig. 3. None of the ten *xis*⁻
mutants isolated by this technique were *hen*⁻. From these two types
of analysis, we conclude that the *hen* gene is most likely distinct
from *xis*, although we cannot exclude a bifunctional protein with
two separate active sites.

CONCLUSION

Recent evidence indicates that the reaction pathways for site-
specific recombination are formally symmetric in catalytic components: *int* and *hen* are required for normal integrative recombination, and *int* and *xis* are required for normal excisive recombination.
However, the requirement for *xis* seems to be more stringent than the

requirement for *hen*. The reaction pathways are notably asymmetric
in their regulatory features: integrative recombination is much
more efficient than excisive recombination in a repressed lysogen.
We do not yet know whether this regulatory asymmetry involves
disparate synthesis of the Int and Hen proteins compared to Xis,
selective breakdown of Xis, or regulatory interactions at the level
of protein activity.

ACKNOWLEDGMENTS

    We thank Allan Campbell and Robert Weisberg for unpublished
information. Our research has been supported by Public Health
Service research grant GM 17078 from the National Institute of
General Medical Sciences.

REFERENCES

Campbell, A. 1962. Episomes. Advan. Genet. <u>11</u>: 101.

Campbell, A. and J. Zissler. 1966. The steric effect in lysogeni-
zation by bacteriophage lambda. III. Superinfection of monolyso-
genic derivatives of a strain diploid for the prophage attachment
site. Virology <u>28</u>: 659.

Chung, S., L. Green and H. Echols. 1974. Mutants of bacteriophage
λ defective in integration but not excision: evidence for an inte-
gration-specific protein in site-specific recombination. Submitted
for publication.

Echols, H., R. Gingery and L. Moore. 1968. Integrative recombination function of bacteriophage λ: evidence for a site-specific
recombination enzyme. J. Mol. Biol. <u>34</u>: 251.

Echols, H. 1970. Integrative and excisive recombination by bacteriophage λ: evidence for an excision-specific recombination protein. J. Mol. Biol. <u>47</u>: 575.

Echols, H. 1971. Lysogeny: Viral repression and site-specific
recombination. Ann. Rev. Biochem. <u>40</u>: 827.

Echols, H. 1972. Developmental pathways for the temperate phage:
lysis vs. lysogeny. Ann. Rev. Genet. <u>6</u>: 157.

Echols, H. 1974. Constitutive integrative recombination by bacteriophage λ. Submitted for publication.

Gingery, R. and H. Echols. 1967. Mutants of bacteriophage λ unable to integrate into the host chromosome. Proc. Nat. Acad. Sci. U.S.A. 58: 1507.

Gingery, R. and H. Echols. 1968. Integration, excision, and transducing particle genesis by bacteriophage λ. Cold Spring Harbor Symp. Quant. Biol. 33: 721.

Gottesman, M. E. and M. B. Yarmolinsky. 1968a. Integration-negative mutants of bacteriophage lambda. J. Mol. Biol. 31: 487.

Gottesman, M. E. and M. B. Yarmolinsky. 1968b. The integration and excision of the bacteriophage lambda genome. Cold Spring Harbor Symp. Quant. Biol. 33: 735.

Gottesman, M. E. and R. A. Weisberg. 1971. Prophage insertion and excision. In (D. Hershey, ed.) The Bacteriophage Lambda. pp. 113-138. Cold Spring Harbor Laboratory, Cold Spring Harbor, New York.

Guarneros, G. and H. Echols. 1970. New mutants of bacteriophage λ with a specific defect in excision from the host chromosome. J. Mol. Biol. 47: 565.

Herskowitz, I. 1973. Control of gene expression in bacteriophage lambda. Ann. Rev. Genet. 7: 289.

Shimada, K. and A. Campbell. 1974. Int-constitutive mutants of bacteriophage lambda. Proc. Nat. Acad. Sci. U.S.A. 71: 237.

Signer, E. R. 1969. Plasmid formation: a new mode of lysogeny by phage λ. Nature 223: 158.

Weil, J. and E. R. Signer. 1968. Recombination in bacteriophage λ. II. Site-specific recombination promoted by the integration system. J. Mol. Biol. 34: 273.

Zissler, J. 1967. Integration-negative (int) mutants of phage λ. Virology 31: 189.

RECOMBINATION OF PHAGE λ DNA *IN VITRO*

Michael Syvanen

Department of Biochemistry, Stanford University School

of Medicine, Stanford, California 94305

Elucidation of the mechanism of genetic recombination at the biochemical level has been hampered by the paucity of recombination-related activities that can be measured *in vitro*. A major difficulty has been the lack of a direct and simple assay for recombinant DNA. I would like to describe conditions in which phage λ DNA recombines *in vitro* and the recombinant DNA is assayed following its assembly into infectious λ particles.

Kaiser and Masuda (1973) have shown that λ DNA added to a cell-free extract of an induced λ lysogen is packaged into infective phage particles. They demonstrated *in vitro* DNA packaging by adding a purified λ *imm*434 DNA to an extract from an induced λ lysogen and by showing the appearance of particles of λ *imm*434 in the extract. λ *imm*434 is identical to λ except for the immunity region; consequently, 434 DNA will package into λ virion protein and, because the 434 operators are insensitive to λ repressor, will make a plaque on a λ lysogen whereas λ itself will not grow in a λ lysogen. This allows one to detect few 434 particles in the presence of the excess of λ particles, which arise from the induced λ lysogen. In the present work, this system was used to detect 434 DNA molecules that had undergone genetic recombination prior to packaging. Specifically, conditions were sought where recombination between the purified 434 DNA added to the extract and the endogenous λ DNA from the induced lysogen did occur.

To demonstrate genetic recombination, 434 DNA with amber mutations in genes *A* and *B* (Fig. 1) was added to an extract of an induced λ lysogen. The extract contained endogenous A^+B^+ λ DNA in the form of circles and linear polymers (Young and Sinsheimer, 1964;

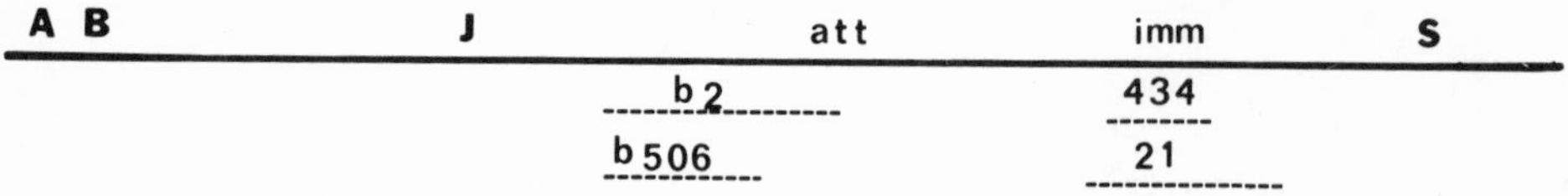

A B	J	att	imm	S

```
                              b 2            434
                       -----------------    --------
                            b 506             21
                       ------------        ----------------
```

Figure 1.   Genetic map of λ showing relevant markers used in this study.

Bode and Kaiser, 1965).   A recombination event between these two kinds of DNA produces am^+ 434 DNA that, when packaged into phage particles, makes a plaque on a sup^0, λ immune host.   When purified A^-B^- 434 DNA was added to the *in vitro* system and incubation was carried out at 37°C, very few 434 am^+ particles were made.   However, if the mixture was first allowed to incubate at 23°C, significant numbers of 434 am^+ particles were formed (Fig. 2).   It has been shown that these 434 am^+ plaques represent particles containing a single 434 am^+ chromosome in a normal capsid.

The recombination activity in the extract is independent of either the host Rec system or the λ-specific Red system.   The extracts described above are made from lysogenic rec^+ bacteria that carry a λ red^+ prophage.   However, extracts prepared from induced $recA^-$ bacteria with a λ $redB^-$ prophage also show *in vitro* recombination (Table 1).   Thus it appears unlikely that one of these two generalized recombination systems (Signer, 1971) is exclusively responsible for the activity.

Table 1.   Recombination does not require Red or Rec

Lysogen	Frequency (%) of am^+ 434 recombinants
rec^+ (λ red^+)	1.2, 3.1, 2.6, 0.3
$recA^-$ (λ red^-)	0.7, 5.0, 1.0, 0.5

Extracts were prepared 1 hr after inducing either W3101 (λ cIts857 Sam7) (top row) or W3101 $recA$ 2463 (λredβ 5 cIts857 Sam7) (bottom entry).   To 50 μl of extract was added 1 to 4 μl of DNA (200 μg/ml) extracted from A^-B^- 434 particles.   The mixtures were incubated 60 min at 23°C before transferring to 37°C.   Other steps are those given in Fig. 2.

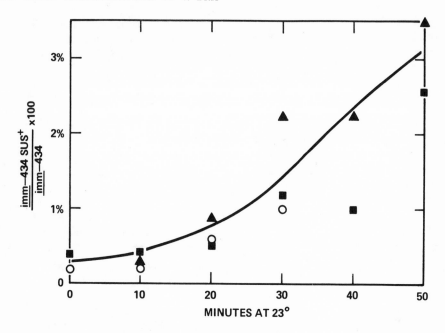

Figure 2. Appearance of *in vitro* recombinants. Extracts were prepared from the heat-induced lysogen W3101 (λ *c*Its857 *S*am7) according
to Kaiser and Masuda (1973). The A^-B^- 434 DNA was extracted with
phenol from a purified stock of λ *A*am32 *B*aml *hy imm* 434 *C*ts56.   To
50 μl of extract was added 0.5 μg of A^-B^- 434 DNA (o—o) or 0.25 μg
of DNA (■ — ■), (▲ — ▲). After incubation of the mixture at
23°C for the given time the mixtures were incubated at 37°C for 1
hr, after which DNase I at 5 μg/ml was added. The total number of
434 particles in the extract was determined by plating on Y mel
(λ) (contains *sup* F) and the number of *am*$^+$ 434 particles were determined by plating on the *sup*^{o} strain W3101 (λ *A*am32).

RECOMBINATION OF CIRCULAR 434 DNA

In a variation of the assay for *in vitro* recombination, advantage was taken of the fact that cyclic monomers do not package directly into infectious phage particles. It has been shown that the
DNA substrate for the packaging reaction is a polymeric, multichromosomal molecule; circular or linear monomers do not package directly.
However, if a monomer circle can recombine with another DNA molecule
and thereby become part of a polymeric structure, it should become a
substrate for packaging. Thus, when circular A^-B^- 434 DNA was added
to the extract the number of 434 phage particles was greatly reduced.
For example, polymeric 434 DNA gave rise to 200,000 plaques per μg
of DNA, compared to 3,000 plaques per μg of circular DNA. However,

among the 434 plaques that did appear from the circular DNA, 70-90%
were am^+, as shown in the top line of Table 2. This suggests that
recombination is an obligatory step in the formation of 434 particles from the circular DNA.

Table 2. Genetic crossover shows map preference

Genotype of exog-enous circular DNA	Genotype of endog-enous DNA	In vitro packaged imm 434 phage	
		Genotype	Frequency
A^-B^- imm 434 S^+	imm λ S^-	am^+	77%
		A^-B^-	23%
		S^-	0/70
A^-B^- imm 434 S^+	J^- imm λ S^-	J^-	61%
		A^-B^-	31%
		am^+	7%
		S^-	0/92

Circular A^-B^- 434 DNA was isolated from endo I$^-$ bacteria which
had been infected with λ Aam32 Bam1 imm434 in the presence of chloramphenicol according to Wang (1969). When the extract was prepared
from the induced lysogen, which carried a prophage with the Jam27
allele (second line), 10 µl of extract prepared from W3101 (λ Eam4
cIts857 Sam7) was added after the addition of DNase I as a source
of phage tails. In each case the DNase-resistant 434 particles were
detected by plating on Y mel (λ) (first line) or Y mel (λ Jam27)
(second line). After one single-plaque isolation, individual plaques
were tested for the ability to plate on Y mel, C600, or W3101. All
phage plate on Y mel (contains sup F); the A^-, B^-, or J^- but not S^-
will plate on C600 (contains sup D); and only am^+ will plate on
W3101 (sup^0). J^- 434 and A^-B^- 434 were distinguished by complementation on the sup^0 lysogen W3101 (λA$^-$) and W3101 (λJ$^-$). The 7% am^+
434 phage produced in the second entry of the table are probably
due to A^-B^- 434 which recombined with the prophage during the first
plating on Y mel (λ Jam27).

SITE SPECIFICITY OF *IN VITRO* RECOMBINATION

Because the recombination observed appears independent of general recombination, it was of interest to see whether it was due to the prophage attachment-site-specific recombination, which is known to be mediated by the λ Int system (Echols *et al.*, 1968). The generation of 434 *am*+ phage from A^-B^- 434 circular DNA indicates that crossing-over occurred between *B* and *imm* (see Fig. 1). To test whether recombination was specific to the attachment site of the λ chromosome, additional crosses were conducted. As shown in Table 2, when the λ DNA in the extract contained an amber mutation in gene *S*, all of 434 packaged were S^+. Therefore, the crossover event that integrates the circular DNA molecule into some higher aggregate occurs between gene *B* and the immunity region but not between gene *S* and immunity (see Fig. 1). When the 434 DNA circles were added to an extract that contained polymeric λ DNA with the *J*am27 allele, as in the experiment presented in the second line of Table 2, very few 434 *am*+ particles were recovered; the majority were J^-. Thus the crossover event frequently occurs between *J* and *imm* but rarely between *B* and *J*. These results strongly suggest that *in vitro* recombination occurs at the attachment site.

RECOMBINANT PHAGE PARTICLES CONTAIN A SINGLE CHROMOSOME

OF NORMAL LENGTH

Recombinants are detected as plaques on sup^- lambda lysogens. To show that the particles responsible for these plaques are, in fact, true haploid recombinants and not some type of aberrant particle containing two phage chromosomes that recombine in the indicator bacteria, the distribution of the recombinant particles in a CsCl sedimentation equilibrium gradient was measured as shown in Fig. 3. Normal phage particles have a characteristic buoyant density that measures their DNA and protein contents (Davidson and Szybalski, 1971). Since the chromosome of λ *imm* 434 is 2% shorter than $λ^+$, 434 particles have a slightly lower density than λ particles. The distribution of λ *b*221 particles (whose DNA is 22% shorter than λ b^+) is also given in the figure; these were added as a density reference. Figure 3 shows that the 434 particles produced *in vitro* have a slightly lower density than the λ particles, as expected for native 434 particles. Furthermore, the 434 *am*+ particles (*i. e.*, the recombinants made *in vitro*) show the same distribution through this region. This result indicates that the 434 *am*+ recombinant is a phage particle containing a single 434 chromosome and a normal amount of protein.

This important point was tested in another way with an extract of cells lysogenic for λ *b*506. The *b*506 deletion is located just to

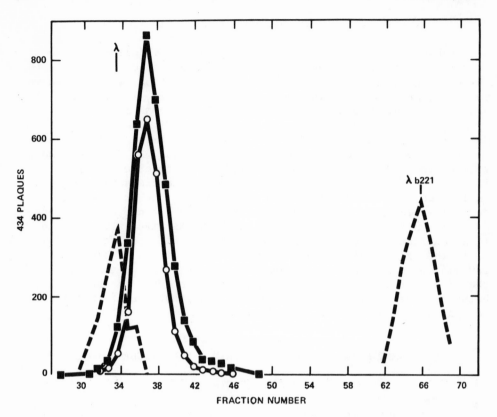

Figure 3.   Density distribution of *in vitro* recombinants in a CsCl
equilibrium gradient.   Phage titers are given as a function of fraction number, where the larger fraction number gives lower densities
in the gradient.   0.07 ml of circular A^-B^- 434 DNA (at 10 µg/ml)
was added to 1.7 ml of extract containing λ *CI* 857 *S*am7 DNA.   After
1 hr at 23°C followed by 1 hr at 37°C, the total volume was brought
to 4.19 ml with buffer (20 mM Tris, 10 mM $MgCl_2$, pH 7.6), when 3.11
g of CsCl was added.   The sample was centrifuged at 20,000 rpm for
48 hr, at 5°C, in an SW 39 rotor.   The tube was pierced through the
bottom, and 5-drop fractions were collected into 0.1 ml each of T br.
Total number of 434 phage in 0.05 ml of each fraction (■ — ■) or
the number of am^+ 434 (o — o) in 0.05 ml is given versus fraction
number.   (----------) gives the distribution of phage λ found in the
extract and the λ *b*221 added as a reference.

the left of the attachment site on the λ chromosome (Parkinson, 1971).
If *in vitro* recombination is *att* specific, all 434 am^+ recombinants
should also be *b*506.   Thus when A^-B^- 434 circular DNA is recombined
and packaged in an extract whose endogenous DNA is A^+B^+ *b*506, the

434 am^+ recombinant particles should have a lower density than
either the A^-B^- 434 or λ b506 parents. This expected result is in
fact obtained (Fig. 4). There are two peaks of 434 plaque-formers,
one at a higher density than λ b506 and one at a lower density.
The 434 am^+ recombinant particles occupy the peak of lower density,
the region of the gradient where b506 434 particles are expected.

The high-density *imm* 434 peak contains nonrecombinant am^-
particles. They may have arisen by the 434 DNA circles that recombine with one another or perhaps by some direct packaging mechanism
that remains to be understood. The peak of 434 am^+ plaques in Fig.
4 has a shoulder toward higher density. These high-density 434 am^+
plaques probably do not represent recombinant particles made *in vitro*; more likely they are caused by recombination between λ b506
and A^-B^- 434 on the assay plate. The shoulder occurs where the
higher-density *imm* 434 peak (solid squares) overlaps the λ b506,
which rises to a height of 9 X 10^{11}/ml. Because the *imm* 434 particles are at a much lower concentration, plating at a dilution
appropriate for the *imm* 434 results in mixed infection with A^-B^-
434 and λ b506. For example, in fractions 36 and 37 the multiplicity of λ b506 particles to indicator bacteria was 40 and 60. This
means that in those fractions every A^-B^- 434 particle infects a
cell that is also infected with many λ b506 particles; consequently,
the probability of recombination occurring under these conditions

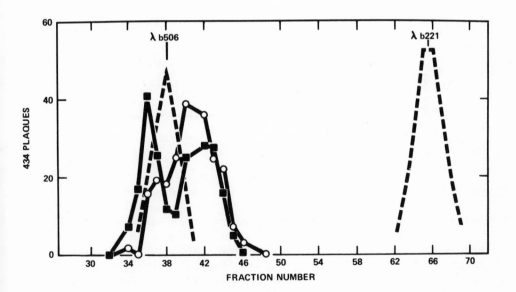

Figure 4. 0.04 ml of circular A^-B^- 434 DNA was added to 1.1 ml of
extract derived from a lysogen whose prophage contains λ b506 *CI*
857 *S*am7. Other steps are the same as in Fig. 3.

is high.   Reconstruction experiments are consistent with this
interpretation.   The main peak of am^+ 434 particles (open circles)
cannot be explained by recombination on the indicator bacteria.
This fact further supports the notion that the *in vitro* recombinants do indeed contain a single chromosome packaged in normal λ
proteins.   It also shows that genetic crossover occurs in the
region between the *b*506 deletion and *imm*, which is consistent with
an *att*-specific recombination event.

CONCLUSION

It is clear that recombinant bacteriophage are produced in
the cell-free extract.   When polymeric 434 DNA is mixed with the
extract, a few percent of the 434 particles are recombinants.   When
circular 434 DNA is used, most of the 434 particles evidence recombination.   The simplest explanation for this arises from the fact

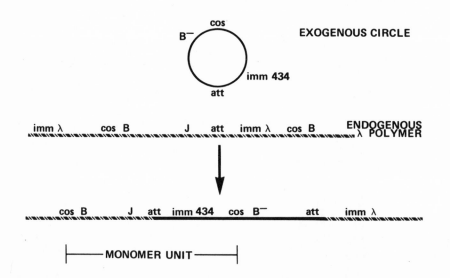

Figure 5.   Mechanism for conversion of the 434 chromosome from
a circular to a polymeric structure.   The exogenous 434 circle will
not package directly into infectious particles.   But when the 434
circle recombines through *att* with the endogenous λ DNA, the 434
marker becomes associated with a polymeric molecule from which
it can be packaged into phage protein.   Because unit-length monomers
are packaged between two *cos* sites, the 434 immunity region will be
combined with DNA sequences from the λ DNA that lie to the left of
att.   Thus when the endogenous λ DNA is am^+ in its left arm, the
434 will be am^+, whereas if the λ DNA is J^- the final 434 particle
will be J^- (see Table 2).

that circular monomers of λ DNA do not package directly into particles; packageable DNA must be multichromosomal. This is not a
property unique to the *in vitro* system; Szpirer and Brachet (1970),
Enquist and Skalka (1973), and Stahl *et al.* (1972) have also shown
this to be true for λ DNA packaging in an infected bacterium. One
way for the circular monomers to become polymeric is for them to
recombine with other DNA. Figure 5 outlines how this might occur.
The genetic evidence suggests that crossing-over is at the attachment site (*att*); thus, in Fig. 5 the circular 434 monomer is shown
to integrate into a λ polymer through *att*. The unique cohesive ends
of λ are contained in the *cos* region; a monomeric unit between two
cos sites is packaged into a phage particle. Thus it can be seen
that the 434 marker will segregate with markers to the left of *att*
on the endogenous λ chromosome but not with markers on the right of
att. Attachment-site-specific recombination would suggest that
the λ Int system is responsible for the activity observed here.
Experiments are in progress to test directly the requirement of
λ Int protein for this *in vitro* recombination.

ACKNOWLEDGMENT

I would like to thank Dale Kaiser for his many helpful suggestions during the course of this work. This investigation was supported by a fellowship from the California Division of the American
Cancer Society and by Public Health Service Grant # PHS AI 04509-13.

REFERENCES

Bode, V. C. and D. Kaiser. 1965. Changes in the structure and
activity of λ DNA in a superinfected immune bacterium. J. Mol.
Biol. 14: 399.

Davidson, N. and W. Szybalski. 1971. Physical and chemical characteristics of lambda DNA. In (A. D. Hershey, ed.) The Bacteriophage Lambda. pp. 45-82. Cold Spring Harbor Laboratory, Cold
Spring Harbor, New York.

Echols, H., R. Gingery and L. Moore. 1968. Integrative recombination function of bacteriophage λ: Evidence for a site-specific
recombination enzyme. J. Mol. Biol. 34: 251.

Enquist, L. and A. Skalka. 1973. Replication of bacteriophage λ
DNA dependent on the function of host and viral genes. I. Interaction of *red, gam* and *rec*. J. Mol. Biol. 34: 251.

Kaiser, D. and T. Masuda. 1973. *In vitro* assembly of bacteriophage
lambda heads. Proc. Nat. Acad. Sci. U.S.A. 70: 260.

Parkinson, J. S.   1971.   Deletion mutants of bacteriophage lambda
II.   Genetic properties of *att*-defective mutants.   J. Mol. Biol.
<u>56</u>: 385.

Signer, E.   1971.   General recombination.   In (A. D. Hershey, ed.)
The Bacteriophage Lambda.   pp. 139-174.   Cold Spring Harbor Laboratory, Cold Spring Harbor, New York.

Stahl, F., K. McMilin, M. Stahl, R. Malone and Y. Nozu.   1972.   A
role for recombination in the production of "free-loader" lambda
bacteriophage particles.   J. Mol. Biol. <u>68</u>: 57.

Szpirer, J. and P. Brachet.   1970.   Relations physiologiques entre
les phages tempérés λ et φ80. Molec. Gen. Genet. <u>108</u>: 78.

Wang, J. C.   1969.Degree of superhelicity of covalently closed cyclic
DNA's from *Escherichia coli*.   J. Mol. Biol. <u>43</u>: 263.

Young, E. and R. Sinsheimer.   1964.   Novel intra-cellular forms of
lambda DNA.   J. Mol. Biol. <u>10</u>: 562.

chi MUTATIONS OF PHAGE LAMBDA

David Henderson and Jon Weil

Department of Molecular Biology, Vanderbilt University,

Nashville, Tennessee 37235

INTRODUCTION

Results of experiments carried out in a number of laboratories demonstrate the interdependence of replication, recombination, and maturation in phage lambda (see, for example, the review by Stahl *et al.*, 1973, and references cited there). The experiments summarized in this report relate to the role of recombination promoted by the *Escherichia coli* Rec system in the growth of deletion mutants of lambda that have lost the genes between *att* and *cIII* (Fig. 1). A detailed description of this work will be presented elsewhere (Henderson and Weil, manuscript in preparation).

The deletions studied were isolated on the basis of their ability to grow on a lysogen of the unrelated phage P2 (Spi⁻ phenotype; Lindahl *et al.*, 1970). The generation of this phenotype requires the loss of at least three lambda functions: *del*, *gam*, and *exo* or *bet* (Zissler *et al.*, 1971a; Barta *et al.*, 1974) (see Fig. 1). Phage that have lost *gam* and either *exo* or *bet* are unable to grow on *rec*A bacteria (Fec⁻ phenotype; Manly *et al.*, 1969; Zissler *et al.*, 1971b). Such phage are, however, able to grow on *rec*B, *rec*C, and *rec*A *rec*B mutants, and an interaction is therefore implied between the products of the *rec*B and *rec*C genes and either *exo*, *bet*, or *gam* protein (Zissler *et al.*, 1971b). The *rec*B and *rec*C genes are known to cooperate in the production of a nuclease, RecBC nuclease (Oishi, 1969; Barbour and Clark, 1970), whose activity is normally controlled by the *rec*A gene (Willetts and Clark, 1969; Hout *et al.*, 1970). Experiments *in vivo* (Unger and Clark, 1972; Unger *et al.*, 1972) and *in vitro*, using purified proteins (Sakaki *et al.*, 1973), have now demonstrated that *gam* protein complexes with and inactivates RecBC nuclease.

89

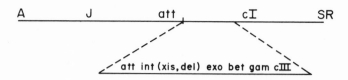

Figure 1. Genetic map of lambda, approximately to scale. The expanded portion shows the region between the prophage attachment
site, *att*, and *cIII* removed by the Spi⁻ deletions referred to in
the text.

     Enquist and Skalka (1973) examined the pattern of DNA replica-
tion in infections involving combinations of mutations in host and
phage recombination genes. They concluded that the failure of
lambda to grow under Fec⁻ conditions (*red⁻gam⁻* phage in a *rec*A host)
results from the failure to produce DNA structures that can be incorporated into mature virions, *i.e.* concatemers or multimeric
circles (Stahl *et al.*, 1973). They found that Fec⁻ infections
accumulate monomeric circular genomes and suggested that the absence
of the *gam* protein blocks the transition from early "theta form"
to late "rolling circle" DNA replication, presumably because there
is an intermediate structure sensitive to the RecBC nuclease. At
the same time, loss of both the Red and Rec recombination systems
prevents the formation of multimeric DNA by recombination. It
would be anticipated that Spi⁻ phage would show a pattern of replication similar to *red⁻gam⁻* phage, although it should be realized
that the *del* gene may also play a role in DNA synthesis (Barta and
Zissler, 1974).

DETECTION OF *chi* MUTANTS

     When first isolated, the Spi⁻ deletions made extremely small
plaques. When grown lytically, these phage gave rise to heterogeneous stocks containing a variable proportion of large plaque-
forming phage. These large plaque formers were shown to carry the
same deletion as the minute plaque formers and an additional "suppressor" mutation, apparently selected because of the growth advantage it confers. Since we discovered these suppressor mutations,
similar mutants have been detected in Frank Stahl's laboratory and
have been shown to introduce a "hot spot" for Rec-promoted recombination (Lam *et al.*, 1974). At the suggestion of these authors, we
shall call the suppressing mutations *chi*.

GENETIC LOCATION OF *chi* MUTATIONS

     Three independently isolated *chi* mutants were found to recom-
bine with each other, indicating that they occur at different sites

in the genome. The formal analysis of crosses involving pairs of *chi* mutations suggests that two of the isolates tested could be separated by as much as 60% of the genome, with one mapping near the *J* gene and the other near *R* (Fig. 1). However, since *chi* mutations affect recombination in the vicinity of the mutation, it is unclear whether this behavior reflects "marker effects" or relates to the true map location of the *chi* mutations.

EFFECTS OF Spi⁻ DELETIONS AND *chi* ON PHAGE DEVELOPMENT

Measurements of burst size following single infection of appropriate bacterial hosts were performed. In a rec^+ host, the burst size of the Spi⁻ deletion *b*1319 was about 20% that of wild-type, while λ*b*1319 *chi*3 had a burst equal to that of wild-type phage. In a *rec*A*rec*B or *rec*B host, the burst of wild-type phage was unaffected, but both λ*b*1319 and λ*b*1319 *chi*3 had low bursts. This indicates that *chi*3 is dependent on a functional RecBC recombination pathway for its activity. A phage carrying only *chi*3 was indistinguishable from wild type.

We also measured DNA synthesis in a rec^+ host and found that λ*b*1319 has a reduced level of synthesis. This is raised by about 50% in λ*b*1319 *chi*3, which still makes less DNA than wild type. There is an approximately equal effect on synthesis of endolysin. Production of serum blocking protein (SBP) was also measured and found to be affected differently. λ*b*1319 alone produces more SBP than wild-type phage, and *chi*3 reduces the level to that of wild type.

POSSIBLE MECHANISM OF *chi* ACTION

The results of our burst size and DNA synthesis experiments are consistent with the model for *chi* action proposed by Lam *et al.* (1974), who suggested that *chi* increases the amount of maturable DNA by enhancing recombination. The substrate for this recombination is assumed to be the circular DNA accumulated as a result of the RecBC nuclease block to late replication (see Introduction). We have observed that the effect of *chi* in increasing burst size is larger than that in enhancing DNA synthesis. This suggests that *chi* may stimulate recombination events that require only small amounts of concomitant DNA synthesis to produce maturable DNA. We have not examined the DNA produced in detail and are therefore unable to say whether the increased synthesis we observe in λ*b*1319 *chi*3 compared to λ*b*1319 infections results only from synthesis associated with completion of recombinant molecules or whether *chi*3 also allows the transition of some circles into late replication.

It is less clear how the results of the endolysin and SBP measurements should be interpreted. In particular, the significance of the differential effects on these two proteins is not known. It should be noted, however, that Brown and Cohen (1974) have described a lambda function that increases the specificity of the host RNA polymerase for lambda DNA. This function is controlled by the region of the genome deleted in our mutants, and one might therefore expect to find quantitative or qualitative differences in transcription during the growth of these phage. In addition, the *chi*-enhanced DNA synthesis may affect late protein production either through gene dosage or by more direct effects on transcription.

chi MUTATIONS IN SUBSTITUTION MUTANTS

We found it striking that the previously isolated Spi⁻ λ*pbio*'s had not been observed to carry *chi* mutations. A possible explanation for this was suggested by McMilin *et al*. (1974). They found that *bio*1 and *bio*69 carry a recombination "hot spot" near the center of the genome, in contrast to two deletion mutants (*b*1319 and *b*1453) obtained from us which have hot spots near the right end. This could be interpreted to mean that there is a hot spot (*chi*) within or near the *bio* DNA substitution.

We have performed a number of crosses to try to detect segregation of *chi* from λ*bio*1, λ*bio*10, and λ*bio*256 but have failed to find *chi*⁺ (minute plaque) segregants. We have also isolated a new Spi⁻ substitution mutant, λ*b*1262, which carries unknown DNA, presumably of bacterial origin. This phage was a minute plaque former when first isolated and subsequently picked up a *chi* mutation that cannot be crossed out. We interpret these results to mean that the *bio* substitutions and *b*1262 carry a *chi* in the *E. coli* DNA. It is assumed that a *chi* exists in the *E. coli* genome near *bio*, since the *pbio* phage seem never to have made small plaques. The behavior of *b*1262 demonstrates that the potential for generating new *chi* sites is probably not restricted to lambda DNA.

ACKNOWLEDGMENTS

This work was supported by research grant number GB27602 from the National Science Foundation to J.W. and in part by NSF grant BG8109 to Dr. Frank Stahl. We are most grateful to Frank Stahl, Ken McMilin and Stephen Lam for communication of their results prior to publication.

REFERENCES

Barbour, S. D. and A. J. Clark. 1970. Biochemical and genetic studies of recombination proficiency in *E. coli* I. Enzymatic activity associated with *rec*B$^+$ and *rec*C$^+$ genes. Proc. Nat. Acad. Sci. U.S.A. <u>65</u>: 955.

Barta, K. and J. Zissler. 1974. The role of genetic recombination in DNA replication of phage lambda II. An effect in DNA replication by gene delta. Manuscript submitted for publication.

Barta, K., P. Tavernier and J. Zissler. 1974. The role of genetic recombination in DNA replication of phage lambda I. Genetic characterization of the delta gene. Manuscript submitted for publication.

Brown, A. and S. N. Cohen. 1974. Effects of λ development on template specificity of *Escherichia coli* RNA polymerase. Biochim. Biophys. Acta <u>335</u>: 123.

Enquist, L. W. and A. Skalka. 1973. Replication of bacteriophage λ DNA dependent on the function of host and viral genes. I. Interaction of *red, gam* and *rec*. J. Mol. Biol. <u>75</u>: 185.

Hout, A., P. Van de Putte, A. J. R. De Jonge, A. Schuite and R. A. Oosterbaan. 1970. Interference between the *rec*A product and an ATP-dependent exonuclease in extracts of *E. coli*. Biochim. Biophys. Acta <u>224</u>: 285.

Lam, S. T., M. M. Stahl, K. D. McMilin and F. W. Stahl. 1974. Rec-mediated recombinational hot spot activity in bacteriophage lambda II. A mutation which causes hot spot activity. Genetics, in press.

Lindahl, G., G. Sironi, H. Bialy and R. Calendar. 1970. Bacteriophage λ: Abortive infection of bacteria lysogenic for phage P2. Proc. Nat. Acad. Sci. U.S.A. <u>66</u>: 587.

Manly, K. F., E. R. Signer and C. M. Radding. 1969. Non-essential functions of bacteriophage lambda. Virology <u>37</u>: 177.

McMilin, K. D., M. M. Stahl and F. W. Stahl. 1974. Rec-mediated recombinational hot spot activity in bacteriophage lambda I. Hot spot activity associated with Spi$^-$ deletions and *bio* substitutions. Genetics, in press.

Oishi, M. 1969. An ATP dependent DNase from *E. coli* with a possible role in genetic recombination. Proc. Nat. Acad. Sci. U.S.A. <u>64</u>: 1292.

Sakaki, Y., A. E. Karu, S. Linn and H. Echols. 1973. Purification and properties of the γ-protein specified by bacteriophage λ: An inhibitor of the host RecBC recombination enzyme. Proc. Nat. Acad. Sci. U.S.A. 70: 2215.

Stahl, F. W., S. Chung, J. Crasemann, D. Faulds, J. Haemer, S. Lam, R. E. Malone, K. D. McMilin, Y. Nozu, J. Siegel, J. Strathern and M. Stahl. 1973. Recombinaton, replication, and maturation on phage lambda. In (C. F. Fox and W. S. Robinson, eds.) Virus Research. p. 487. Academic Press, New York.

Unger, R. C. and A. J. Clark. 1972. Interaction of the recombination pathways of bacteriophage λ and its host E. coli K12: Effects on exonuclease V activity. J. Mol. Biol. 70: 539.

Unger, R. C., H. Ecols and A. J. Clark. 1972. Interaction of the recombination pathways of bacteriophage λ and host E. coli: Effects on λ recombination. J. Mol. Biol. 70: 531.

Willetts, N. S. and A. J. Clark. 1969. Characteristics of some multiply recombination-deficient strains of Escherichia coli. J. Bacteriol. 100: 231.

Zissler, J., E. Signer and F. Schaefer. 1971a. The role of recombination in growth of bacteriophage lambda II. Inhibition of growth by prophage P2. In (A. D. Hershey, ed.) The Bacteriophage Lambda. p. 469. Cold Spring Harbor Laboratory, Cold Spring Harbor, New York.

Zissler, J., E. Signer and F. Schaefer. 1971b. The role of recombination in growth of bacteriophage lambda I. The gamma gene. In (A. D. Hershey, ed.) The Bacteriophage Lambda. p. 455. Cold Spring Harbor Laboratory, Cold Spring Harbor, New York.

IN VITRO STUDIES OF THE *gam* GENE PRODUCT OF BACTERIOPHAGE λ

Alexander Karu, Yoshiyuke Sakaki*, Harrison Echols and
Stuart Linn

*Department of Biochemistry and Department of Molecular
Biology, University of California, Berkeley, California
94720*

About six years have elapsed since it was established that the
recB and *recC* genes of *Escherichia coli* specify a complex DNase-
ATPase, the RecBC enzyme. Although this enzyme has been extensively
purified, and a great deal is known of its catalytic properties and
its preference for certain forms of DNA *in vitro*, its biochemical
activity *in vivo* is still unknown. However, considerable evidence
has accumulated indicating that this enzyme is antagonistic to the
normal pathway for phage λ DNA replication, and that as a consequence, phage λ has evolved a means to regulate the RecBC enzyme.

Zissler and his co-workers (1971a,b) identified a λ gene, *gam*,
which is essential for the growth of λ in the absence of the general
recombination pathways of phage and bacterium (*i.e.*, *red*⁻ phage and
a *recA*⁻ bacterial host). An active *gam* gene is also essential for
growth on a *polA*⁻ host, and for the capacity of phage P2 to prevent
growth of λ. These phenotypes, summarized in Table 1, may be explained in part by the hypothesis that the *gam* gene is responsible
for an inhibition of the host RecBC enzyme (Lindahl *et al.*, 1970).
Indeed, Unger and Clark (1972) observed the disappearance of RecBC
enzyme activity from crude extracts of cells which had been infected
with λ carrying an active *gam* gene. In this report, we summarize

---

* Present address: The Mitsubishi-Kasei Institute of Life
Sciences, 11 Minamiooya, Machida-shi, Tokyo, Japan.

Table 1. Consequences of *gam* mutations in bacteriophage λ

Growth Properties

A. Fec⁻ phenotype: *gam⁻red⁻* phage do not form plaques on *recA⁻*
    hosts, but they do form plaques on *recA⁻recB⁻* hosts (Zissler
    et al., 1971a).

B. Spi⁻ phenotype: *gam⁺red⁻del⁻* phage do not form plaques on P2
    lysogens, but *gam⁻red⁻del⁻* phage do (Zissler *et al.*, 1971b;
    Barta *et al.*, 1974; Sironi *et al.*, 1971).

C. Feb⁻ phenotype: *gam⁻* phage do not form plaques on *polA⁻* hosts
    (Zissler *et al.*, 1971a).

Recombinational Properties

A. Recombination mediated by the host RecBC pathway is more
    efficient for phage in *gam⁻* than in *gam⁺* infections (Unger
    et al., 1972).

B. In *recA⁻* hosts recombination mediated by the phage Red pathway
    is slightly less efficient for *gam⁻* than for *gam⁺* phage
    (Zissler *et al.*, 1971a).

---

recent results from our laboratories that show that this disappearance is due to an inhibitor specified by the *gam* gene, the "γ-
protein," and we describe some of the properties of the purified
protein (Sakaki *et al.*, 1973). Finally, a discussion of the possible
biochemical bases for the biological effects listed in Table 1 is
presented.

IDENTIFICATION AND PURIFICATION OF THE *gam* GENE PRODUCT

    We initially identified the *gam* gene product by comparison of
partially purified extracts of induced cells lysogenic for *gam⁺* or
gam⁻ prophages, or cells infected with various deletion mutants of
λ spanning the *gam* gene. Brij-lysozyme lysates were prepared from
these cells and sedimented through glycerol gradients, and the
gradient fractions were assayed for the ability to inhibit the duplex exonuclease activity of purified RecBC enzyme. One of the
inhibitory activities in these gradients was present exclusively in
lysates from *gam⁺* inductions and infections. This activity was
abolished by nonsense mutations or deletions of the *gam* gene, and
the material in this peak was thermolabile in extracts from cells
infected with a temperature-sensitive *gam* mutant (Sakaki *et al.*,
1973). These results indicate that *gam* is the structural gene for
this inhibitor.

To isolate the γ-protein, a double lysogen, *E. coli* K-12 *gal⁻ endI⁻ recB⁻ recC⁻* (*cI857x13,λimm434gal⁺c⁺*) was constructed. The λ phage is heat-inducible and lysis-defective, and the Cro⁻ pheno-type of the *x13* mutation provides for overproduction of proteins from the recombination region of the λ genome, including *gam*. The *recB, recC,* and *endI* mutations facilitate assays of the inhibitor. Cells are grown at 32°C to mid-log phase, shifted to 42°C for 1 hr, and then harvested for the purification. The purification procedure is rather involved (Sakaki *et al.*, 1973) and yields only about 2.5 mg of the protein, purified between 1000- and 50000-fold, from 200 liters of mid-log-phase culture.

PHYSICAL PROPERTIES OF γ-PROTEIN

Analysis of the most purified fractions of γ-protein by non-denaturing or sodium dodecyl sulfate (SDS) polyacrylamide gel elec-trophoresis reveals one major protein species containing about 80% of the stain (see Fig. 3, below). Activity inhibitory for the RecBC enzyme can be recovered from a nondenaturing gel as a single peak that co-migrates with the major protein band. When the inhibi-tory material eluted from the nondenaturing gel is put onto SDS-polyacrylamide gels, it migrates as a single polypeptide of molecu-lar weight 16,500. When a preparation of γ-protein is put directly on an SDS gel, the major protein species migrates to the same posi-tion. The rate of sedimentation of the inhibitory activity through a glycerol gradient and its migration through Sephadex columns both suggest that it exists as a single species of molecular weight approximately 33,000. Taken together, these results demonstrate that the *gam* gene product is a protein of approximately 33,000 daltons which is made up of two subunits of equal molecular weight (Sakaki *et al.*, 1973).

The purified γ-protein is stable for several months at -20°C; however, it is inactivated when heated to 95°C.

FUNCTIONAL PROPERTIES OF γ-PROTEIN *IN VITRO*

γ-Protein by itself has no detectable exo- or endonuclease activity. It has no ATPase activity, nor does it appear to bind ATP, or transfer label from [^{14}C]ATP or [γ-^{32}P]ATP to the RecBC enzyme.

Specificity of Inhibition

The RecBC enzyme has been shown to catalyze several reactions (Goldmark and Linn, 1972; Karu *et al.*, 1973). These include an ATP-dependent exonuclease active on duplex or single-stranded linear

DNA, an ATP-stimulated endonuclease active on single-stranded DNA,
and a DNA-dependent ATPase. All of these activities are inhibited
to roughly the same extent by γ-protein. Although the rates of
uninhibited RecBC nuclease reactions are quite dependent upon the
ATP concentration (Goldmark and Linn, 1972), the effectiveness of
inhibition by γ-protein was independent of the ATP level. It is
noteworthy that the endonuclease activity is inhibited even in the
absence of ATP, and that the ATPase is inhibited in the absence of
nuclease activity when cross-linked DNA--a nondigestible cofactor
for the ATPase--is present (Sakaki *et al.*, 1973). γ-Protein also
inhibits the formation of the sedimentable reaction intermediates
observed during the digestion of duplex DNA by the RecBC enzyme
(Karu *et al.*, 1973).

γ-Protein is a highly specific inhibitor of the RecBC enzyme.
λ Exonuclease is not significantly inhibited by high levels of γ-
protein, nor are *E. coli* exonuclease I, exonuclease II (the 3'→5'
exonuclease of DNA polymerase I), or exonuclease III. Also, the
DNA-dependent ATPase of the *E. coli* B restriction enzyme is unaffected by γ-protein. Thus, γ-protein is not a general ATPase or inhibitor of DNases.

Factors Affecting the Inhibition

No lag or anomalous reaction kinetics are observed during RecBC
enzyme reactions in the presence of γ-protein, only a reduced reaction rate. Preliminary kinetic studies indicate that the inhibition is noncompetitive--*i.e.*, that γ-protein renders molecules of
RecBC enzyme completely unavailable for reaction, but the residual,
active enzyme has normal affinities for ATP and DNA.

If γ-protein is added to a reaction already in progress, virtually no inhibition occurs. Instead, γ-protein must be mixed with
RecBC enzyme before substrate is added. Highest levels of inhibition
are observed if enzyme and inhibitor are mixed 5 to 10 min prior to
the addition of DNA to a reaction mixture (Fig. 1). This preincubation is generally conducted at 37°C, but it is nearly as effective
at temperatures as low as 15°C. Inhibition is further enhanced
roughly twofold if ATP is present during the preincubation; the
enhancement is independent of the concentration of ATP from 20 µM
to 3.5 mM.

Inhibition of RecBC enzyme appears to be directly proportional
to the amount of γ-protein present until 60-70% of the activity is
inhibited (Fig. 2). Beyond this point, additional γ-protein does
not give proportionately greater inhibition, and we have not observed complete inhibition using highly purified γ-protein. This is
true for every concentration of RecBC enzyme and γ-protein tested.
There are several conceivable explanations for the inability of γ-

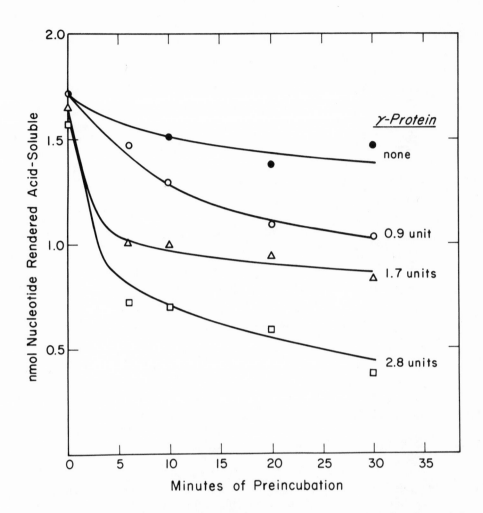

Figure 1.   Inhibition of RecBC exonuclease after incubation with
γ-protein.   γ-Protein [a Sephadex G-100 fraction prepared from
Fraction VII described by Sakaki *et al*. (1973)] was mixed with
RecBC enzyme [2.3 units of Fraction IX described by Goldmark and
Linn (1972)] in 0.09 ml containing 10 mM Tris·HCl (pH 8.2), 3 mM
KPO_4 (pH 6.8), 10 mM $MgCl_2$, 1.1 mM dithiothreitol, 0.27 mM ATP,
0.55 mg/ml of acetylated bovine serum albumin (Goldmark and Linn,
1972) and 20% glycerol.   After preincubation at 37°C as shown,
6.3 nmol of duplex *E. coli* [^{3}H]DNA [in 0.06 ml 10 mM Tris·HCl (pH
8.2) – 10 mM $MgCl_2$] was added; incubation was continued for 30 min
at 37°C, then the amount of DNA nucleotide rendered acid-soluble
was determined (Goldmark and Linn, 1972).   One unit of γ-protein
inhibits one unit of RecBC DNase in the assay described by Sakaki
et al. (1973).

A. KARU *ET AL.*

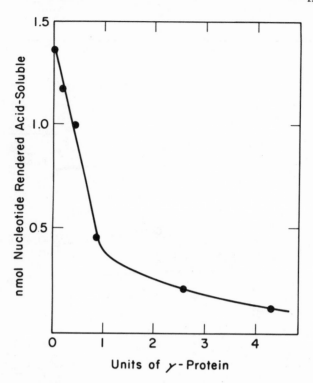

Figure 2. Inhibition of RecBC exonuclease by various levels of γ-protein. γ-Protein was added to 1.4 units of RecBC enzyme; the mixtures were preincubated for 10 min at 37°C, then DNA was added and acid-soluble nucleotide was determined after 30 min at 37°C.

protein to give total inhibition. A fraction of enzyme molecules might be resistant to inhibition, or our preparations might contain some damaged γ-protein which competes with active γ-protein for the enzyme. Alternatively, the effect may be due to an equilibrium between bound and free inhibitor, if inhibition requires actual physical association of γ-protein with the enzyme. Regardless of the actual reason, the existence of residual activity might be relevant to the genetic data that indicate a low level of RecBC-mediated recombination in infections by λ *gam*[+] phage (Shulman *et al.*, 1970; Unger *et al.*, 1972).

Possible Mechanisms for the Action of γ-Protein

We have attempted to distinguish whether inhibition of γ-protein might involve a catalytic modification or a noncatalytic physical interaction with RecBC enzyme. Most evidence supports the latter

Table 2. *In vitro* reversal at the nonpermissive temperature of γ^{ts}
inhibition of RecBC enzyme

| | ATP-dependent exonuclease in lysates (nmoles nucleotide rendered acid-soluble/mg protein) | |
Infecting phage	Lysate preincubated 10 min at 29°C; assayed at 29°C	Lysate preincubated 10 min at 42°C; assayed at 29°C
γ^+	ND	ND
γ^{37}	ND	15.9

E coli rec[+] was grown at 37°C to a cell density of 7.7 X 10^8
cells/ml, then harvested by centrifugation and resuspended in one-
tenth volume of 10 mM Tris·HCl (pH 8.0) = 10 mM $MgCl_2$. Aliquots
were infected with λ*bio72* (*gam*[+]) or λ*bio72gamts37* at a multiplicity
of 5 and, after 10 min at 4°C, diluted tenfold with broth at 29°C.
Control samples were harvested after 15 min at 29°C. Brij-lysozyme
lysates (Sakaki *et al.*, 1973) were prepared, then assayed as described in Fig. 1, except that 10 nmol of *E. coli* tRNA was present
to inhibit endonuclease I, and preincubation and assay temperatures
were as shown. The ATP-dependent activity was obtained by subtract-
ing the values obtained from assays from which ATP was omitted. The
specific activities of the ATP-dependent exonuclease in the samples
not incubated in broth after infection were 7.9 and 11.7 for the
gam[+] and *gam37* samples, respectively. ND = no detectable stimulation of exonuclease by ATP added to the assay.

mechanism. First, the inhibition is reversible if a thermolabile
γ-protein is denatured. When extracts are prepared from *rec*[+] cells
15 min after infection at the permissive temperature with the thermo-
sensitive λ *gam37*, no RecBC enzyme is detected in assays done at the
permissive temperature. However, RecBC exonuclease activity re-
appears in the extract if the assay is preceded by incubation at
42°C, the nonpermissive temperature for the *gam37* product (Table 2).
Activity does *not* reappear in λ[+] extracts under the same conditions.
A similar but less pronounced restoration of RecBC exonuclease is
also obtained in experiments in which λ *gam37*-infected cells are
shifted to the nonpermissive temperature *in vivo* in the presence
of chloramphenicol, and extracts are then prepared from these cells
and assayed at the permissive temperature. These results imply
that the enzyme and inhibitor form a protein-protein complex.

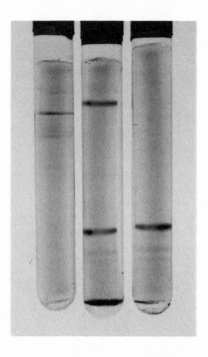

Figure 3.   Alteration of the electrophoretic mobility of RecBC
enzyme in the presence of γ-protein.   RecBC enzyme (580 units of
Fraction IX) and 580 units of γ-protein (prepared as in the legend
to Fig. 1) were mixed in 0.55 ml 10 mM KPO_4 (pH 6.8), 64 μM EDTA,
64 μM dithiothreitol, 3.6 mM 2-mercaptoethanol, 37% glycerol.
Control samples contained only one of the proteins.   After 10 min
at 4°C, 0.06 ml of 50 mM 2-mercaptoethanol, 0.235 M $Tris \cdot H_3PO_4$
(pH 6.8), 0.0009% bromphenol blue was added, and the samples were
subjected to electrophoresis in 7.5% polyacrylamide gels, essentially as described by Davis (1964).   The gels were cut at the position
of the bromphenol blue dye, stained with Coomassie Brilliant Blue
R-250, then destained electrophoretically.   *Left*, RecBC enzyme;
center, RecBC enzyme plus γ-protein; *right*, γ-protein.   The mobility
of the RecBC enzyme relative to the marker dye was 0.21 in the
absence of γ-protein (*left*) and 0.18 in the presence of γ-protein
(*center*).   γ-Protein is the major band in the center and right gels,
with a relative mobility of 0.71.

In another type of experiment, when excess γ-protein and RecBC
enzyme are mixed, virtually all of the enzyme is converted to a form
which migrates more slowly than RecBC enzyme alone in nondenaturing
polyacrylamide gels (Fig. 3).   When material from the new band is
eluted from the gel, denatured and subjected to electrophoresis in
SDS-polyacrylamide gels, two polypeptides are found that migrate
identically to the subunits of uninhibited RecBC enzyme.   This

indicates that no obvious proteolysis accompanies the enzyme-inhibitor interaction. Although the slowly migrating species might arise by the formation of a stable enzyme-inhibitor complex, we have been unable to detect the subunit characteristic of the γ-protein by SDS-polyacrylamide gel electrophoresis of this material (perhaps because the relatively low molecular weight of γ-protein makes detection difficult, or perhaps because the association of enzyme and inhibitor is not sufficiently tight to survive the electrophoresis).

These experiments and the other observations we have noted above provide no evidence that γ-protein inhibits the RecBC enzyme by catalyzing a protein modification reaction. Rather, they suggest that γ-protein may act by binding to RecBC enzyme. Work is in progress to test this binding hypothesis.

ROLE OF THE γ-PROTEIN *IN VIVO*

The *in vitro* properties of γ-protein appear consistent with most of the biological effects of *gam* mutations listed in Table 1. Enquist and Skalka (1973) have provided a biochemical rationale for the Fec⁻ phenotype. They found that in a Fec⁻ phage infection (*red⁻gam⁻* phage in a *recA⁻* host) circular replicative intermediates of phage DNA are produced, but the linear concatemers characteristic of late infection are not. This finding suggests that the transition from an "early" to a "late" mode of phage DNA replication is not accomplished if active RecBC enzyme is present. The direct role of RecBC enzyme is supported by the observation that linear concatemers are produced after infection of a *recA⁻recB⁻* host by *red⁻gam⁻* phage (*i.e.*, when the RecBC enzyme is removed by mutation) (Enquist and Skalka, 1973). Since a multi-length λ DNA molecule appears to be necessary for effective encapsulation (Stahl *et al.*, 1972; Enquist and Skalka, 1973), the production of phage progeny presumably requires either a replicative route to concatemers, which depends on γ-protein, or a recombinational route to multi-length molecules, which depends on the Red or Rec pathway.* Thus, *red⁻gam⁻* phage are unable to produce a substantial yield of progeny in a *recA⁻* host.

The Feb⁻ phenotype may be a formal corollary to Fec⁻, since Skalka and Enquist (personal communication) found that production of

---

* In addition to the potential for multimer formation by recombination of two circles, Stahl *et al.* (1973) and Skalka (personal communication) have pointed out that λ recombination enzymes might potentiate concatemer formation through a capacity of recombination intermediates to serve also as replication intermediates (Boon and Zinder, 1969); for example, to initiate rolling-circle replication.

linear concatemers is inefficient when *gam⁻* λ infects a *polA⁻* host.
This implies that the recombinational route to multi-length molecules fails when RecBC enzyme is fully active and DNA polymerase I
is not; whether this further implies a destructive attack on gapped
molecules by RecBC nuclease, or some more subtle interaction, remains to be established.

The more complex Spi⁻ phenotype can be explained in part by
the work of Lindahl *et al.* (1970), which demonstrated that phage P2
expresses a function lethal to *recB⁻* or *recC⁻* cells. Since λ *gam⁺*
phage establish a RecBC⁻ phenotype in an infected cell, the presence
of prophage P2 might be lethal to λ as well as the cell. However,
the involvement of the *red* and *del* mutations in this phenotype remains unexplained (Zissler *et al.*, 1971b; Barta *et al.*, 1974; Barta
and Zissler, 1974).

With regard to the recombinational properties of *gam* mutants,
the inhibition of RecBC enzyme by γ-protein provides an obvious
direct explanation for the lower contribution of the RecBC pathway
to recombination by *gam⁺*, as opposed to *gam⁻* phage. On the other
hand, a residual level of RecBC-mediated recombination by *gam⁺* phage
is observed consistent with the residual RecBC enzyme activity we
find even when excess γ-protein is present *in vitro*.

One property of *gam* mutants which is not consistent with the
known properties of γ-protein, however, is the lower efficiency of
phage recombination attributable to the phage Red pathway in the
case of *gam⁻* mutants. Inhibition of λ exonuclease by γ-protein
would provide one explanation for this phenomenon, but we have observed no such effect. Perhaps further study of the effects of γ-
protein *in vitro* upon products of the phage *red* genes will clarify
this question. However, it must be recognized that investigation
of the recombinational properties of *gam⁻* phage *in vivo* is handi-
capped by the growth effects of *gam⁻* mutations under the *red⁻* or
recA⁻ conditions used to eliminate the phage or host recombinational
pathway. Thus, the relationship between recombination frequency
among phage progeny may not necessarily reflect the frequency of
the primary recombination event.

CONCLUSION

The γ-protein of phage λ is a specific inhibitor of the host
RecBC enzyme. The mechanism of inhibition is most likely a direct
protein-protein interaction. The inhibitory activity of γ-protein
appears to be essential for the normal late stage of λ replication
in vivo.

ACKNOWLEDGMENTS

We wish to thank Drs. Lynn Enquist, Ann Skalka, and James Zissler for communicating their results prior to publication, James Zissler for phage strains and helpful discussion, and Vivian MacKay for providing RecBC enzyme. This investigation was supported in part by grants GM 17078 and GM 19020 from the National Institute of General Medical Sciences, and Contract No. AT(04-3)-34 from the United States Atomic Energy Commission. A. K. is a Postdoctoral Fellow (grant CA 52887) of the National Cancer Institute.

REFERENCES

Barta, K. and J. Zissler. 1974. The role of genetic recombination in DNA replication of phage lambda. II. An effect in DNA replication by gene delta. J. Virol. in press.

Barta, K., P. Tavernier and J. Zissler. 1974. The role of genetic recombination in DNA replication of phage lambda. I. Gene characterization of the delta gene. J. Virol. in press.

Boon, T. and N. D. Zinder. 1969. A mechanism for genetic recombination generating one parent and one recombinant. Proc. Nat. Acad. Sci. U.S.A. 64: 573.

Davis, B. J. 1964. Disk electrophoresis. II. Method and application to human proteins. Ann. N.Y. Acad. Sci. 121: 404.

Enquist, L. W. and A. Skalka. 1973. Replication of bacteriophage λ DNA dependent on the function of host and viral genes. I. Interaction of *red*, *gam*, and *rec*. J. Mol. Biol. 75: 185.

Goldmark, P. J. and S. Linn. 1972. Purification and properties of the RecBC DNase of *Escherichia coli* K-12. J. Biol. Chem. 247: 1849.

Karu, A. E., V. MacKay, P. Goldmark and S. Linn. 1973. The RecBC deoxyribonuclease of *Escherichia coli* K-12: substrate specificity and reaction intermediates. J. Biol. Chem. 248: 4874.

Lindahl, G., G. Sironi, H. Bialy and R. Calendar. 1970. Bacteriophage lambda: abortive infection of bacteria lysogenic for phage P2. Proc. Nat. Acad. Sci. U.S.A. 66: 587.

Sakaki, Y., A. E. Karu, S. Linn and H. Echols. 1973. Purification and properties of the γ-protein specified by bacteriophage λ: an inhibitor of the host RecBC recombination enzyme. Proc. Nat. Acad. Sci. U.S.A. 70: 2215.

Shulman, M. J., L. M. Hallick, H. Echols and E. R. Signer. 1970. Properties of recombination-deficient mutants of bacteriophage lambda. J. Mol. Biol. 52: 501.

Sironi, G., H. Bialy, H. A. Lozeron and R. Calendar. 1971. Bacteriophage P2: Interaction with phage lambda and with recombination-deficient bacteria. Virology 46: 387.

Stahl, F. W., S. Chung, J. Crasemann, D. Faulds, J. Haemer, S. Lam, R. E. Malone, K. D. McMilin, Y. Nozu, J. Siegel, J. Strathern and M. M. Stahl. 1973. Recombination, replication, and maturation in phage lambda. In (C. F. Fox and W. S. Robinson, eds) Virus Research. p. 487. Academic Press, New York.

Stahl, F. W., K. D. McMilin, M. M. Stahl, R. E. Malone, Y. Nozu and V. E. A. Russo. 1972. A role for recombination in the production of "free-loader" lambda bacteriophage particles. J. Mol. Biol. 68: 57.

Unger, R. C. and A. J. Clark. 1972. Interaction of the recombination pathways of bacteriophage λ and its host *Escherichia coli* K-12: Effects on exonuclease V activity. J. Mol. Biol. 70: 539.

Unger, R. C., H. Echols and A. J. Clark. 1972. Interaction of the recombination pathways of bacteriophage λ and host *Escherichia coli* K-12: Effects on λ recombination. J. Mol. Biol. 70: 531.

Zissler, J., E. Signer and F. Schaefer. 1971a. The role of recombination in growth of bacteriophage lambda. I. The gamma gene. In (A. D. Hershey, ed.) The Bacteriophage Lambda. p. 455. Cold Spring Harbor Laboratory, New York.

Zissler, J., E. Signer and F. Schaefer. 1971b. The role of recombination in growth of bacteriophage lambda. II. Inhibition of growth by prophage P2. In (A. D. Hershey, ed.) The Bacteriophage Lambda. p. 469. Cold Spring Harbor Laboratory, New York.

TRANSDUCTION OF $recB^-$ HOSTS IS PROMOTED BY λ red^+ FUNCTION

Robert A. Weisberg and Nat Sternberg

Laboratory of Molecular Genetics, NICHD, NIH,

Bethesda, Maryland 20014

The $redB$ and $redX$ genes of bacteriophage λ specify a recombination pathway that efficiently recombines phage genomes in lytically infected $recA^-$ and $recB^-$ cells (see Signer, 1971, for a review). However, the red genes do not promote efficient specialized transduction of a $recA^-$ host (Manly $et\ al.$, 1969; Mizuuchi and Fukasawa, 1969; Gottesman $et\ al.$, 1974; H. Echols, personal communication). We report here that the red pathway does promote efficient transduction of $recB^-$ hosts.

We have measured λ-mediated transduction of gal and $proA$. We see (Table 1) that $recB^-$ cells are transduced almost as efficiently as $recB^+$ when red^+ functions are provided. In fact, the remaining difference between them might be due to the lower viability of $recB^-$ strains (Willets and Mount, 1969). Transduction of gal in rec^+ hosts is stimulated about 15-fold by red^+ functions, whereas $proA$ transduction is stimulated little if at all. We have no explanation of this difference.

Transduction of both gal and $proA$ is reduced more than 100-fold in $recA^-$ and $recA^-B^-$ hosts even in red^+ conditions. (However, we do see very inefficient red-promoted gal transduction of $recA^-$ and $recA^-B^-$ strains.) This inefficient red-promoted transduction of $recA^-$ hosts contrasts with the efficient red-promoted phage recombination seen in these cells. This contrast cannot be explained simply by assuming that the expression of the $redB$ and $redX$ genes is insufficient for recombination in infected cells undergoing the temperate response: such an assumption is contradicted by our finding of red-promoted transduction of $recB^-$ strains. Instead, we suggest that λ specifies a function that replaces $recA^+$ for phage recombination and whose expression is lethal to the cell.

Table 1. λ-mediated transduction of *gal* and *proA*

Recombination Genes		*Pro*A$^+$ transductions (X 10^5) per ml	*Gal*$^+$ transductants (X 10^4) per infected cell
Phage	Host		
+	+	310	2,200
red$^-$	+	240	150
+	*rec*A$^-$	≤ 1	17
red$^-$	*rec*A$^-$	≤ 1	≤ 0.5
+	*rec*B$^-$	190	420
red$^-$	*rec*B$^-$	≤ 1	0.27
+	*rec*A$^-$B$^-$	≤ 1	7.7
red$^-$	*rec*A$^-$B$^-$	≤ 1	≤ 0.02

*Pro*A transduction: Lysates of *proA*$^+$ transducing paticles were prepared by inducing a *rec*A *su*$^-$ (λ *c*I857 *b*2 *red*3 *Sam*7) lysogen. *Pro*A transduction by such a lysate occurs exclusively by substitution (unpublished results, see Campbell, 1964). The recipient strains were derivatives of AB 1157 (*proA*$^-$), and transduction was carried out by plating on minimal–glucose bio-B1 plates containing all the amino acids required by the above strain except proline. Lambda *c*I857 or λ *c*I857 *red*3 helper phage was added at a virus:cell ratio of 5:10.

Gal transduction: The lysate used was prepared by induction of *rec*A *su*$^-$ (λ *c*I857 *int am*29 *red*3 *Sam*7). The DNA of the *gal* transducing particles found in this lysate carries only the right cohesive end of λ (Little and Gottesman, 1971) and thus transduce exclusively by substitution (see Campbell, 1964) rather than by addition of a *gal*$^+$ gene to the bacterial genome (unpublished results). Recipient cells were derivatives of strain W3102 and carry the *gal*K2 mutation. Transduction was measured by plating the infected cells on *gal*-TTC plates according to the procedure of Shimada *et al.* (1973). Lambda *c*I857 *int am*29 *red*$^+$ or λ *c*I857 *int am*29 *red*3 helper phage was added at a virus:cell ratio of 5:10, and transducing phage were added at virus:cell ratio much less than 1. The number of transducing phage particles was determined by measuring the absorbance at 260 nm of a purified lysate.

REFERENCES

Campbell, A. 1964. Transduction. In (I. C. Gunsalus and R. Y. Stanier, eds.) The Bacteria, vol. 5, p. 49. Academic Press, New York.

Gottesman, M. M, M. E. Gottesman, S. Gottesman and M. Gellert. 1974. Characterization of λ reverse as an *E. coli* phage carrying a unique set of host derived recombination functions. J. Mol. Biol., submitted.

Little, J. and M. E. Gottesman. 1971. Defective lambda particles whose DNA carries only a single cohesive end. In (A. D. Hershey, ed.) The Bacteriophage λ. p. 371. Cold Spring Harbor Laboratory, New York.

Manly, K., E. Signer and C. Radding. 1969. Nonessential functions of bacteriophage λ. Virology 37: 177.

Mizuuchi, K. and T. Fukasawa. 1969. Chromosome mobilization in *rec*-merodiploids of *Escherichia coli* K12 following infection with bacteriophage λ. Virology 39: 467.

Shimada, K., R. Weisberg and M. E. Gottesman. 1973. Prophage lambda at unusual chromosomal locations II. Mutations induced by bacteriophage lambda in *Escherichia coli* K12. J. Mol. Biol. 80: 297.

Signer, E. 1971. General recombination. In (A. D. Hershey, ed.) The Bacteriophage λ. p. 139. Cold Spring Harbor Laboratory, New York.

Willets, N. and D. Mount. 1969. Genetic analysis of recombination-deficient mutants of *Escherichia coli* carrying *rec* mutations co-transducible with *thy*A. J. Bacteriol. 100: 405.

TRANSFORMATION AND TRANSDUCTION OF *ESCHERICHIA COLI:* THE

NATURE OF RECOMBINANTS FORMED BY Rec, RecF, AND λ Red

Wilfried Wackernagel[*] and Charles M. Radding[†]

Abteilung Biologie, Lehrstuhl Biologie der Mikroorgan-

ismen, Ruhr-Universitat, 463 Bochum, West Germany, and

†Departments of Medicine and Molecular Biophysics and

Biochemistry, Yale University, New Haven, Connecticut 06510

Genetic transformation of *Escherichia coli* is possible when
two requirements are met: (1) the recipient strain lacks exonuclease V, due to a mutation in *recB* or *recC*, but has recovered
proficiency for recombination by virtue of a second suppressing
mutation, *sbcA* or *sbcB*; and (2) the uptake of DNA is facilitated
by treatment of the recipient cells with $CaCl_2$ (Oishi and Cosloy,
1972; Wackernagel, 1973). However, compared with other bacteria,
the frequency of transformation of *E. coli* is low, usually about
one cell in 10^6. In an effort to improve this frequency we turned
to a source of DNA that is both uniform and enriched for specific
markers, namely the specialized transducing variants of phage λ.
Our initial observations on transformation by λ *gal bio* DNA and our
efforts to vary its genetic control suggested that certain questions
might be approached more readily by studying transduction. We
report here observations on transformation and transduction mediated
by the RecBC and RecF pathways of *E. coli* (for review see Clark,
1973) and the Red system of phage λ (for review see Radding, 1973).
These experiments have provided an opportunity to examine the properties of recombination mediated by the λ Red system without the
possible complications introduced by maturation of phage particles.

RESULTS

Variations in the Genetic Control of Transformation

111

The source of DNA for these experiments was λ *gal*8 *bio*256 *cI*857 (Table 1), a nondefective derivative that carries the galactose and biotin operons of *E. coli* but lacks the genes for the site-specific (Int) and general (Red) recombination systems of λ. In some experiments, the λ Red system was provided by infection with a helper phage, λ *b*538 *red*$^+$ *cI*857 *cro*27, from which the λ attachment site (*att*^{λ}) and the *int* gene have been deleted (Parkinson, 1971).

When JC7623, *recBC sbcB*, was transformed with intact or sheared DNA from λ *gal bio*, Gal$^+$ transformants arose at a frequency of 1.5 to 3 X 10^{-5} per viable cell, which is 30 to 60 times higher than that observed under similar conditions with *E. coli* DNA (Table 2; Wackernagel, 1973). This increase in the frequency of transformation is similar in magnitude to the 80-fold enrichment of the *gal* genes in DNA from λ *gal bio* over those in DNA from *E. coli*. In the recombination-deficient strain AB2470, *recB*, transformation by intact DNA from λ *gal bio* was about 10 times higher than the background, but about 100 times lower than in *recBC sbcB* (Table 2).

In the absence of helper phage, most Gal$^+$ transformants of *recB* inherited λ immunity (*imm*^{λ}), whereas most transformants of *recBC sbcB* did not (Table 2). Infection of recipient cells with helper phage, which were (*att int*)^Δ *red*$^+$ *cI*857 *cro*, prior to the addition of DNA stimulated transformation by intact λ *gal bio* DNA about 20-fold in *recBC sbcB* and 1000-fold in *recB*. The helper, which cannot integrate efficiently by itself (Parkinson, 1971), qualitatively changed the transformation of *recBC sbcB*, causing the frequent incorporation of *imm*^{λ}.

Shearing of λ *gal bio* DNA had no discernible effect on the frequency of Gal$^+$ transformation of *recBC sbcB*, whereas the frequency was reduced by shearing in those instances in which *imm*^{λ} was usually incorporated (Table 2). Both the insensitivity of transformation to shearing and the absence of *imm*^{λ} suggest that the mechanism by which donor DNA is integrated into the recipient genome in *recBC sbcB* is different from that occurring in *recB* or in either strain infected with helper.

Variations in the Genetic Control of Transduction

Experiments on transduction were designed along lines similar to those described above for transformation: (1) the transducing phage was the same λ *gal bio* that lacks recombination genes of its own, and (2) in certain experiments the helper phage, λ (*att int*)^Δ *red*$^+$ *cI*857 *cro*, was used to provide the Red system.

A survey of transduction in various strains is presented in Table 3. The highest frequencies of transduction were observed with the two recombination-proficient strains, *rec*$^+$ and *recBC sbcB*.

Table 1. Bacteria and phages

Strains	Relevant genotype	Source or reference
E. coli K12		
AB1157	*galK2*	Howard‒Flanders and Boyce, 1966
AB2463	*galK2 recA13*	Howard‒Flanders and Boyce, 1966
AB2470	*galK2 recB21*	Howard‒Flanders and Boyce, 1966
JC7623	*galK2 recB21C22 sbcB15*	Kushner *et al.*, 1971
QR23	*gal bioA*	Manly *et al.*, 1969
QR9	*gal bioA recA*	Manly *et al.*, 1969
Phage λ		
gal8 bio256 cI857	*gal⁺ chlDᐃ bio⁺ attᴮ*	Feiss *et al.*, 1972;
	(int, red, gam)ᐃ	M. Gottesman, personal communication
λ *b538 cI857 cro27*	*(attλ int)ᐃ red⁺*	Parkinson, 1971;
λ *b538 red3 cI857 cro27*	*(attλ int)ᐃ red⁻*	this paper

Table 2. Transformation of *E. coli* with DNA of λ *gal bio int⁻ red⁻*

DNA	Helper	recBC sbcB		recB	
		Frequency (X 10^{-5})	imm^λ	Frequency (X 10^{-5})	imm^λ
0	0	0.0003	—	0.0009	—
λ	0	1.5	0/12	0.008	9/9
λ/2	0	1.4	0/14	0.0009	—
λ/4	0	2.8	0/8	0.0009	—
λ	+	31	16/22	9.1	19/20
λ/2	+	28	6/16	0.3	18/20
λ/4	+	0.15	9/28	0.03	17/20

Transforming DNA was isolated by phenol extraction of [³H]thymine-labeled λ *gal*8 *bio*256 *cI*857. To obtain 1/2-length fragments, this DNA at a concentration of 80 μg/ml was forced through a #22 hypodermic needle three times. To obtain 1/4-length fragments, the sheared DNA was forced through a #27 needle 10 times. The fragment size was determined by sucrose gradient centrifugation, using ³²P-labeled λ *c*71 DNA as a reference. Competent cells were obtained by treatment of growing cells with $CaCl_2$ as described earlier (Wackernagel, 1973). Helper phage, twice purified on CsCl gradients, was adsorbed to recipient cells (m.o.i. = 5) during 8 min of incubation at 30°C in 10 mM Tris-HCl, pH 7.5, and 20 mM $MgSO_4$, prior to treatment with $CaCl_2$. Transformation assays were performed as described (Wackernagel, 1973). All assays contained 4 μg of transforming DNA. Gal⁺ transformants were selected on minimal medium containing galactose instead of glucose. Transformants were purified by single-colony isolation on selective medium and checked for *imm*^λ by streaking across λ *c*71 and λ *vir* on an agar plate.

The frequency in *recB* was 10-20% of that in *rec⁺*. Even in *recA*, in which the frequency was only 5 X 10^{-4} times that observed in *rec⁺*, transductants appeared at least 1000 times more often than spontaneous revertants. Thus, under these circumstances recombination was observed at a high frequency in *recB* (0.23%) and at a low but

Table 3.   Transduction by λ *gal bio* (*int red*)

E. coli strain	Helper λ (*att int*) *red*$^+$ *cro*$^-$	Survival (%)	Gal$^+$ %	Gal$^+$ *imm*$^\lambda$ (%)
rec$^+$	0	20	3	100
	+	47	3	100
recB	0	16	0.23	92
	+	56	0.6	100
recA	0	16	0.0015	—
	+	23	0.12	82
recBC sbcB	0	32	5.8	21
	+	68	4.0	96

Cells were grown in complete broth at 37°C to a density of 3 to 4 X 10^8 per ml. After centrifugation the cells were resuspended in the same volume of 10 mM Tris-HCl (pH 7.5)-20 mM MgSO$_4$ and infected with the transducing phage at a multiplicity of 5 (15 min adsorption at 30°C). In experiments with helper phage, cells were simultaneously infected with helper at a multiplicity of 5. Selection of Gal$^+$ clones and the test for λ immunity were as described in the legend to Table 2. The strains used in these experiments were AB1157 (*rec*$^+$), AB2470 (*recB*), AB2463 (*recA*), and JC7623 (*recBC sbcB*) (see Table 1). The frequency of spontaneous Gal$^+$ colonies in every strain was less than 2 X 10^{-8}.

---

significant frequency in *recA* (0.0015%). The low frequency in *recA* made this strain suitable for investigating the possibility of transduction mediated by the general recombination system of phage λ (Red). Transduction of *recA* by λ *gal bio* was stimulated 80-fold by the addition of the *red*$^+$ helper phage. The stimulation by helper was related to the Red system by experiments in which *red*$^-$ helper was shown to be 1/10 to 1/300 as efficient as *red*$^+$ in promoting transduction (Table 4). A similar stimulation of transduction by *red*$^+$ helper was observed in a *recAB* recipient and in a *recA* recipient in which the λ attachment site was deleted (data not shown).

Table 4.   Transduction mediated by λ Red

Experiment	Helper	Gal$^+$ per 10^6 cells	red^+/red^-
1	red^+	240	48
	red^-	5	
2	red^+	220	9
	red^-	25	
3	red^+	830	69
	red^-	12	
4	red^+	190	19
	red^-	10	
5	red^+	1200	300
	red^-	4	

A $recA^-$ gal^- bio^- strain (QR9, Table 1) was transduced by λ gal bio in the presence of helper phage which was either red^+ (λ b538 cI857 cro27) or red^- (λ b538 red3 cI857 cro27).   The cells were infected at a multiplicity of 5 each of the transducing phage and the helper phage.   After adsorption, the infected cells were incubated in broth for 20 min at 39°C, followed by 20 min at 30°C. Washed infected cells were plated on selective medium.

Inheritance of imm^λ $chlD$ and bio by Gal$^+$ Transductants

In addition to the selected marker, gal, three others were scored in the experiments on transduction.   Inheritance of the marker imm^λ, which is in DNA that is not homologous to the recipient genome, measures the addition of λ genes by recombination in the homologous gal or bio regions.   The $chlD$ gene, which is located between gal and bio, is deleted from the transducing phage λ gal8 bio256 (Feiss et al., 1972).   Loss of the chl^+ allele from the recipient is readily scored. Bio provided a third marker that was useful in assessing the possibility of multiple exchanges.

Two classes of transductants were observed.   Most Gal$^+$ trans-ductants of rec^+ and $recB$, or of $recA$ infected by red^+ helper, inherited imm^λ.   Further analysis of the transductants produced under the control of Rec or Red showed that most were ChlD$^+$ and Bio$^+$ (Table 5).   By contrast, most transductants of $recBC$ $sbcB$ did not

Table 5.   Segregation of markers among Gal$^+$ transductants

System	Imm$^\lambda$	Chl		Bio		Totals
		+	-	+	-	
Rec	+	192	0	191	1	192
	-	0	1	0	1	1
Red	+	227	2	220	9	229
	-					0
RecF	+	7	0			7
	-	172	88			260

Gal$^+$ transductants were isolated and scored for λ immunity as described in the legends to the previous tables. The *bio* marker was scored by spotting a suspension of cells on minimal medium containing avidin (Manly *et al.*, 1969). The *chl* marker was scored by the test for nitrate reductase activity (Adhya *et al.*, 1968). The strains used for these experiments were QR23 (*rec$^+$*), JC7623 (*recBC sbcB*), and QR9 (*recA$^-$*), which was infected by transducing phage and helper as described in the legend to Table 4. Data were pooled from several experiments.

---

inherit *imm$^\lambda$*, and many had lost the *chlD$^+$* allele originally present in the recipient genome. (A *bio$^-$* allele was not available for scoring in this strain.)

Diploidy of Gal$^+$ Transductants Produced by Red-Mediated Recombination

All of the Gal$^+$ *imm$^\lambda$* transductants produced by Red-mediated recombination carried the temperature-sensitive allele of the λ repressor, *cI857*. Separate clones were cured of λ by superinfection with *b2 imm^{434}* and selection of colonies that survived at 39°C. Of 49 clones, 43 segregated both Gal$^+$ and Gal$^-$ cured progeny. This shows that most of the Red-mediated transductants were heterozygous and hence diploid for Gal.

DISCUSSION

Consistent with earlier results (Wackernagel, 1973), these experiments show that transformation in *E. coli* can be put under the genetic control of several systems of recombination, including (1) RecF, (2) some residual activity present in recB, and (3) probably λ Red. The use of DNA from specialized transducing variants of λ improves the efficiency of transformation and provides a well-defined source of DNA. Similar observations on transformation of *recBC sbcB* by DNA from transducing derivatives of phages 80 and λ have been published recently by Oishi and Cosloy (1974).

For some kinds of information about recombination it is easier to study transduction than transformation. In order of decreasing frequency, transduction was observed in the following systems: Rec⁺, RecF⁺ > *recB⁻* > λ Red⁺ > *recA⁻*.

In these experiments, any stable association of the donor *gal⁺* allele with the recipient cell was selected. In *recBC sbcB* this clearly involved recombination in the *gal* region. In the Red-mediated system, the production of some Gal⁺ Bio⁻ transductants and the inheritance of Gal⁺ by some cured derivatives may be taken as evidence of recombination in the *gal bio* region. Echols (personal communication) has observed transduction of *rec⁺* and *recA* strains by λ *gal int⁻ red⁻* and λ *gal int⁻ red⁺*, respectively, at frequencies that are similar to those reported here. In experiments with transducing particles, the DNA of which presumably remains linear in the recipient, Weisberg and Sternberg (this symposium) have observed more pronounced stimulation of transduction by the Red system, particularly in *recB*.

In *recBC sbcB*, both transformants and transductants differed strikingly from those produced in other strains, with respect to the frequency with which *imm^λ* was incorporated. This difference was examined in more detail by observing the inheritance of other markers. Gal⁺ transductants of *recBC sbcB* usually did not inherit *imm^λ* from the donor and frequently did not inherit *chl⁺* from the recipient. These observations suggest that a segment of the recipient genome was replaced by a segment of the donor genome through an even number of exchanges, which may or may not have been reciprocal. By contrast, Gal⁺ transductants issuing from recombination promoted by Rec or Red usually inherited *chl⁺* from the recipient as well as *imm^λ* and *bio⁺* from the donor. These data are most readily explained by supposing that a single reciprocal exchange added the circular donor genome to the recipient to produce a partially diploid recombinant (Fig. 1a). The data do not support more complicated explanations for the frequent inheritance of *imm^λ*, such as exchanges involving duplications of the recipient and transducing genomes (Fig. 1b), for the following reasons:

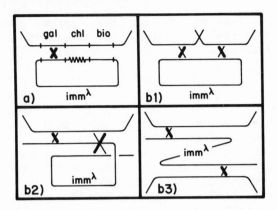

Figure 1. Possible explanations for the incorporation of imm^λ by general recombination between λ *gal* chl^Δ *bio* and the chromosome of *E. coli*. (a) A single reciprocal exchange between one chromosome of λ and one of *E. coli*. (b) Multiple exchanges, which may or may not be reciprocal, between single or duplicated chromosomes. In (b2) and (b3) the λ chromosome may be either a circular or linear concatemer in which imm^λ is flanked by identical copies of the *gal* and *bio* regions. In the cases illustrated by (b1) and (b3), a third crossover is required to restore the integrity of a single *E. coli* chromosome (see Hill *et al.*, 1969).

---

(1) Unless special assumptions are made, interactions involving duplicated genomes might equally often produce nonimmune as immune transductants (Fig. 1b). One such assumption, namely selection on the basis of λ immunity, is made less tenable by the observations on the transductants of *recBC sbcB*, which were mostly nonimmune.

(2) Gal$^+$ transductants produced by double exchanges involving concatemers of the transducing genome might be expected to have lost *chlD$^+$* at a frequency that depends upon the relative lengths of the *gal* and *bio* regions. For example, if these regions were of similar length, half of the transductants that inherited imm^λ should have lost *chl$^+$* by an exchange on each side of the latter (see Fig. 1, b2 and b3). But few Gal$^+$ imm^λ transductants lost *chl$^+$* (Table 5).

(3) In the *rec$^+$* and *recA$^-$* strains used in the experiments shown in Table 5 the *bio* mutation is in the A gene, at the end of the *bio* region that is proximal to *gal* (Shulman and Gottesman, 1973; and unpublished observations). Thus if Gal$^+$ imm^λ transductants were produced by double exchanges between one transducing genome and two copies of the recipient genome (Fig. 1, b1) they might inherit the *bio$^-$* allele in as many as half of the instances, assuming (1) that

the two exchanges required are equally likely anywhere within the
gal-bio region and (2) that *gal* and *bio* are of similar length.
But few of the Gal$^+$ transductants produced by Rec or Red recombination were Bio$^-$.

Our results are consonant with earlier observations on exchanges
between episome and chromosome which showed that Rec-mediated
recombination is often reciprocal with respect to widely spaced
markers (Meselson, 1967; Herman, 1968). We interpret our observations on Red-mediated recombination to mean that it may sometimes
be reciprocal for distant markers. The reciprocity of recombination
observed in transduction contrasts with the nonreciprocity observed
in phage crosses (Weil, 1969; Sarthy and Meselson, personal communication), but these results are not necessarily in conflict. On the
one hand, in spite of a contrary argument that we made above, it
remains possible that transduction of some strains may select
reciprocal recombinants by selecting for immunity. On the other
hand, the maturation of phage λ is subject to different selective
forces (Stahl *et al.*, 1972; Enquist and Skalka, 1973). For example, only one λ genome in a dimeric circle appears to get packaged,
a phenomenon which could reduce the recovery of reciprocal recombinants (Ross and Freifelder, in preparation; Freifelder *et al.*,
1974). From observations of another experimental situation that
does not require phage maturation, namely the formation of double
lysogens in the absence of Int, Freifelder and Levine (personal
communication) have also inferred that recombination mediated by
Red may sometimes be reciprocal. The possible operation of selective forces both in transduction and in phage crosses makes it
difficult to assess the true frequency of reciprocity or nonreciprocity. The question is an important one for the further understanding of λ recombination.

ACKNOWLEDGMENTS

We are grateful to Dr. Max Gottesman for supplying us with λ
gal bio. We are indebted to K. Wackernagel and Dr. N. Lundh and
J. Beckendorf for expert technical assistance. This work was supported by Deutsche Forschungsgemeinschaft and by Grant ACS NP 90
from the American Cancer Society, and Grant 268 from the Jane Coffin
Childs Memorial Fund for Medical Research.

REFERENCES

Adhya, S., P. Cleary and A. Campbell. 1968. A deletion analysis
of prophage lambda and adjacent genetic regions. Proc. Nat. Acad.
Sci. U.S.A. <u>61</u>: 956.

Clark, A. J.   1973.   Recombination deficient mutants of *E. coli*
and other bacteria.   Ann. Rev. Genet. 7: 67.

Enquist, L. W. and A. Skalka.   1973.   Replication of bacteriophage
λ DNA dependent on the function of host and viral genes I.   The
"fec⁻" defect.   J. Mol. Biol. 75: 185.

Feiss, M., S. Adhya and D. L. Court.   1972.   Isolation of plaque-
forming, galactose-transducing strains of phage lambda.   Genetics
71: 189.

Freifelder, D., L. Chud and E. E. Levine.   1974.   Requirement for
maturation of *Escherichia coli* bacteriophage lambda.   J. Mol. Biol.
83: 503.

Herman, R. K.   1968.   Identification of recombinant chromosomes and
F-merogenotes in merodiploids of *Escherichia coli*.   J. Bacteriol.
96: 173.

Hill, C. W., D. Schiffer and P. Berg.   1969.   Transduction of mero-
ploidy: Induced duplication of recipient genes.   J. Bacteriol. 99:
274.

Howard-Flanders, P. and R. P. Boyce.   1966.   DNA repair and genetic
recombination: Studies on mutants of *Escherichia coli* defective in
these processes.   Radiat. Res. 6 (suppl.): 156.

Kushner, S. R., H. Nagishi, A. Templin and A. J. Clark.   1971.
Genetic recombination in *Escherichia coli*:   The role of exonuclease
I.   Proc. Nat. Acad. Sci. U.S.A. 68: 824.

Manly, K. F., E. R. Signer and C. M. Radding.   1969.   Nonessential
functions of bacteriophage λ.   Virology 37: 177.

Meselson, M.   1967.   Reciprocal recombination in prophage lambda.
J. Cell Physiol. 70: 113.

Oishi, M. and S. D. Cosloy.   1972.   The genetic and biochemical
basis of the transformability of *Escherichia coli* K12.   Biochem.
Biophys. Res. Commun. 49: 1568.

Oishi, M. and S. D. Cosloy.   1974.   Specialized transformation in
Escherichia coli K12.   Nature 248: 112.

Parkinson, J. S.   1971.   Deletion mutants of bacteriophage λ: II.
Genetic properties of att-defective mutants.   J. Mol. Biol. 56: 385.

Radding, C. M.   1973.   Molecular mechanisms in recombination.   Ann.
Rev. Genet. 7: 87.

122   W. WACKERNAGEL AND C. RADDING

Shulman, M. and M. Gottesman. 1973. Attachment site mutants of
bacteriophage lambda. J. Mol. Biol. 81: 461.

Stahl, F. W., K. D. McMilin, M. M. Stahl, R. E. Malone, Y. Nozu
and V. E. A. Russo. 1972. A role for recombination in the
production of "free-loader" lambda bacteriophage particles. J.
Mol. Biol. 68: 57.

Wackernagel, W. 1973. Genetic transformation in *E. coli:* The
inhibitory role of the *recBC* DNAse. Biochem. Biophys. Res. Commun.
51: 306.

Weil, J. 1969. Reciprocal and non-reciprocal recombination in
bacteriophage λ. J. Mol. Biol. 43: 351.

The RecE PATHWAY OF BACTERIAL RECOMBINATION

Jane R. Gillen and Alvin J. Clark

Department of Molecular Biology, University of California,

Berkeley, California 94720

There appear to be three pathways of recombination active or potentially active in strains of *Escherichia coli* (Clark, 1971, 1973). The operation of two of these three pathways has so far been associated with nuclease activities. The RecBC pathway makes use of exonuclease V (ExoV), the product of the *recB* and *recC* genes (see *e.g.* Goldmark and Linn, 1972). The RecE pathway does not use ExoV; it proceeds in cells that contain exonuclease VIII (ExoVIII). The RecF pathway also does not use ExoV. The RecF pathway appears to be inhibited by exonuclease I (ExoI) in that it operates at high efficiency only when ExoI is mutationally inactivated by *sbcB* mutations. Here we wish to consider the role that ExoVIII may play in the RecE pathway, particularly in comparison with the roles that can be postulated for ExoV in the RecBC pathway and for the exonuclease of lambda (Exoλ) in the Red recombination system of lambda.

sbcA MUTATIONS AND THE PRESENCE OF ExoVIII

sbcA mutations were first described by Barbour *et al.* (1970) by virtue of their ability to suppress indirectly the recombination and repair deficiencies associated with *recB* and *recC* mutations. Thus, triply mutant *sbcA⁻ recB⁻ recC⁻* strains were as proficient in recombination and repair as wild-type *sbcA⁺ recB⁺ recC⁺* strains. In the wild-type strains, the ATP-dependent nuclease ExoV is associated with the recombination and repair proficiency; in the triply mutant strains, ExoV could not be detected. Instead, an ATP-independent exonuclease was found. The properties of this enzyme, now called ExoVIII, are summarized in the next section.

Recent experiments by Lloyd and Barbour (in preparation) show that the *sbcA* gene appears to be located near *trp*, at 29' on the standard map of *E. coli*. Furthermore, these workers have information which leads them to claim that *sbcA⁺* is dominant to *sbcA⁻*. Dominance of *sbcA⁺* is consistent with the view expressed previously (Clark, 1971) that *sbcA* regulates the structural gene for ExoVIII, which is defined to be *recE*, and that *sbcA* mutations derepress *recE*.

COMPARISON OF ExoVIII WITH ExoV AND Exoλ

In Vitro Properties

The purification and some of the properties of ExoVIII, described in detail in a separate publication (Kushner *et al.*, 1974), are summarized in Table 1. In brief, the enzyme has a sub-unit molecular weight of about 1.3×10^5. (Later experiments by the present authors have shown that the molecular weight of the active enzyme may also be 1.3×10^5). Partially purified preparations show no endonuclease activity on single-stranded circular DNA and a marked preference for the enzyme to act on linear native rather than linear denatured DNA. The enzyme is completely independent of ATP for its action. Except for the subunit molecular weight, ExoVIII most closely resembles Exoλ, the product of the *redX* gene of lambda. This enzyme is known to be necessary for general recombination of phage lambda, and its properties have been studied extensively *in vitro*. It remains to be determined whether or not the products of action of ExoVIII resemble those formed by Exoλ and whether or not the direction of exonucleolytic digestion is 5' to 3', as is that of Exoλ.

Although the size of ExoVIII is similar to that of the subunits of ExoV, which are about 1.3×10^5 and 1.4×10^5 daltons, the activities of ExoV are quite different. ExoV, the hallmark of the RecBC pathway, is a multifunctional enzyme that acts as an ATP-stimulated endonuclease on single-stranded DNA and as an ATP-dependent exonuclease equally well on native and denatured DNA. It also has a DNA-dependent ATPase. Recently, S. Kushner and I. R. Lehman (personal communication) have obtained evidence leading them to suggest that the exonucleolytic activity on native DNA is necessary for recombination. Whether or not the other activities are also necessary cannot be determined from their evidence. In another line of investigation on ExoV, stimulated by the findings of Friedman and Smith (1973) on an ExoV analog from *Haemophilus influenzae*, MacKay and Linn (1974) obtained electron micrographs of intermediates formed during the exonucleolytic action of ExoV on native DNA. These structures appear to be double-stranded molecules with extensive single-stranded ends. If these structures represent intermediates in the action of the native DNA exonuclease activity

Table 1. Comparison of the properties of three nucleases associated with recombination

	ExoV	ExoVIII	Exoλ
Structural gene(s)	*recB, recC*	*recE*	*redX*
Molecular weight (enzyme)	2.7×10^5	1.3×10^5	1.0×10^5
Exonuclease activity ratio $\dfrac{\text{Native DNA}}{\text{Denatured DNA}}$	1	≥ 150	350
Direction of action on native DNA	$5' \rightleftharpoons 3'$	unknown	$5' \rightarrow 3'$
Endonuclease activity on denatured DNA	+	−	−
Dependence on ATP — Exonuclease activity	+	−	−
Dependence on ATP — Endonuclease activity	±	−	−
Action initiated at nicks	−	unknown	−

Data for exonuclease V (ExoV) are from Goldmark and Linn (1972). Data for exonuclease VIII (ExoVIII) are from Kushner *et al.* (1974), and Gillen and Clark (unpublished results). Data for exonuclease of λ (Exoλ) are from Little (1967), Carter and Radding (1971), and Radding (personal communication).

of ExoV in recombination, then it seems plausible to expect ExoV to act presynaptically by opening up single-stranded regions of native DNAs for base pairing interaction. It should be noted that ExoV does not act to degrade covalently closed or "nicked" double-stranded circular DNA molecules; however, it does degrade double-stranded circular DNA molecules containing a gap that can be as short as 5 nucleotides (Karu *et al.*, 1973). At present, it is not clear how the enzyme acts on such gapped molecules, but at least

one hypothesis provides for essentially reversible opening of the
molecule (Fig. 1). Such action would be advantageous in the presynaptic preparations of the bacterial chromosome or plasmids for
recombination.

Lambda Recombinant Frequencies

We have performed several experiments dealing with the recombination of lambda to determine whether ExoVIII behaves *in vivo*

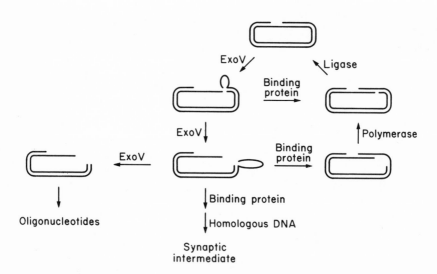

Figure 1.   Diagram of a possible presynaptic role for ExoV, using
the mechanism of ExoV action proposed by MacKay and Linn (1974).   A
circular element of DNA is shown carrying a gap of five or more
nucleotides in one of the strands.   ExoV may bind to the end of the
gap and nick the unbroken strand about a hundred nucleotides away.
It then may continue to nick the same strand at intervals of about
a hundred nucleotides.   Alternatively, the overlapping single strands
may renature in the presence of binding protein.   Following renaturation, ligase with or without polymerase would be expected to restore
the circular element to its original form.   A second alternative is
that the broken molecule may interact with homologous DNA to produce
a synaptic intermediate in recombination.   This alternative is also
expected to require the presence of a binding protein.   In the
absence of binding protein, such as in the *in vitro* experiments of
Karu *et al*. (1973), the single strand to which ExoV is bound may be
subject to attack, preventing restoration of the circular element to
its original form.   In this event, the element is degraded to
oligonucleotides.

like ExoV or like Exoλ. Previous experiments (Clark, 1974; Table 2) showed that recombination between the *A* and *J* genes in the left arm of lambda proceeds just as well by the RecE system as by the Red system of lambda. Recombinant frequencies were essentially the same whether the parental phage were *red*+ *gam*+ or *red*- *gam*- (achieved by a *bio10* substitution) or were crossed in a *recB*+ *recC*+ *sbcA*+ or *recB*- *recC*- *sbcA*- host. When *red*- *gam*- lambda parents were used in a strain which was *recB*- *recC*- *sbcA*-, only ExoVIII of the three nucleases (ExoVIII, ExoV, Exoλ) was present to participate in recombination. Since the frequencies of *A*+*J*+ recombinants were the same in both crosses, we concluded that lambda recombination using ExoVIII was as effective as lambda recombination using Exoλ.

Even more striking was the fact that the ExoVIII-promoted recombination of lambda in the *A* to *J* region was independent of the *recA* and *recF* functions, as is Exoλ (Red) recombination (Table 2). In contrast, bacterial recombination by the RecE pathway utilizes *recF* and is absolutely dependent on *recA* function (Table 2).

Table 2. Dependence on *recA* and *recF* of bacterial and lambda recombinant frequencies in ExoV- ExoVIII+ ExoI+ strains

		Recombinant frequencies (%) in		
		E. coli	Lambda (*A-J*)	
recA	*recF*	TL+[Sm^R]	*red*+*gam*+	*red*-*gam*-
+	+	4	4.9	3.3
-	+	<6 X 10^{-5}	4.5	2.9
+	-	6 X 10^{-2}	3.6	2.6

Bacterial recombinants were produced in 60-min interrupted matings using Hayes Hfr strain JC158 as donor. Threonine- and leucine-independent, streptomycin-resistant progeny were selected. *susA*- *susJ*+ and *susA*+ *susJ*- strains of wild-type lambda or λ*bio10* were crossed, and *sus*+ recombinants were detected by standard methods (Unger *et al.*, 1972). Experimental results are averages of two or more experiments.

Additional experiments have now been done in which recombinant frequencies for the intervals A to cI and cI to R have been determined, using phage carrying red-3 and gam-210 point mutations (see Table 3). These experiments show that ExoVIII-promoted lambda recombination in the A to cI and the cI to R regions is somewhat dependent on $recA$ function. Furthermore, in the $recA^-$ ExoVIII$^+$ strains, the presence of ExoV seems to inhibit recombinant production. Removal of ExoVIII from the $recA^-$ ExoV$^+$ background results in a drastically lowered frequency of recombinants for the cI to R interval and a lesser reduction for recombinants in the A to cI interval. The presence of A to cI recombinants in this case reveals the contribution of int-mediated recombination in the A to cI interval under the conditions of these experiments. In the wild-type $E.\ coli$ strain, in which there is functional $recA$ product but no ExoVIII, recombinant frequencies are once again high. One might expect the recombinant frequencies for the A to cI and cI to

Table 3. The effects of $recA$, ExoV, and ExoVIII on lambda recombinant frequencies in the intervals A to cI and cI to R

Host			Recombinant frequencies (%) for lambda	
$recA$	ExoV	ExoVIII	A to cI	cI to R
+	−	+	5.4	2.5
−	−	+	2.0	0.74
−	+	+	0.27	0.064
−	+	−	0.15	0.003
+	+	−	5.2	0.83

A diagram of the crosses is presented in Fig. 3. One parental phage was $Ats14\ cI26\ R^+$ and the other was $A^+\ cI^+\ Rts2$. Both phages carried red-3 and gam-210.

The crosses were performed as described by Unger $et\ al.$ (1972), except that they were performed at 42°C to reduce int-mediated recombination; recombinant phage were detected at 42°C, and total phage were detected at 30°C. Clear-plaque recombinants were formed by recombination in the A to cI interval, and turbid-plaque recombinants were formed by recombination in the cI to R interval.

R intervals to be the same in $recA^+$ ExoV$^+$ ExoVIII$^-$ and $recA^+$ ExoV$^-$ ExoVIII$^+$ strains, as they are for the A to J interval (Clark, 1974). This expectation is fulfilled for the A to cI interval but not for the cI to R interval, for which the recombinant frequency is threefold higher in the ExoVIII$^+$ strain. We are led to suspect that there may be a ExoVIII- and $recA$-mediated recombination "hot spot" in the cI to R region.

The Degree of Association of DNA Replication with Lambda Recombination

Further evidence that ExoVIII acts like Exoλ *in vivo* comes from an experiment done with Frank and Mary Stahl. The Stahls had discovered that Red recombination at the ends of the λ chromosome, *e.g.* between cI and R, was relatively independent of DNA synthesis compared to recombination in the middle of the λ chromosome, *e.g.* between J and cI (Stahl *et al.*, 1972). This phenomenon had been observed under conditions of a partial block to replication of the parent phages by the presence of immunity repressor.

The parental phages, $susJ^-$ cI^+ R^+ and J^+ cI^- $susR^-$, were labeled with heavy isotopes prior to mixed infection. The J^+R^+ recombinants detected on a nonpermissive host were either cI^+ (*i.e.* turbid plaque formers) if recombination occurred in the central J to cI interval, or cI^- (*i.e.* clear plaque formers) if recombination occurred in the right hand cI to R interval. Replication of these parents was inhibited by the presence of an appropriately marked homoimmune prophage, and chromosomes derived from these parents were matured with the assistance of a heteroimmune helper, also appropriately marked. In one case the helper carried the gene for Exoλ^+ into a host which was ExoVIII$^-$ and ExoV$^-$. In the other case the helper carried the gene for Exoλ^- into a host which was ExoVIII$^+$ and ExoV$^-$. Thus, in the first case recombination is correlated with the presence of Exoλ and in the second with the presence of ExoVIII. (The crosses were conducted under Int$^-$ conditions, eliminating the possibility of site-specific recombination in the J to cI interval.) The cross was performed in light medium so that, after centrifugation of the progeny to equilibrium in cesium formate, the density of the recombinant peaks indicated the amount of replication that those phage had undergone. Under Exoλ^+ ExoVIII$^-$ conditions the distribution of cI^- and cI^+ phages was as shown in Fig. 2a. These results are similar to those obtained by Stahl *et al.* (1972) and support their conclusion that, for the Red system, recombination between cI and R tends to occur in the absence of replication. Exactly the same results were obtained under the Exoλ^- ExoVIII$^+$ conditions (Fig. 2b). Thus it would not be surprising to discover that Exoλ and ExoVIII are functionally identical.

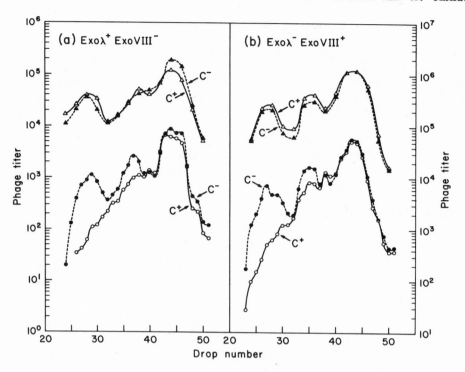

Figure 2. The density distributions of i^λ progeny from the cross of density-labeled parents $susJ6$ cI^+ R^+ and J^+ cI^- $susR5$ performed in hosts in which replication of i^λ phage was largely blocked by lambda repressor produced by a $susJ6$ $susR5$ $red-3$ i^λ prophage. Recombination and maturation functions were provided by an i^{434} helper phage which was $susJ6$ $susR5$ $int6$.   (a) Data obtained when the helper phage was red^+ (Exoλ^+) and the host was $recB^-$ $recC^-$ ExoVIII$^-$ (JC5519).   (b) Data obtained when the helper phage was $red-3$ (Exoλ^-) and the host was $recB^-$ $recC^-$ ExoVIII$^+$ (JC8679).   The titers refer to the estimated number of phage of each type in the 1-ml volume of broth into which single-drop fractions from the ce-sium formate density gradient were collected. ($\bullet$—$\bullet$) c^- sus^+ recombinants; (o—o) c^+ sus^+ recombinants; ($\blacktriangle$ — $\blacktriangle$) total c^- i^λ phage; ($\triangle$ — $\triangle$) total c^+ i^λ phage.

chi "Hotspotting"

Crossover hot-spot instigator mutations of lambda, called chi mutations, have been described by McMilin et $al.$ (1974) and by Lam et $al.$ (1974).   The effect of these mutations appears to be depend-ent on a functional $recB$ (and presumably $recC$) gene (Lam et $al.$, 1974).   Since the phages used to detect the chi effect were red^- gam^-, they were defective in Exoλ and in the ability to inhibit

ExoV. Thus the *chi* effect may be a characteristic of the mode of *in vivo* action of ExoV. To determine whether or not ExoVIII shows this same characteristic action, we performed crosses in several bacterial hosts with *chi*[+] and *chi*[-] strains generously provided by F. W. Stahl. The results are shown in Table 4. We present these results in a different form from that used by Lam *et al.* (1974), to emphasize the finding that in wild-type hosts, with ExoV present, the level of recombination in the *cI* to *R* region carrying *chi*[-] is greater than in the *cI* to *R* region carrying *chi*[+]. The phages we used were of the genotypes shown in Fig. 3. Each phage carried a temperature-sensitive mutation, and temperature-resistant recombinants were selected.

The basic *chi* phenomenon is illustrated by the data in the first line of Table 4. The recombinant frequency for the *cI* to *R* interval is sixfold higher in the *chi*[-] cross than in the *chi*[+] cross, whereas the recombinant frequencies for the *A* to *cI* interval are essentially the same (slightly reduced for the *chi*[-] cross). In the second line, the host strain lacks ExoV, and consequently the observed recombinant frequencies for the *cI* to *R* interval are the same whether *chi* is mutant or not. When the host lacks ExoV but contains ExoVIII (line 3), there is also no difference between the *chi*[+] and *chi*[-] recombinant frequencies in the *cI* to *R* interval, although this frequency is unusually high. Thus ExoVIII does not appear to have the characteristic *in vivo* action of ExoV in

Table 4. A^+R^+ recombinant frequencies of *chi*[+] and *chi*[-] lambda phage measured in various hosts

ExoV[a]	ExoVIII[a]	*chi*[+] X *chi*[+]		*chi*[-] X *chi*[-]	
		A to *cI*	*cI* to *R*	*A* to *cI*	*cI* to *R*
+	−	5.2	0.83	3.5	5.0
−	−	0.54	0.12	0.51	0.11
−	+	5.4	2.5	4.4	2.2
+	+	4.4	1.6	3.7	4.0

[a] These crosses are diagrammed in Fig. 3 and further described in Table 3. For Table 4, *chi*[+] and *chi*[-] derivatives of each parental phage were used.

mediating the *chi* hotspot phenomenon. The last line in Table 4
shows that the ExoV-mediated *chi* effect is still observed in the
presence of ExoVIII. It seems clear that in this situation ExoVIII
does not affect recombinant production in the way that ExoV does.

λ*rev* CARRIES *recE*

In 1971, Zissler *et al.* reported the existence of rare
"mutants" of a plaque-forming *bio*-transducing derivative of lambda
phage. These rare mutants, called λ*rev* (short for λ*reverse*), were
detected by their ability to form plaques on a *recA⁻ recB⁺ recC⁺*
host. The *bio* substitution strain from which λ*rev* derived was
unable to form plaques on the same host because of the deletion of
the *redX* and *gam* genes. Recently, one of Zissler's λ*rev* strains
has been compared with two other λ*rev* strains of different and
independent origin (Gottesman *et al.*, 1974). By genetic experiments
and heteroduplex mapping, each of the λ*rev* strains was found to
carry a deletion of lambda DNA from 45 to 71 on the standard map of
lambda (Davidson and Szybalski, 1971). In place of the deleted
region, all three phages carry "substitutions of non-λ DNA which
are indistinguishable in extent, location, and base sequence"
(Gottesman *et al.*, 1974). The substitutions are expected to have
derived from the bacterial chromosome.

λ*rev* strains are able to grow on *recA⁻ recB⁺ recC⁺* strains
presumably because they are able to circumvent the inhibition of
replication produced by ExoV. Wild-type lambda has two methods of
doing this: one is the inhibition of ExoV by the *gam* protein
(Sakaki *et al.*, 1973), and the other is the synthesis of functional
Exoλ and beta protein. It is therefore possible that λ*rev* has
gained one or the other of these ways of counteracting ExoV. It
cannot be that λ*rev* has regained all the functions of wild-type
lambda, however, since λ*rev* is insensitive to the inhibition of
multiplication experienced by λ^+ in a lysogen for phage P2. The
sensitivity to P2 inhibition is produced in wild-type lambda by the
gamma protein, functional Exoλ and beta protein, and what may be a
del gene product. It was found by Gottesman *et al.* (1974) that
λ*rev*-infected cells contain an ATP-independent nuclease (*i.e.*
Exoλ*rev*), which is not inactivated by antiserum to Exoλ and hence
is not identical to Exoλ. Exoλ*rev* might, however, be functionally
similar to Exoλ, since λ*rev* is capable of multiplying in *recA⁻ recB⁺*
recC⁺ strains. We have found that this nuclease is very similar to
ExoVIII. Exoλ*rev* is eluted from DEAE-cellulose at pH 7.2 by the
same molarity of NaCl and in the same relative position to ExoI as
ExoVIII. Furthermore, we have found that the optimum Mg^{2+} concentration for the action of Exoλ*rev* is 0.02 M, exactly that of ExoVIII.
In addition, Exoλ*rev* sediments in a glycerol gradient as if it had
a molecular weight of 1.3×10^5, exactly that determined for ExoVIII
under identical conditions. Finally, we have been able to identify

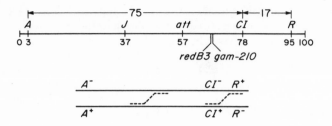

Figure 3. Diagrams of the genetic map of lambda and the recombinant types expected in an A^- cI^- R^+ by A^+ cI^+ R^- cross. Distances
in percent of the lambda chromosome are shown between A and cI and
cI and R. The phage used in the cross carried *red-3* and *gam-210*.
The results of the crosses performed are shown in Table 3.

bands corresponding to Exoλ*rev* and ExoVIII which have the same
electrophoretic retardation factor in a polyacrylamide gel containing 0.1% sodium dodecyl sulfate. Thus it seems very likely to
us that Exoλ*rev* and ExoVIII are one and the same. Further evidence
on this point will be obtained by immunological means.

    It seems likely, therefore, that lambda is able to incorporate
at some frequency a portion of the *E. coli* chromosome carrying *recE*,
the gene determining ExoVIII. Given the functional similarity of
ExoVIII to Exoλ, it is not impossible that the chromosomal region
picked up by λ*rev* derives from a (possibly cryptic) prophage. The
hypothesis that *sbcA* is a regulator gene for *recE* is consistent
with this idea. At present we do not know whether *sbcA* is carried
by λ*rev*. λ*rev* apparently lacks a *gam* function (Gottesman *et al.*,
1974). It may be that the presence of *recE* and the absence of a
gam-type gene results in the combined abilities of λ*rev* to grow in
recA⁻ recB⁺ recC⁺ and P2-lysogenic strains.

                 GENETIC ANALYSIS OF THE RecE PATHWAY

    A genetic analysis of the RecE pathway is now underway. It is
too early at this time to report on the nature of the 10 or so Rec⁻
mutants thus far obtained from a *sbcA⁻ recB⁻ recC⁻* strain. We
have already reported findings (see Clark, 1974), on conjugational
progeny of *sbcA⁻ recB⁻ recC⁻* strains which have inherited *recA⁻*
or *recF⁻*. These data are summarized in Table 2. It is seen that
both *recA⁻* and *recF⁻* derivatives are markedly reduced in ability
to form TL⁺ [Sm^R] (threonine- and leucine-independent, streptomycin-
resistant) progeny following conjugation with JC158, a derivative
of HfrH. The same strains are, however, fully capable of forming
TL⁺ [Sm^R] progeny when the donor carries the *thr⁺ leu⁺* genes on an

F-prime plasmid (data not shown). Thus it appears that the RecE
pathway of bacterial recombination uses both *recA* and *recF*. In
this regard, it appears to overlap the RecF pathway. We have also
constructed a *recL⁻ sbcA⁻ recB⁻ recC⁻* strain. In this case, however, the frequency of TL⁺ [Sm^R] recombinants appears normal following conjugation with the Hfr JC158. It seems reasonable, therefore, to conclude that *recL* acts in the RecF pathway of bacterial
recombination and not in the RecE pathway.

The participation of ExoVIII in the RecE pathway of bacterial
recombination wants proof at present. We hope to be able to detect
recE⁻ mutants in order to obtain this proof. The functional similarity of ExoVIII and Exoλ might lead us to expect the molecular
details of the RecE and the Red pathways of recombination to be
identical. This expectation may be fulfilled, however, only for
lambda recombination, because the results in Table 2 show that
neither *recA* nor *recF* mutations have an effect on the recombination
of *red⁻ gam⁻* lambda strains commensurate with their effects on conjugational recombination. We expect there to be molecular differences between lambda recombination and ExoVIII-mediated bacterial
recombination.

ACKNOWLEDGMENTS

The density-labeled lambda crosses described here were made
possible by the hospitality and generosity of Frank and Mary Stahl.
We are also indebted to the Stahls and Jean Crasemann for providing
us with *chi⁻* and *chi⁺* lambda strains. We thank Haruko Nagaishi,
Stuart Linn and his group, and Rosemary Paterson for help with the
enzyme purifications. This work was supported by AI-05371-12 from
the N.I.H.

During much of this investigation, J.R.G. was a Predoctoral
Trainee on Training Grant AI-120-WOFSY from the N.I.H.

REFERENCES

Barbour, S. D., H. Nagaishi, A. Templin and A. J. Clark. 1970.
Biochemical and genetic studies of recombination proficiency in
Escherichia coli. II. Rec⁺ revertants caused by indirect suppres-
sion of Rec⁻ mutations. Proc. Nat. Acad. Sci. U.S.A. <u>67</u>: 128.

Clark, A. J. 1971. Toward a metabolic interpretation of genetic
recombination of *E. coli* and its phages. Ann. Rev. Microbiol. <u>25</u>:
438.

Clark, A. J. 1973. Recombination deficient mutants of *E. coli* and
other bacteria. Ann. Rev. Genet. <u>7</u>: 67.

Clark, A. J. 1974. Progress toward a metabolic interpretation of genetic recombination of *Escherichia coli* and bacteriophage lambda. Genetics (Suppl.), in press.

Carter, D. M. and C. M. Radding. 1971. The role of exonuclease and β protein of phage λ in genetic recombination. J. Biol. Chem. 246: 2502.

Davidson, N. and W. Szybalski. 1971. Physical and chemical characteristics of lambda DNA. In (A. D. Hershey, ed.) The Bacteriophage Lambda. p. 45. Cold Spring Harbor Laboratory, Cold Spring Harbor, New York.

Friedman, E. A. and H. O. Smith. 1973. Production of possible recombination intermediates by an ATP-dependent DNAase. Nature New Biol. 241: 54.

Goldmark, P. J. and S. Linn. 1972. Purification and properties of the *recBC* DNase of *Escherichia coli* K-12. J. Biol. Chem. 247: 1849.

Gottesman, M. M., M. E. Gottesman, S. Gottesman and M. Gellert. 1974. Characterization of λ*reverse* as an *E. coli* phage carrying a unique set of host-derived recombination functions. J. Mol. Biol., in press.

Karu, A. E., V. MacKay, P. J. Goldmark and S. Linn. 1973. The *recBC* deoxyribonuclease of *Escherichia coli* K-12. Substrate specificity and reaction intermediates. ·J. Biol. Chem. 248: 4874.

Kushner, S., H. Nagaishi and A. J. Clark. 1974. Isolation of exonuclease VIII: The enzyme associated with the *sbcA* indirect suppressor. Proc. Nat. Acad. Sci. U.S.A., in press.

Lam, S. T., M. M. Stahl, K. D. McMilin and F. W. Stahl. 1974. Rec mediated recombinational hot spot activity in bacteriophage lambda. II. A mutation which causes hot spot activity. Genetics, in press.

Little, J. W. 1967. An exonuclease induced by bacteriophage λ. II. Nature of the enzymatic reaction. J. Biol. Chem. 242: 679.

MacKay, V. and S. Linn. 1974. The mechanism of degradation of duplex DNA by the *recBC* enzyme of *Escherichia coli* K-12. J. Mol. Biol., in press.

McMilin, K. D., M. M. Stahl and F. W. Stahl. 1974. Rec mediated recombinational hot spot activity in bacteriophage lambda. I. Hot spot activity associated with Spi⁻ deletions and *bio* substitutions. Genetics, in press.

Sakaki, Y., A. E. Karu, S. Linn and H. Echols. 1973. Purification and properties of the γ-protein specified by bacteriophage λ: an inhibitor of the host RecBC recombination enzyme. Proc. Nat. Acad. Sci. U.S.A. 70: 2215.

Stahl, F. W., K. D. McMilin, M. M. Stahl, R. E. Malone, Y. Nozu and V. E. A. Russo. 1972. A role for recombination in the production of "free-loader" lambda bacteriophage particles. J. Mol. Biol. 68: 57.

Unger, R. C., H. Echols and A. J. Clark. 1972. Interaction of the recombination pathways of bacteriophage λ and host *Escherichia coli:* Effects on λ recombination. J. Mol. Biol. 70: 531.

Zissler, J., E. Signer and F. Schaeffer. 1971. The role of recombination in growth of bacteriophage lambda. I. The gamma gene. In (A. D. Hershey, ed.) The Bacteriophage Lambda. p. 455. Cold Spring Harbor Laboratory, Cold Spring Harbor, New York.

ISOLATION OF THE ENZYME ASSOCIATED WITH THE *sbcA* INDIRECT

SUPPRESSOR

Sidney R. Kushner[*†], Haruko Nagaishi[†] and A. J. Clark[†]

*Department of Biochemistry, Stanford University School

of Medicine, Stanford, California 94305 and †Department

of Molecular Biology, University of California, Berkeley,

California 94720

recB and/or recC deficiency in *Escherichia coli* K-12 is indirectly suppressed in the presence of *sbcA⁻* mutations. Such strains remain genotypically *recB* and/or *recC* deficient but become recombination proficient and resistant to ultraviolet light. Barbour *et al.* (1970) showed that strains carrying *sbcA⁻* mutations contained increased levels of an ATP-independent DNase. Since the product of the *recB-recC* genes (exonuclease V) is a multifunctional DNase that requires ATP for the hydrolysis of double-stranded DNA (Goldmark and Linn, 1972), characterization of the ATP-independent nuclease found in *sbcA⁻* strains might provide an important clue to the *in vivo* function of the *recB-recC* gene products.

In this communication we show by genetic and enzymatic tests that the nuclease present in *sbcA⁻* strains is not exonuclease III, exonuclease V, DNA polymerase I, or lambda exonuclease. Electrophoretic analysis of purified fractions suggests that this enzyme, which we call exonuclease VIII, is probably not present in unsuppressed strains. In its partially purified form, exonuclease VIII preferentially digests double-stranded DNA over heat-denatured single-stranded DNA.

---

†Present address: Department of Biochemistry, University of Georgia, Athens, Georgia 30602.

PURIFICATION OF THE ENZYME ASSOCIATED WITH THE *sbcA⁻* INDIRECT SUPPRESSOR

The ATP-independent nuclease found in *sbcA⁻* strains was assayed by measuring the release of radioactively labeled nucleotides from double-stranded DNA. The strain JC7693 *(recB21, sbcB15, and sbcA9)* was used as an enzyme source. A purification procedure, which involved a Brij-58 lysis, streptomycin sulfate precipitation, ammonium sulfate precipitation, and DEAE- and DNA-cellulose chromatography, resulted in approximately a 700-fold purification. A similar purification was carried out on an isogenic strain (JC7722) that was *sbcA⁺*. A summary of these two purifications is given in Table 1. A more detailed description of the purification is published elsewhere (Kushner *et al.*, 1974).

The enzyme obtained from JC7693 has an absolute requirement for Mg^{++}, with optimal activity at 20 mM, and exhibits a pH optimum of 8.0 in Tris-HCl buffer. Activity on double-stranded DNA is unaffected by addition of ATP between 20 and 200 μM.

IDENTIFICATION OF EXONUCLEASE VIII

The appearance of high levels of an ATP-independent exonuclease in cells carrying *sbcA⁻* mutations could be explained by some alteration in preexisting cellular enzymes. Modifcation of the *recB* and/or *recC* subunit could produce an enzyme of altered specificity. The fact that strains carrying *sbcA⁻* alleles lack all the activities associated with exonuclease V, that they carry genotypically unaltered *recB21* and/or *recC22* mutations, and that the *sbcA⁻* alleles do not map in the *thyA-argA* region tend to rule out this possibility.

Other enzymes that might be candidates for alteration include exonuclease III (Richardson and Kornberg, 1964) and the 5'→3' exonuclease activity associated with DNA polymerase I (Richardson *et al.*, 1964). Strains carrying *sbcA⁺* or *sbcA9* alleles contained identical levels of DNA polymerase I and exonuclease III as assayed in crude lysates. When antiserum prepared against purified DNA polymerase I was added to the crude lysates, both strains exhibited a 20% decrease in activity on double-stranded DNA. Subsequent antiserum tests on Fraction VI produced no effect.

In order to determine more precisely whether exonuclease III might be involved, a partial purification of the ATP-independent nuclease was undertaken, with the early fractions being assayed for the specific 3'-phosphatase associated with exonuclease III. As shown in Table 2, less than 4% of the exonuclease III activity was precipitated in the ammonium sulfate step. On the basis of these results, the nuclease appearing in *sbcA⁻* strains was

Table 1. Purification of exonuclease VIII from JC7722 (*sbcA*$^+$) and JC7693 (*sbcA9*)

Fraction	JC7693			JC7722		
	Units/ml	Protein (mg/ml)	Specific activity	Units/ml	Protein (mg/ml)	Specific activity
Crude lysate (I)	172	7.5	23	86	10.0	8.6
Crude supernatant (II)	165	5.0	33	124	6.0	20.7
Streptomycin supernatant (III)	148	2.7	55	101	2.3	44
Ammonium sulfate (IV)	1842	10.7	172	89	7.1	12.5
Concentrated DEAE- cellulose (V)	12345	10.7	1154	41	3.0	13.7
DNA-cellulose (VI)	874	0.05	17480	—	—	—

Exonuclease VIII was purified from both strains as described by Kushner *et al.* (1974). Exonuclease VIII was assayed by measuring nucleotide release from ^{32}P-labeled double-stranded DNA. The incubation mixture (0.3 ml) contained 10 mM Tris, pH 8.0, 20 mM MgCl$_2$, 10 mM 2-mercaptoethanol, 24 μM labeled *E. coli* B DNA, and enzyme. After incubation for 30 min at 37°C, 0.2 ml of salmon sperm DNA (2.5 mg/ml) and 0.3 ml of 7% cold perchloric acid were added. The acid-soluble supernatant fraction was counted in a toluene Triton X-100 scintillator. One unit of exonuclease VIII is defined as that amount of protein which catalyzes the release of 1.0 nmole of nucleotide in 30 min at 37°C.

Table 2.   Fate of exonuclease III in exonuclease VIII purification
procedure

Fraction	Exonuclease III		Exonuclease activity	
	Specific activity	Percent recovery	Specific activity	Percent recovery
Streptomycin supernatant (III) [a]	8.8	100	33.2	100
Ammonium sulfate precipitate	1.2	3.6	120.2	74
Ammonium sulfate supernatant	17.5	117	18.5	24

Exonuclease VIII was assayed as described in Table 1.   Exonuclease III was assayed as 3'-DNA phosphatase (Richardson and
Kornberg, 1964).

[a] Fraction numbers correspond to those in Table 1.

considered a new enzyme and called exonuclease VIII.

Since the *sbcA*⁻ indirect suppressor is found in only certain
genetic backgrounds (Templin *et al.*, 1972), it has been suggested
that perhaps exonuclease VIII is carried on a cryptic prophage
that is derepressed during mutagenesis.   Bacteriophage lambda is
known to carry genetic information for an exonuclease involved in
phage recombination.   In order to test whether exonuclease VIII
might in fact be this enzyme or some closely related species, Fraction VI was treated with antiserum prepared against crystalline
lambda exonuclease.   Less than a 10% loss in activity was observed.
While this finding suggests that exonuclease VIII is not lambda
exonuclease, it does not eliminate the possibility that the enzyme
is of cryptic prophage origin.

Although the results indicated that exonuclease VIII is not a
modified preexisting cellular enzyme, it was of interest to determine whether low levels of this activity were present in unsuppressed strains.   In order to determine this, the purification
procedure used for JC7693 (*sbcA9*) was carried out on JC7722 (*sbcA+*).
In Fig. 1 are shown the DEAE-cellulose elution profiles obtained

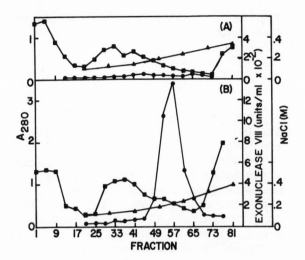

Figure 1.   DEAE-cellulose elution profiles from $sbcA^+$ (A) and
$sbcA9$ (B) strains.   A linear gradient from 0.15 M to 0.5 M NaCl
in a buffer containing 50 mM Tris-HCl, pH 7.2, and 1 mM dithiothreitol was applied to each column.   Exonuclease VIII was assayed
as described in Table 1. ■——■, optical density at 280 nm;
●—●, activity of exonuclease VIII; ▲——▲, NaCl concentration in
eluting buffer.

---

from these two purifications.   Fractions that eluted at the same
NaCl concentrations as exonuclease VIII were pooled and concentrated with $(NH_4)_2SO_4$.   The low level of activity present in concentrated material from JC7722 was assayed against single- and double-
stranded DNA.   In contrast to exonuclease VIII, which preferred
double-stranded DNA by a 9-to-1 ratio at this stage, the material
obtained from JC7722 showed a marked preference for single-stranded
DNA.

In addition, the concentrated DEAE-cellulose fractions were
run on 5% polyacrylamide gels containing 0.1% sodium dodecyl
sulfate.   The banding patterns obtained from JC7722 ($sbcA^+$) and
JC7693 ($sbcA9$) were identical except for the absence of a band
corresponding to a molecular weight of 122,000 in the gel obtained
with the $sbcA^+$ strain.   The DNA-cellulose fraction from JC7693
($sbcA9$) showed a marked enrichment for this band.

Since exonuclease VIII apparently replaces the multifunctional
$recBC$ nuclease, the purified enzyme was tested for its activity on
a variety of DNA substrates.   The enzyme shows a 20- to 50-fold
preference for native over heat-denatured DNA.   Unlike the $recBC$
nuclease, purified exonuclease VIII showed negligible activity on

single-stranded closed circular DNA in the presence or absence of ATP. It also contained only trace levels of 3'-DNA phosphatase activity.

DISCUSSION

Loss of the *recB-recC* gene products results in recombination deficiency, UV sensitivity, and decreased cell viability. The *recBC* nuclease degrades both single- and double-stranded DNA in the presence of ATP. It also digests single-stranded closed circular DNA in an ATP-stimulated reaction (Goldmark and Linn, 1972). The presence of exonuclease VIII reverses the observed pleiotropic effects associated with *recB* and/or *recC* deficiency. From the evidence presented in this communication, exonuclease VIII appears not only to be a new enzyme but also to have only an exonuclease function. While the search for intermediates involved in repair and recombination produced by the *recBC* enzyme has been hampered by the presence of multiple catalytic activities, this problem does not seem to hold true for exonuclease VIII. A detailed analysis of the substrate specificity of exonuclease VIII should lead to the prediction of the types of DNA intermediates that may be involved in repair and recombination. It should be pointed out, however, that while the presence of exonuclease VIII is sufficient to allow recombination to occur in *recB*- and/or *recC*-deficient strains, the process may be entirely different from that occurring in wild-type cells.

ACKNOWLEDGMENTS

One of us (S. R. K.) wishes to thank Dr. I. R. Lehman for providing facilities for carrying out certain experiments. This work was supported in part by Public Health Service Research grant no. AI-05371 from the National Institute of Allergy and Infectious Diseases and a Postdoctoral Fellowship from the National Institute of General Medical Sciences (GM-47038-03).

REFERENCES

Barbour, S. D., H. Nagaishi, A. Templin and A. J. Clark. 1970. Biochemical and genetic studies of recombination proficiency in *Escherichia coli* II. *Rec+* revertants caused by indirect suppression of *rec-* mutations. Proc. Nat. Acad. Sci. U.S.A. <u>67</u>: 128.

Goldmark, P. J. and S. Linn. 1972. Purification and properties of the *recBC* DNase of *Escherichia coli*. J. Biol. Chem. <u>247</u>: 1849.

Kushner, S. R., H. Nagaishi and A. J. Clark. 1974. Isolation of

exonuclease VIII: The enzyme associated with the *sbcA* indirect
suppressor. Proc. Nat. Acad. Sci. U.S.A. in press.

Richardson, C. C. and A. Kornberg. 1964. A deoxyribonucleic acid
phosphatase-exonuclease from *Escherichia coli*. I. Purification
of the enzyme and characterization of the phosphatase activity.
J. Biol. Chem. 239: 242.

Richardson, C. C., C. L. Schildkraut, H. V. Aposhian and A. Kornberg. 1964. Enzymatic synthesis of deoxyribonucleic acid. XIV.
Further purification and properties of deoxyribonucleic acid polymerase of *Escherichia coli*. J. Biol. Chem. 239: 222.

Templin, A., S. R. Kushner and A. J. Clark. 1972. Genetic analysis of mutations indirectly suppressing *recB* and *recC* mutations.
Genetics 72: 205.

TRANSFORMATION-MEDIATED RECOMBINATION IN *ESCHERICHIA COLI*

M. Oishi, S. D. Cosloy and S. K. Basu

The Public Health Research Institute of the City of

New York, Inc., New York, New York 10016

Recently generalized and specialized transformation systems in an *Escherichia coli* K12 strain have been established (Oishi and Cosloy, 1972, 1974; Cosloy and Oishi, 1973a,b; Wackernagel, 1973). Among various factors that affect the frequency of transformation, the status of the recombination pathways in the recipient cells, especially that of *recBrecC* DNase (ATP-dependent DNase), seemed to have the most striking effect on the transformation. We report here some of the basic characteristics of the transformation system in *E. coli*, with special emphasis on the recombination process involved, and discuss the effect of *recBrecC* DNase on the mode of genetic recombination. (The effect of *recBrecC* Dnase on transformation and transduction is also described by Wackernagel and Radding in this volume.)

GENERAL CHARACTERISTICS OF THE TRANSFORMATION SYSTEM IN *E. COLI*

When a multi-auxotrophic *E. coli* K12 strain (JC7623), which lacks the *recBrecC* Dnase (*recB⁻recC⁻*) and exonuclease I (*sbcB⁻*) (Kushner *et al.*, 1971) was treated with $CaCl_2$ and exposed to DNA isolated from a prototrophic *E. coli* strain, a significant number ($\sim 10^{-6}$) of transformants of various chromosomal markers appeared on the selective plates (Table 1). The transforming activity in the DNA preparation was lost upon heating (100°C, 5 min), DNase treatment or sonication but was not affected by RNase or Pronase treatment. The active material had the buoyant density of *E. coli* DNA (1.710 g/ml). These results indicate that the active component in the DNA preparation is the double-stranded DNA. Furthermore, the

145

Table 1.   Transformation of various chromosomal genetic markers.
Transformation was performed as described previously (Cosloy and
Oishi, 1973a), using unsheared donor DNA (10 µg/0.5 ml) and strain
JC7623 as recipient.   The number of transformants was the sum of
the transformants produced on four plates with 1.7 X 10^8 total recipient cells.   For DNase treatment, the DNA (100 µg/ml in 15 mM
NaCl, 1.5 mM Na_3-citrate, and 5 mM $CaCl_2$) was incubated with pancreatic DNase (2 µg/ml, Worthington Biochemical Co.) for 20 min at
37°C.

Donor DNA (genotype)	Number of Transformants				
	Leu^+	His^+	Arg^+	Pro^+	Thr^+
HfrC6 (*$leu^+his^+arg^+pro^+thr^+$*)	347	200	225	135	268
HfrC6 (*$leu^+his^+arg^+pro^+thr^+$*) with DNase pre-treatment)	0	1	1	0	24
MO617 (F⁻, *$leu^+his^-arg^-pro^-thr^-$*)	146	0	4	–	–
No DNA	0	2	1	0	20

genetic linkage of approximately 40% found for *leu* and *ara* markers
with high-molecular-weight donor DNA (30 to 300 X 10^6) was reduced
to 2 to 6% with use of sheared low-molecular-weight donor DNA (8 X
10^6).   Thus, physical breakage of the DNA molecules caused loss of
the genetic linkage originally observed, supporting the interpretation that the biologically active fraction in the DNA preparation
must be DNA itself.

Transformation was also obtained with DNA isolated from specialized transducing phages carrying a particular chromosomal segment (Oishi and Cosloy, 1974).   Such a specialized transformation
system should be advantageous for studies of molecular mechanisms
of recombination in transformation, because all the donor DNA molecules are homogeneous in genetic composition and molecular size.
Table 2 demonstrates specialized transformation for a *trpB* marker
with DNA (sheared and unsheared) isolated from φ80pt(*$trpA^+B^+C^+$*),
λpt(*$trpA^+B^+C^+D^+E^+$*), and control donors.   These phages carry all or
part of the tryptophan operon from the *E. coli* chromosome, in place
of a phage chromosome segment that includes the *int-red* region.
This *int⁻red⁻* condition of the phages eliminated the phage recombination system, which might have complicated studies of the host
recombination system.   Transformation with such phage DNA is, of
course, restricted to the particular genetic marker (*$trpB^+$*), but
the transformation frequency is much higher (10^{-5} to 10^{-4}) than that
observed with total bacterial chromosome DNA.   This higher efficien-

Table 2. Specialized transformation of the *trpB* mutation with DNA from various sources. Transformation was performed as described previously (Oishi and Cosloy, 1974), using MO671 (Oishi and Cosloy, 1974) as the recipient cells and DNA at a concentration of 5 µg per tube (0.5 ml). The average molecular weight of sheared DNA from various phages was in the range of 8 to 9 X 10^6. The number of transformants is the sum of Trp$^+$ colonies produced with a total of 1.9 X 10^7 viable recipient cells.

Source of DNA (genotype)	No. of Transformants
None	0
ϕ80pt($trpA^+B^+C^+$)	1012
ϕ80pt($trpA^+B^+C^+$), sheared	1333
ϕ80pt($trpA^+B^-C^+$)	1
ϕ80pt($trpA^+B^-C^+$), sheared	1
ϕ80pt($trpD^+E^+$)	0
ϕ80pt($trpD^+E^+$), sheared	0
ϕ80	0
ϕ80, sheared	0
λpt($trpA^+B^+C^+D^+E^+$)	648
λpt($trpA^+B^+C^+D^+E^+$), sheared	770
λ(cI26)	0
λ(cI26), sheared	3

cy approaches what one might expect, since concentration of the *trpB* gene in the ϕ80pt DNA (also λpt DNA) preparation is approximately 80-fold higher than that in the bacterial chromosome DNA preparation.

This specialized transformation system was extended to the transformation of an episomal marker (Oishi and Cosloy, 1974). A transformable strain (MO646) was constructed harboring an F' carrying the *trp* operon (containing a *trpB* mutation) plus adjacent chromosomal regions, including the *tonB* locus. The *trp* operon and *tonB* locus were deleted from the bacterial chromosome. When this strain was used as recipient for ϕ80pt($A^+B^+C^+$) and λpt($A^+B^+C^+D^+E^+$) donor DNA, Trp$^+$ transformants emerged (Table 3). Since the F'-bearing recipient cells (MO646) contained a large deletion on the chromosome ranging from the *tonB* locus through the entire *trp* operon, the Trp$^+$

Table 3.   Specialized transformation of *trpB* mutation on F' episome.
Transformation was performed as described previously (Oishi and Cosloy, 1974).   Because of the temperature sensitivity of the F' replication, the cells (MO640 and MO646) were grown at 35°C and the selective plates were incubated at 30°C following the transformation.
The molecular weights of sheared DNA used here were 8.5 X 10^6 and
8.9 X 10^6 for φ80pt and λpt DNA, respectively.   DNA was added at a
concentration of 10 μg per tube (0.5 ml).   Trp⁺ transformants were
scored and the transformation frequency was calculated according to
the total number of 9.4 X 10^6 and 2.7 X 10^7 recipient cells produced
by MO640 and MO646, respectively.

Strain	Relevant genotype	DNA source	Transformation frequency (Trp+/10^7 cells)
MO646	F' *tonB⁺trpB⁻*/Δ*tonBtrpABCDE*	None	<0.1
		φ80pt(*trpA⁺B⁺C⁺*)	51.1
		φ80pt(*trpA⁺B⁺C⁺*), (sheared)	29.3
		λpt(*trpA⁺B⁺C⁺D⁺E⁺*)	73.3
		λpt(*trpA⁺B⁺C⁺D⁺E⁺*), (sheared)	78.1
MO640	Δ*tonBtrpABCDE*	None	<0.1
		φ80pt(*trpA⁺B⁺C⁺*)	<0.1
		φ80pt(*trpA⁺B⁺C⁺*), (sheared)	<0.1
		λpt(*trpA⁺B⁺C⁺D⁺E⁺*)	<0.1
		λpt(*trpA⁺B⁺C⁺D⁺E⁺*), (sheared)	<0.1

transformants seemed likely to be the products of recombination
between the homologous *trp* regions on the F' DNA and the φ80pt or
λpt donor DNA.   This was confirmed by our findings that (1) no Trp⁺
transformants were obtained when recipients (MO640) harboring the
same large chromosomal deletion but lacking the episome were used
(Table 3), and (2) the Trp⁺ character along with the associated
chromium resistance phenotype determined by *tonB⁺* can be transferred
from Trp⁺ transformants to a recombination-deficient F⁻ strain.

Compared to transformation of other bacteria, three features appear to be important in the *E. coli* generalized and specialized transformation systems. One is the absolute requirement for $CaCl_2$ treatment of recipient cells to facilitate the uptake of donor DNA (Mandel and Higa, 1970). The second is the effect of the molecular weight of donor DNA on the transformation frequency. The maximum transformation of a single genetic marker was obtained with donor DNA whose molecular weight ranged from 1 to 3 X 10^7. Higher- or lower-molecular-weight donor DNA reduced the transformation frequency drastically. The third feature is the importance of the intracellular status of recombination-related DNases such as *recBrecC* DNase. This is discussed in the next section.

THE NATURE OF RECOMBINATION PROCESS IN TRANSFORMATION

The involvement of a recombination process in *E. coli* transformation was originally inferred from the stability of the acquired genetic characters in the transformants. We further investigated this in the following experiments. In generalized transformation, a recipient strain ($leu^-ara^+his^+$) is transformed with DNA derived from a strain possessing leu^+, ara^-, and his^- markers. The *leu* marker is cotransformable with *ara* but not with *his*. Leu$^+$ transformants were selected and tested to determine whether they had incorporated the donor's ara^- marker. It was found that 34% of Leu$^+$ transformants were Ara$^-$ but none of Leu$^+$ was His$^-$. The transformation to a negative phenotype (Ara$^-$) makes it reasonable to conclude that the donor marker integrates into the homologous site on the recipient chromosome by recombination, replacing the preexisting marker. In specialized transformation of a $trpB^-$ mutation with sheared ϕ80pt($trpA^+B^+C^+$) DNA, the following results were obtained: (1) the original $trpB^-$ marker was not present in Trp$^+$ transformants; (2) all Trp$^+$ transformants were stable in their acquired Trp$^+$ character; (3) all Trp$^+$ transformants were sensitive to ϕ80 and did not produce any phage particles upon UV irradiation. These results indicate that the mechanism of specialized transformation involves recombination, which replaced the preexisting trp^- marker by the trp^+ allele provided by the ϕ80pt donor DNA. Such a recombination by substitution is similar to what occurs in generalized transformation and is in sharp contrast to specialized transduction with ϕ80pt (Oka *et al.*, 1971) and to transformation with $\lambda dgal$ DNA (Kaiser and Hogness, 1961), in which the entire ϕ80pt and $\lambda dgal$ phage genomes are integrated into the host chromosome through recombination by addition.

In order to investigate further the nature of the recombination process involved in these transformations, we compared the nature of transformation in strains with various combinations of recombination pathways. As demonstrated by Clark and his associates (Clark, 1973),

Table 4. Effect of various *rec* alleles on transformability. Transformation was performed as described previously (Cosloy and Oishi,
1973b) using HfrC6 DNA (M.W. 8 - 16 X 10^6) as donor DNA at a concentration of 10 μg per 0.5 ml. Leu$^+$ (A) and Gal$^+$ (B) transformants
from four plates were scored and the transformation frequency was
calculated according to the number of recipient cells used (1 - 3
X 10^8 per plate).

Strain	Phenotype (*rec* pathway)	Genotype	Transformation frequency (transformants/ 10^8 cells)
(A)			
JC7623	Rec$^+$(*recF*)	*recB⁻recC⁻sbcB⁻recA⁺*	105
MO626	Rec$^+$(*recBC*)	*recB⁺recC⁺sbcB⁺recA⁺*	2
MO627	Rec$^+$(*recF recBC*)	*recB⁺recC⁺sbcB⁻recA⁺*	20
JC5519	Rec$^-$	*recB⁻recC⁻sncB⁺recA⁺*	<1
JC7903	Rec$^-$	*recB⁻recC⁻sbcB⁻recA⁻*	<1
(B)			
JC5176	Rec$^+$(*recE*)	*recB⁻recC⁻sbcA⁻recA⁺*	97
HF4733	Rec$^+$(*recBC*)	*recB⁺recC⁺sbcA⁻recA⁺*	<1
SDB1311	Rec$^+$(*recE recBC*)	*recB⁺recC⁺sbcA⁻recA⁺*	17
JC4584	Rec$^-$	*recB⁻recC⁻sbcA⁺recA⁺*	<1

E. coli K12 can possess either one or both of two recombination pathways, *recBC* and *recF*. As shown in Table 4(A), the highest frequency
of transformation was obtained in the strain originally studied
(JC7623 *recB⁻recC⁻sbcB⁻*), in which the *recF* pathway functions as the
sole recombination pathway without participation of the *recBrecC*
gene product (*recBrecC* DNase). In contrast, little if any transformability was found in a wild-type strain (MO626 *recB⁺recC⁺sbcB⁺*)
with the *recBC* pathway as the principle means of recombination. In
the strain (MO627 *recB⁺recC⁺sbcB⁻*) in which both *rec* pathways exist,
the frequency was approximately 20% of that observed in JC7623. The
two Rec$^-$ strains (JC5519 *recB⁻recC⁻sbcB⁺*, JC7903 *recB⁻recC⁻sbcB⁻*
recA⁻) showed absolutely no transformability. Essentially the same
results were obtained with specialized transformation. These results demonstrated the following points: First, the recombination
process involved in the transformation in *E. coli* K12 is cata-

lyzed not by the *recBC* pathway but by the *recF* pathway. The involvement of *recF* pathway in transformation was further confirmed by Kato and Clark (personal communication), who demonstrated that mutations in the *recF* pathway caused loss or drastic reduction of transformability. Second, the presence of *recBrecC* DNase in the cells seemed to have an adverse effect on transformation efficiency (this is discussed below).

Barbour *et al.* (1970) reported another indirect suppressor mutation (*sbcA⁻*) of the *recB⁻recC⁻* mutation. This suppressor mutation has been characterized as another recombination pathway, termed the *recE* pathway, which functions without the *recBrecC* DNase (Clark, 1973). The *sbcA⁻* mutation is believed to cause the appearance of a new type of DNase. As seen in Table 4(B), the strain (JC5176 *recB⁻recC⁻sbcA⁻*) with only the *recE* pathway functioning was transformable, indicating that the *recE* recombination pathway also serves for transformation. Again, the presence of *recBrecC* enzyme in such a strain (SDB1311 *recB⁺recC⁺sbcA⁻*) reduced the transformation efficiency considerably.

These results indicate that in *E. coli* at least two recombination pathways (*recF* and *recE*) can function as the recombination pathways for transformation but not the *recBC* pathway, which is the major *rec* pathway in wild-type cells.

THE EFFECT OF *recBrecC* DNase ON THE MODE OF GENETIC RECOMBINATION

One interesting question arising from these experiments is the role of *recBrecC* Dnase on genetic recombination. The adverse effect on transformation of the presence of DNase in the cells suggests that either the donor DNA, which consists of linear DNA molecules, or intermediates of transformation process are highly susceptible to degradation by the DNase. In this respect, it is interesting to note that *in vitro* the DNase attacks linear DNA molecules extensively but cannot act on circular DNA molecules even with "nicks" (or gaps). These results raise the possibility that in wild-type cells this DNase might affect the mode of recombination by selectively destroying DNA molecules that have a particular type of molecular structure. We therefore examined the effect of the *recBrecC* DNase on the two major modes of recombination (substitution and addition). In contrast to substitution, which involves some type of removal and replacement procedure, recombination by addition is generally believed to involve addition of circular donor DNA to the recipient by a reciprocal crossover process, as proposed by Campbell (1962) for prophage integration and excision.

Transduction with the *trpB* marker was performed by specialized transducing phages such as φ80pt(*trpA⁺B⁺C⁺*) and λpt(*trpA⁺B⁺C⁺D⁺E⁺*).

In this transduction system, the same donor DNA could participate in either (or both) of the two types of host recombination mechanisms. Generally two classes of Trp$^+$ recombinants are observed in a single transduction experiment. One class consists of Trp$^+$ recombinants lysogenized by the donor phage (addition) and the other consists of Trp$^+$ recombinants that are the products of substitution-type recombination as found in the specialized transformation. Oka *et al.*, (1971) studied the former type of recombinant and demonstrated that the entire ϕ80pt genome integrates exclusively at the *trp* operon of *E. coli* by the reciprocal recombination mechanism. Recombinants of the latter type are also commonly observed in transduction by these phages. Therefore, testing Trp$^+$ recombinants for the absence or presence of phage-specific characteristics, such as phage immunity and inducibility, provided a simple and convenient method for distinguishing the two classes.

We have compared these characteristics in the Trp$^+$ recombinants obtained from three isogenic Rec$^+$ (*trpB*$^-$) recipient strains. One (MO650 *trpB*$^-$*recB*$^+$*recC*$^+$*sbcB*$^+$) is a wild-type strain that possesses a recombination pathway dependent upon *recBrecC* DNase (*recBC* pathway). The second recipient (MO639 *trpB*$^-$*recB*$^-$*recC*$^-$*sbcB*$^-$) possesses only the *recF* recombination pathway, which functions without *recBrecC* DNase. The third was a strain (MO649 *trpB*$^-$*recB*$^+$*recC*$^+$*sbcB*$^-$) that possesses two recombination pathways (*recBC* and *recF*). Table 5 presents the results of transduction experiments involving MO650, MO639, and MO649 with ϕ80pt (*trpA*$^+$*B*$^+$*C*$^+$) and λpt60-3(*trpA*$^+$*B*$^+$*C*$^+$*D*$^+$*E*$^+$). In the wild type (MO650), where only the *recBC* pathway is functioning, from 10 to 20% (13.5% for ϕ80pt, 17.0% for λpt) of Trp$^+$ recombinants were ϕ80pt or λpt lysogens, suggesting that they are the products of addition-type recombination. The rest (86.5% for ϕ80pt, 83.0% for λpt) were sensitive to donor phages, and presumably the products of substitution-type recombination. In contrast, in MO639, where the *recF* pathway functions without *recBrecC* DNase, the proportion of Trp$^+$ recombinants that are ϕ80pt or λpt lysogens is drastically reduced to less than 1% of the total Trp$^+$ recombinants, and more than 99% of the Trp$^+$ recombinants are the products of substitution-type recombination. In the third strain (MO649), in which *recBC* DNase was present as well as the *recF* pathway, the proportion of Trp$^+$ recombinants that harbored ϕ80pt or λpt was at the same level as that of the wild-type strain.

These results demonstrate that the presence of the *recBrecC* DNase in the cells affects the fate of donor DNA and the ratio of the two types of recombinants. Two possibilities may be considered: (1) Recombination events via the *recF* pathway produce only substitution-type recombination, whereas the *recBrecC* pathway catalyzes both types (substitution and addition). (2) The increase in the proportion of addition-type recombinants observed with the recipients having *recBrecC* DNase (*recB*$^+$*recC*$^+$*sbcB*$^+$;*recB*$^+$*recC*$^+$*sbcB*$^-$) may be due

Table 5. Transduction of *trpB* marker by φ80pt and λpt. Transductions were performed according to Oka *et al.* (1971) with slight modifications. All the Trp[+] transductants subject to the characterization were purified by two series of single-colony isolations on Difco Bacto Penassay agar plates. More than 99% of the original Trp[+] transductants remained Trp[+] after the purification steps. The presence of the phage-specific characteristics in the Trp[+] recombinants was demonstrated by both the ability to produce the phages upon ultraviolet irradiation and immunity to clear-plaque mutants of the homologous phages (φ80c and λcI26). All the Trp[+] recombinants immune to the homologous phages produced phages, whereas all sensitive recombinants produced no phage.

Donor	Recipient (genotype)	Frequency of Trp[+] transductants	Trp[+] transductants harboring the donor phage	
			Fraction	Frequency (%)
φ80pt	MO639 (*recB⁻recC⁻sbcB⁻*)	1.5×10^{-3}	1/149	0.7
	MO649 (*recB⁺recC⁺sbcB⁻*)	3.7×10^{-4}	15/150	10.0
	MO650 (*recB⁺recC⁺sbcB⁺*)	3.1×10^{-4}	21/155	13.5
λpt60–3	MO639 (*recB⁻recC⁻sbcB⁻*)	5.4×10^{-3}	1/155	0.6
	MO649 (*recB⁺recC⁺sbcB⁻*)	1.8×10^{-3}	17/155	11.0
	MO650 (*recB⁺recC⁺sbcB⁺*)	5.6×10^{-4}	27/155	17.0

to decreased availability of a particular type of donor DNA molecule necessary for substitutional recombination, *i.e.* the selective degradation of linear molecules by *recBrecC* DNase. Presumably such linear DNA molecules would have been the substrate or intermediates for substitution-type recombination. The surviving circular DNA molecules would then take part in the addition-type recombination process. We believe the second possibility is the case for the following reasons: (1) A reduction of transduction frequency (3- to 10-fold) is always observed in recipient cells with *recBrecC* DNase (see Table 5). (2) The frequency with which Trp[+] of lysogens spontaneously segregate Trp⁻ cells due to loss of the phage was equal in the three recipient strains (1.5 - 2%), regardless of their recombination pathways. Although a definite answer to this problem must await further investigation, it is quite clear that the status of a single enzyme (*recBrecC* DNase) in the cells affects the fate of donor DNA molecules and thus changes the pattern of genetic recombination.

ACKNOWLEDGMENT

This work was supported by grants from USPHS (GM21073) and
NSF (GB14313).

REFERENCES

Barbour, S. D., H. Nagaishi, A. Templin and A. J. Clark. 1970.
Biochemical and genetic studies of recombination proficiency in
Escherichia coli, II *rec*⁺ revertants caused by indirect suppression
of *rec*⁻ mutations. Proc. Nat. Acad. Sci. U.S.A. 67: 128.

Campbell, A. L. 1962. Episomes. Advan. Genet. 11: 101.

Clark, A. J. 1973. Recombination deficient mutants of *E. coli* and
other bacteria. Ann. Rev. Genet. 7: 67.

Cosloy, S. D. and M. Oishi. 1973a. Genetic transformation in
Escherichia coli K12. Proc. Nat. Acad. Sci. U.S.A. 70: 84.

Cosloy, S. D. and M. Oishi. 1973b. The nature of the transformation process in *Escherichia coli* K12. Molec. Gen. Genet. 124: 1.

Kaiser, A. D. and D. S. Hogness. 1960. The transformation of
Escherichia coli with deoxyribonucleic acid isolated from bacteriophage λ*dg*. J. Mol. Biol. 2: 392.

Kushner, S. R., H. Nagaishi, A. Templin and A. J. Clark. 1971.
Genetic recombination in *Escherichia coli*: the role of exonuclease
I. Proc. Nat. Acad. Sci. U.S.A. 68: 824.

Mandel, M. and A. Higa. 1970. Calcium-dependent bacteriophage
DNA infection. J. Mol. Biol. 53: 159.

Oishi, M. and S. D. Cosloy. 1972. The genetic and biochemical
basis of the transformability of *Escherichia coli* K12. Biochem.
Biophys. Res. Commun. 49: 1568.

Oishi, M. and S. D. Cosloy. 1974. Specialized transformation in
Escherichia coli K12. Nature 248: 112.

Oka, A., H. Ozeki and J. Inselburg. 1971. Integration and excision
of ɸ80pt prophage in *Escherichia coli* I. Replacement of tryptophan
genes of ɸ80pt with the host alleles through the lysogenic process.
Virology 46: 556.

Wackernagel, W. 1973. Genetic transformation in *E. coli*: the
inhibitory role of the *recBC* DNase. Biochem. Biophys. Res. Commun.
51: 306.

TRANSFORMATION OF *ESCHERICHIA COLI* BY RECOMBINANT PLASMID

REPLICONS CONSTRUCTED *IN VITRO*

Stanley N. Cohen

Department of Medicine, Stanford University School of

Medicine, Stanford, California 94305

Treatment of *Escherichia coli* with calcium chloride renders
this bacterial species competent for transfection by purified
bacteriophage DNA (Mandel and Higa, 1970) and for transformation
by plasmid (Cohen *et al.*, 1972) or *E. coli* chromosomal (Cosloy
and Oishi, 1973; Wackernagel, 1973) DNA. Transformation of *E. coli*
by plasmid DNA, which unlike chromosomal DNA does not require a
recipient strain defective in the *rec*BC nuclease, has proved to be
a useful tool for investigating the genetic and molecular properties
of discrete plasmid species, and for introducing nonconjugative
plasmids into specific *E. coli* hosts in the absence of transducing
phage or conjugally proficient transfer plasmids (Cohen *et al.*,
1972; Cohen and Chang, 1973; van Embden and Cohen, 1973; Lederberg
et al., 1973; Guerry *et al.*, 1974; Oishi and Cosloy, 1974).

The requirements for transformation of *E. coli* by plasmid DNA
(Cohen *et al.*, 1972) are shown in Table 1. Transformation is
accomplished by plasmids of various incompatability groups, and by
closed circular, open (nicked) circular, and catenated forms of
plasmid DNA; however, denaturation or sonication of the DNA destroys
its transforming ability. Transformation efficiency is unaffected
by treatment of plasmid DNA with ribonuclease, Pronase, or phenol
but is abolished by treatment with pancreatic deoxyribonuclease if
carried out prior to the 42°C heat-pulse step responsible for DNA
uptake (Cohen *et al.*, 1972). Transformed bacteria acquire a closed-
circular autonomously replicating DNA species with the characteristics of the parent plasmid (Fig. 1), and plasmid DNA isolated from
such transformants can itself be used to transform other bacteria.

Earlier experiments have shown that some DNA fragments that have
been generated from larger plasmids by shearing (Cohen and Chang,

155

Table 1.   Requirements for transformation by R-factor DNA

DNA species	Transformants/µg DNA
R6-5 (F-like)	
Closed circular	9.2×10^4
+ DNase (before)	<0.3
+ DNase (after)	7.7×10^4
+ RNase (before)	9.6×10^4
+ Pronase (before)	8.1×10^4
Phenol extraction	9.9×10^4
Isolated from transformed bacteria	7.0×10^4
Catenated	3.2×10^4
Open-circular	5.6×10^4
Denatured	<0.3
Sonicated	<0.3
No DNA	---[a]
No bacteria	<0.3
R64-11	
Closed circular	9.4×10^3
No DNA	---[a]
No bacteria	<0.3

Conditions for isolation of plasmid DNA, and for transformation under the various conditions listed in the table have been described elsewhere (Cohen *et al.*, 1972).   Transformation efficiency was determined after a 2-hr incubation in antibiotic-free medium, to allow full expression of drug resistance.   The terms "before" and "after" refer to the period of incubation of plasmid DNA and $CaCl_2$-treated cells at 42°C.

[a] No colonies were observed when 10^9 bacteria were assayed in the absence of DNA.

Figure 1.   Centrifugation analysis of R-factor DNA isolated from transformed cells.   (Top) Tritium-labeled DNA isolated from transformed cells by a detergent-lysis procedure was centrifuged to equilibrium in ethidium bromide.   Fractions were collected and assayed for radioactivity.   After removal of ethidium bromide from the covalently closed circular DNA contained in peak A (fractions 40-43), this DNA was analyzed in a 5-20% linear sucrose gradient in the presence of ^{14}-C-labeled DNA marker.   The DNA species observed have the molecular properties of the transforming plasmid.   Experimental details have been described elsewhere (Cohen *et al.*, 1972).   Note the change in scale in the top figure.

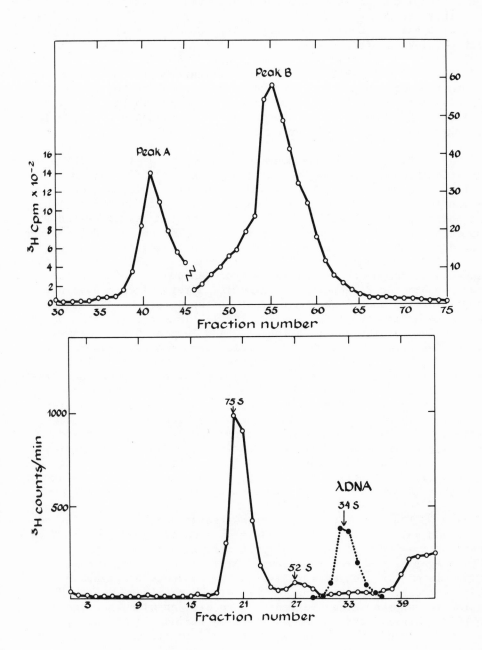

1973) or by treatment with the *Eco*RI restriction endonuclease (Cohen
et al., 1973) can be introduced by transformation into *E. coli*,
where they can recircularize and become functional plasmid replicons.
One such plasmid, (Cohen and Chang, 1973; Cohen *et al.*, 1973), pSC101
which was formed after transformation of *E. coli* by a shear-fragment
of the larger antibiotic resistance plasmid R6-5 (Silver and Cohen,
1972; Sharp *et al.*, 1973) carries genetic information necessary for
its own replication and for expression of resistance to tetracycline.
This plasmid has proved to be of considerable use in the construction
of plasmid chimeras *in vitro* because of the location of its single
cleavage site for the *Eco*RI endonuclease.

The *Eco*RI restriction endonuclease (Hedgepeth *et al.*, 1972)
cleaves double-stranded DNA so as to produce short overlapping
single-strand ends. On a random basis, the nucleotide sequence
cleaved is expected to occur once in every 4,000 to 16,000 nucleotide pairs (Hedgepeth *et al.*, 1972); thus, most *Eco*RI-generated DNA
fragments contain one or more intact genes. The nucleotide sequences
cleaved by the enzyme are unique and self-complementary (Hedgepeth
et al., 1972; Mertz and Davis, 1972; Sgaramella, 1972), so that DNA
fragments produced can associate by hydrogen bonding with either end
of any other *Eco*RI-generated fragment. After hydrogen bonding,
the 3'-hydroxyl and 5'-phosphate ends can be joined by DNA ligase
(Mertz and Davis, 1972; Sgaramella, 1972). Thus the enzyme appeared
to be useful for the construction of DNA molecules having segments
originating from diverse sources. Molecular chimeras produced by
the joining of different *Eco*RI-generated DNA fragments could potentially be introduced into bacterial strains by transformation, provided that at least one of the segments carries a capability for
replication and selection in transformed bacteria. As noted above,
the pSC101 plasmid was especially useful for this purpose, since
insertion of a DNA segment at its single *Eco*RI cleavage site does
not interfere with either its replication functions or expression
of its tetracycline resistance genes. Our initial plasmid construction experiments involved the linkage of this replicon to a fragment
of another "synthetic" antibiotic resistance plasmid, pSC102.

The pSC102 plasmid, which carries resistance to kanamycin, neo-
mycin, and sulfonamide, was formed by reassociation of several *Eco*RI-
generated fragments of the larger plasmid, R6-5 (Cohen *et al.*,
1973). Agarose gel electrophoresis (Fig. 2) demonstrates that the
pSC102 plasmid is cleaved into its three component fragments by the
*Eco*RI restriction endonuclease. The molecular weight of 17.4 X 10^6
for the sum of the three fragments is consistent with the size of
the pSC102 plasmid determined by electron microscopy and sucrose
gradient sedimentation. The pSC101 plasmid is cleaved by the *Eco*RI
restriction endonuclease into a single linear DNA fragment (Fig. 2D),
as noted above.

A mixture of *Eco*RI-cleaved pSC101 and pSC102 plasmid DNA was treated with DNA ligase, and the ligated molecules were used to transform *E. coli*. Transformants that were resistant to both tetracycline and kanamycin contained a new plasmid, pSC105 (Fig. 2A), which contains fragment II of pSC102 (*i.e.* the fragment that carries kanamycin resistance) plus the *Eco*RI-generated fragment that comprises the entire pSC101 tetracycline resistance plasmid.

This procedure for the *in vitro* construction of recombinant plasmid molecules has also proved useful for the formation of plasmids that include DNA derived from different bacterial species. Such experiments have been carried out with a penicillinase-producing plasmid of *Staphylococcus aureus* [pI258, molecular weight ~20 X 10^6 (Rush *et al.*, 1969; Novick and Bouanchaud, 1971; Lindberg and Novick, 1973)]. This plasmid appeared to be especially appropriate for interspecies genome construction, since its properties have been well defined, and it carries several different genetic determinants that were potentially detectable in *E. coli*. Moreover, agarose gel electrophoresis indicated that this plasmid is cleaved into four easily identifiable fragments by the *Eco*RI restriction endonuclease.

Molecular chimeras containing both staphylococcal and *E. coli* DNA were constructed by ligation of a mixture of *Eco*RI-cleaved pSC101 and pI258 DNA, and were used to transform a restrictionless strain of *E. coli* (C600$r_k^-m_k^-$). Selection was carried out for transformants that expressed the penicillin resistance determinant carried by the staphylococcal plasmid, and plasmid DNA isolated from penicillin-resistant transformants was characterized. CsCl gradient analysis of an *E. coli-Staphylococcus* plasmid chimera

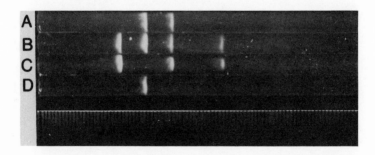

Figure 2. Agarose gel electrophoresis of *Eco*RI digests of plasmids. DNA fragments subjected to electrophoresis in agarose gels as described elsewhere (Cohen *et al.*, 1973) were stained with ethidium bromide, and the fluorescing DNA bands were photographed under long-wavelength ultraviolet light. (A) pSC105 DNA, (B) mixture of pSC101 and pSC102 DNA, (C) pSC102 DNA, (D) pSC101 DNA.

isolated from one such transformant (pSC112) is shown in Fig. 3.
The buoyant density of the intact plasmid chimera (ρ = 1.700
g/cm^3) is intermediate between the buoyant density of the *E. coli*
plasmid (ρ = 1.710) and the density of the staphylococcal plasmid
(ρ = 1.691). Upon treatment with the *Eco*RI endonuclease, the
pSC112 plasmid is cleaved into separate fragments with the buoyant
density characteristics of its component DNA species. Further
study of this plasmid chimera by agarose gel electrophoresis and
electron microscope heteroduplex analysis (Chang and Cohen, 1974)
confirmed that it contains DNA sequences derived from both *E. coli*
and *Staphylococcus*. The staphylococcal genes linked to the pSC101
replicon were shown to be transferrable among different *E. coli*
strains by a conjugally proficient transfer plasmid indigenous to
the Enterobacteriaceae.

In the experiments described thus far, genetic determinants
carried by DNA fragments linked to the pSC101 plasmid replicon were
utilized to select for transformants that contain plasmid chimeras.
More recent experiments (Morrow *et al.*, 1974) involve the *in vitro*
construction of plasmid chimeras containing both prokaryotic and
eukaryotic DNA, and the recovery of recombinant DNA molecules from
transformed *E. coli* in the *absence* of selection for genetic

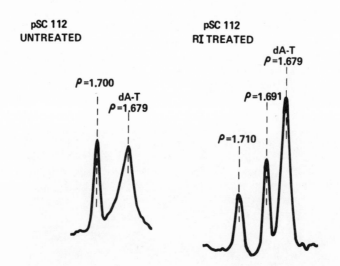

Figure 3.   Analytical ultracentrifugation of the *E. coli-Staphylococcus aureus* plasmid chimera, pSC112. Densitometer tracings are
shown.   (Left) Untreated plasmid chimera, showing a buoyant density intermediate between *E. coli* and *Staphylococcus*.   (Right)
Cleaved plasmid, showing the component *Eco*RI generated fragments.
The experimental conditions have been described elsewhere (Chang
and Cohen, 1974).

properties expressed by the eukaryotic DNA. The amplified ribosomal DNA (rDNA) coding for 18S and 28S ribosomal RNA of *Xenopus*
laevis was used as a source of eukaryotic DNA for these experiments,
since this DNA has been well characterized and can be isolated in
quantity (Dawid *et al.*, 1970; Birnstiel *et al.*, 1971). Moreover,
the repeat unit of *X. laevis* rDNA contains a site susceptible to
cleavage by the *Eco*RI endonuclease, resulting in the production of
DNA fragments of characteristic size (primarily fragments of 3.0,
3.9, and 4.2 X 10^6 daltons) that can be linked to the pSC101 plasmid (Morrow *et al.*, 1974).

A mixture of *Eco*RI-cleaved pSC101 DNA and *X. laevis* rDNA was
ligated and used to transform *E. coli* strain C600 $r_k^- m_k^-$. Tetra-
cycline-resistant transformants were selected, and the plasmid DNA
isolated from 55 separate clones was analyzed by agarose gel electrophoresis, cesium chloride gradient centrifugation, and/or electron microscopy to determine the presence of *X. laevis* rDNA linked
to the pSC101 plasmid replicon. The results of these experiments
are summarized in Table 2. Thirteen of the 55 tetracycline-
resistant clones selected contained one or more *Eco*RI-generated
fragment with the same size as the fragments produced by cleavage
of *X. laevis* rDNA. Moreover, the plasmid chimeras isolated from
E. coli were shown to contain DNA with a buoyant density characteristic of the high G+C base composition of *X. laevis* rDNA.
The observed variation in size of the *Eco*RI generated *X. laevis*
rDNA fragments contained in plasmid chimeras was consistent with
the observed size heterogeneity of fragments generated by *Eco*RI
cleavage of the amplified *X. laevis* rDNA repeat unit (Morrow *et al.*,
1974).

Electron microscope analysis (Fig. 4) of a heteroduplex formed
between *X. laevis* rDNA and one of the plasmid chimeras (*i.e.*, CD42)
listed in Table 2 demonstrates that this plasmid contains DNA
nucleotide sequences present in *X. laevis* rDNA. Moreover, in this
and other heteroduplexes, two separate plasmid DNA molecules were
seen to form duplex regions with a single strand of *X. laevis* rDNA,
consistent with the observation (Wensink and Brown, 1971; Hourcade
et al., 1973) that the rDNA sequences of *X. laevis* are tandemly
repeated.

Plasmid chimeras containing both *E. coli* and *X. laevis* DNA
replicate stably in the bacterial host as part of the pSC101 plasmid replicon, and can be recovered from transformed *E. coli* by
procedures commonly employed for the isolation of bacterial plasmids. Moreoever, ^{3}H-labeled RNA isolated from bacteria harboring
these plasmids hybridizes *in vitro* to amplified *X. laevis* rDNA
isolated directly from the eukaryotic organism (Morrow *et al.*,
1974), indicating that transcription of this eukaryotic DNA occurs
in its prokaryotic host.

Table 2. *X. laevis-E. coli* recombinant plasmids

Plasmid DNA	Molecular weight of *EcoRI* plasmid fragments estimated by gel electrophoresis (X 10^{-6})	Molecular weight from contour length (X 10^{-6})	Buoyant density of intact plasmid in CsCl (g/cm³)	Buoyant density of *EcoRI* generated fragments in CsCl (g/cm³)
CD 4	5.8, 4.2, 3.0	13.6	1.721	1.710, 1.729
CD 7	5.8, 4.2	—	—	—
CD 12, CD 20, CD 45, CD 47, CD 51	5.8, 3.0	—	—	—
CD 14	5.8, 4.2, 3.0	—	—	—
CD 18	5.8, 3.0	9.2	1.720	1.710, 1.728
CD 30	5.8, 3.9	10.0	1.719	1.710, 1.730
CD 35	5.8, 3.9, 3.0	—	—	—
CD 42	5.8, 4.2	10.6	1.720	1.710, 1.730
pSC101	5.8	6.0	1.710	

The procedures employed for plasmid DNA isolation, agarose gel electrophoresis, cesium chloride gradient centrifugation, and calculation of molecular weight and buoyant density of DNA have been described elsewhere (Morrow *et al.*, 1974).

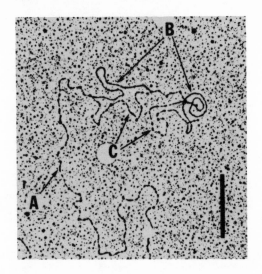

Figure 4.   Electron photomicrograph of heteroduplex of *X. laevis* rDNA and two separate molecules of a tetracycline-resistance plasmid chimera (CD42) isolated from *E. coli*.   (A) Single strand of *X. laevis* rDNA.   (B) Double-stranded regions of homology between plasmid CD42 and *X. laevis* rDNA.   (C) Single-stranded regions corresponding in length to the DNA segment of the CD42 plasmid that was derived from pSC101.   Experimental conditions were as indicated by Morrow *et al*. (1974).

The experiments reviewed here demonstrate that plasmids constructed *in vitro* and containing genes from diverse sources can be introduced by transformation into *E. coli*, where they exist as stable replicons.   The procedures described offer a general approach that utilizes bacterial plasmids for the cloning of a variety of prokaryotic and eukaryotic DNA species in *E. coli*.

ACKNOWLEDGMENT

This paper reviews certain experiments that were done collaboratively with H. W. Boyer, A. C. Y. Chang, H. M. Goodman, R. B. Helling, L. Hsu, and J. F. Morrow, as cited in the text.   The studies carried out in the laboratory of the author were supported by grant AI08619 from the National Institutes of Health and by grant GB30581 from the National Science Foundation.

REFERENCES

Birnstiel, M. L., M. Chipchase and J. Speirs.   1971.   The ribosomal

RNA cistrons.   Prog. Nucl. Res. Mol. Biol. 11: 351.

Chang, A. C. Y. and S. N. Cohen.   1974.   Genome construction between
bacterial species *in vitro*:   replication and expression of *Staphylococcus* plasmid genes in *E. coli*.   Proc. Nat. Acad. Sci. U.S.A.
71 in press.

Cohen, S. N. and A. C. Y. Chang.   1973.   Recircularization and
autonomous replication of a sheared R-factor DNA segment in
Escherichia coli transformants.   Proc. Nat. Acad. Sci. U.S.A. 70:
1293.

Cohen, S. N., A. C. Y. Chang, H. W. Boyer, and R. B. Helling.   1973.
Construction of biologically functional bacterial plasmids *in vitro*.
Proc. Nat. Acad. Sci. U.S.A. 70: 3240.

Cohen, S. N., A. C. Y. Chang and L. Hsu.   1972.   Nonchromosomal
antibiotic resistance in bacteria: genetic transformation of
Escherichia coli by R-factor DNA.   Proc. Nat. Acad. Sci. U.S.A.
69: 2110.

Cosloy, S. D. and M. Oishi.   1973.   Genetic transformation in
Escherichia coli K12.   Proc. Nat. Acad. Sci. U.S.A. 70: 84.

Dawid, I. B., D. D. Brown and R. H. Reeder.   1970.   Composition and
structure of chromosomal and amplified ribosomal DNA's of *Xenopus
laevis*.   J. Mol. Biol. 51: 341.

Guerry, P., J. van Embden and S. Falkow.   1974.   Molecular nature
of two nonconjugative plasmids carrying drug resistance genes.
J. Bacteriol. 117: 619.

Hedgepeth, J., H. M. Goodman and H. W. Boyer.   1972.   DNA nucleotide sequence restricted by the RI endonuclease.   Proc. Nat. Acad.
Sci. U.S.A. 69: 3448.

Hourcade, D., D. Dressler and J. Wolfson.   1973.   The amplification
of ribosomal RNA genes involves a rolling circle intermediate.
Proc. Nat. Acad. Sci. U.S.A. 70: 2926.

Lederberg, E. M., L. L. Brothers and S. N. Cohen.   1973.   Molecular
properties of an F-lac[+]-tetracycline resistance plasmid in *E. coli*
and *Salmonella typhimurium* LT2.   Genetics 74: 5152 (abstract).

Lindberg, M. and R. P. Novick.   1973.   Plasmid-specific transformation in *Staphylococcus aureus*.   J. Bacteriol. 115: 139.

Mandel, M. and A. Higa.   1970.   Calcium-dependent bacteriophage DNA
infection.   J. Mol. Biol. 53: 159.

Mertz, J. E. and R. W. Davis. 1972. Cleavage of DNA by R_I restriction endonuclease generates cohesive ends. Proc. Nat. Acad. Sci. U.S.A. 69: 3370.

Morrow, J. F., S. N. Cohen, A. C. Y. Chang, H. W. Boyer, H. M. Goodman and R. B. Helling. 1974. Replication and transcription of eukaryotic DNA in *Escherichia coli*. Proc. Nat. Acad. Sci. U.S.A. 71 in press.

Novick, R. P. and D. Bouanchaud. 1971. Extrachromosomal nature of drug resistance in *Staphylococcus aureus*. Ann. N. Y. Acad. Sci. 182: 279.

Oishi, M. and S. D. Cosloy. 1974. Specialized transformation in *E. coli* K12. Nature 248: 112.

Rush, M. G., C. N. Gordon, R. N. Novick and R. C. Warner. 1969. Penicillinase plasmid DNA from *Staphylococcus aureus*. Proc. Nat. Acad. Sci. U.S.A. 63: 1304.

Sgaramella, V. 1972. Enzymatic oligomerization of bacteriophage P22 DNA and of linear simian virus 40 DNA. Proc. Nat. Acad. Sci. U.S.A. 69: 3389.

Sharp, P. A., S. N. Cohen and N. Davidson. 1973. Electron microscope heteroduplex studies of sequence relations among plasmids of *Escherichia coli*. II. Structure of drug resistance (R) factors and F factors. J. Mol. Biol. 75: 235.

Silver, R. P. and S. N. Cohen. 1972. Nonchromosomal antibiotic resistance in bacteria. V. Isolation and characterization of R-factor mutants exhibiting temperature-sensitive repression of fertility. J. Bacteriol. 110: 1082.

van Embden, J. and S. N. Cohen. 1973. Molecular and genetic structures of an R factor system consisting of independent transfer and drug resistance plasmids. J. Bacteriol. 116: 699.

Wackernagel, W. 1973. Genetic transformation in *E. coli*: the inhibitory role of the recBC DNAase. Biochem. Biophys. Res. Commun. 51: 306.

Wensink, P. C. and D. D. Brown. 1971. Denaturation map of the ribosomal DNA of *Xenopus laevis*. J. Mol. Biol. 60: 235.

UPTAKE AND INTEGRATION OF TRANSFORMING DNA IN *BACILLUS SUBTILIS*

David Dubnau and Carol Cirigliano

Department of Microbiology, The Public Health Research Institute of the City of New York, Inc., New York, N.Y. 10016

In the past decade, considerable information has accumulated concerning the molecular events that accompany the uptake and integration of transforming DNA by competent bacterial cultures. This article presents our understanding of the molecular events accompanying genetic transformation in *Bacillus subtilis*. The approach employed in our laboratory has been a straightforward one, involving the addition of isotopically and genetically labeled DNA to competent cells and the analysis of extracts of those cells.

BINDING AND THE FORMATION OF DOUBLE-STRAND FRAGMENTS

The first detectable interaction of transforming DNA with competent cells results in the binding of the DNA to the cell surface. When high-molecular-weight *B. subtilis* or T7 phage DNA is used, apparently intact donor molecules are recoverable from the competent cells, demonstrating that any nucleolytic cleavage involved in the binding step either does not result in double-stranded breaks or occurs near the termini of the donor molecules (Fig. 1). The donor DNA bound in this state is completely removed from the cell surface by moderate shearing forces (Dubnau and Cirigliano, 1972b), indicating that the cell-bound DNA is spatially extended and not bound as a coiled mass. Our work does not demonstrate that the DNA is bound at the molecular termini. However, Williams and Green (1972) have shown that transfecting DNA from phage SP82G is bound at or near the molecular ends. The initial binding step is probably not a simple adsorption phenomenon, since it is more than 90% inhibited

167

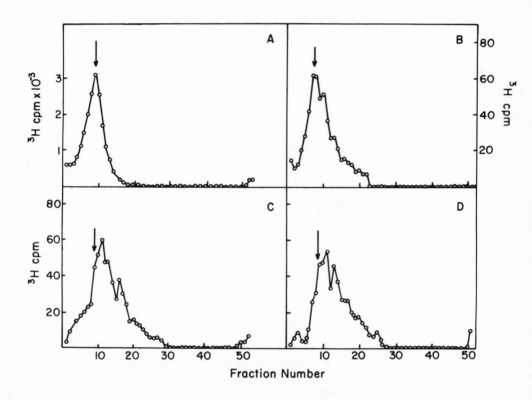

Figure 1.   Fragments derived from ^{3}H-labeled T7 DNA bound to competent cells of *B. subtilis*. ^{3}H-Labeled T7 DNA (1 µg/ml) was
incubated with a competent *B. subtilis* culture (2 X 10^8 cells/ml)
for 20 sec at 37°C.   The culture was then diluted 10-fold into
warm medium containing 200 µg/ml salmon sperm DNA.   At 29 sec (B),
80 sec (C), and 100 sec (D), samples were removed and washed free
of unbound DNA by sedimenting through 15% sucrose + 0.1 M NaCl +
0.1 M EDTA, pH 6.9 (Dubnau and Cirigliano, 1972b).   The cell pellet
was resuspended by gentle maceration with a glass rod and incubated
for 20 min at room temperature with gentle shaking with 2% Sarkosyl-
NL30 plus an equal volume of neutralized water-saturated phenol.
The suspensions were separated by centrifugation and the aqueous
layers were removed and dialyzed against 0.015 M NaCl + 0.0015 M
Na citrate.   This treatment resulted in the release of 90 to 95%
of the radioactivity bound to the cells.   Aliquots of each sample
were cosedimented with ^{14}C-labeled T7 DNA (position indicated by
vertical arrows) in an SW50.1 rotor at 20°C.   Centrifugation was
for 180 min at 44,000 rpm with the brake off.   The sedimentation
profile of the ^{3}H-labeled T7 DNA preparation used in the experiment is shown in A.

in the presence of 10^{-2} M KCN (Dubnau and Cirigliano, unpublished observations). Lacks and Greenberg (1973) have reported that in *Pneumococcus* the initial binding is energy dependent, requiring the presence of glucose.

Following this binding step, a fragmentation of the donor DNA molecules by double-strand cleavage is observed (Dubnau and Cirigliano, 1972a). The distribution of fragments generated by the cells from ^{3}H-labeled T7 DNA is shown in Fig. 1. In the experiment the cell-DNA complexes were diluted ten times into 100-fold excess salmon sperm DNA to slow down further attachments of T7 DNA to the cells. In spite of this treatment the total ^{3}H bound to the cells increased 25% from 30 to 100 seconds. The T7 DNA was rapidly fragmented to yield a skewed distribution of radioactivity, with a major peak at a molecular weight of 20 to 22 X 10^6 and with several minor peaks and shoulders. The distribution suggests that each T7 molecule received, on the average, about one double-strand break. This break may occur randomly or at unique sites on the molecule, accounting for the irregularities that are consistently observed in the sedimentation profiles. The resolution of sucrose gradient centrifugation is insufficient to distinguish between these alternatives. Similar distributions of double-strand fragments are observed when *B. subtilis* donor DNA is used.

We have shown previously that the double-strand fragments are precursors of the donor moiety of the donor-recipient complex (Dubnau and Cirigliano, 1972b; Davidoff-Abelson and Dubnau, 1973b). We do not know whether they are obligatory intermediates in the process of transformation by duplex DNA, and we are currently attempting to isolate nuclease-deficient mutants that may permit us to answer this question. Scher and Dubnau (1973) have described a Mn^{2+}- and Ca^{2+}-dependent endonuclease that is an attractive candidate for an enzyme producing the double-strand fragments. This enzyme is located in the periplasm of the cell and produces a limited number of double-strand cleavages in a variety of DNA substrates including *B. subtilis* and phage T7 DNA. It may be the same as the nuclease activity detected by Haseltine and Fox (1971) in whole cells of *B. subtilis*. The double-strand fragments produced from phage and bacterial DNA are external to the cell membrane. They are accessible to pancreatic deoxyribonuclease (Dubnau and Cirigliano, 1972a) and can be freed from the cells by gentle shaking at room temperature for 20 min with 2% Sarkosyl-NL30 plus phenol. This treatment does not result in the release of recipient cell DNA (Dubnau and Cirigliano, unpublished observations).

Morrison and Guild (1973) have shown that, in *Pneumococcus*, donor DNA bound to the cell surface in a DNase-sensitive state also receives double-strand breaks before it enters the cell and is converted to single-stranded DNA.

Fragmentation of transforming DNA may facilitate transformation at two subsequent steps by increasing the availability of molecule ends. Molecular ends may be required to initiate synapsis with the recipient chromosome. They may also be required for the next step in the process, which involves the conversion to single-strand DNA.

CONVERSION TO SINGLE-STRAND DNA

Beginning about 1 to 2 min after the addition of transforming DNA to competent cells, acid-soluble donor-derived material is released into the cell medium, largely as 5'-mononucleotides (Dubnau and Cirigliano, 1972a). Beginning at about the same time, high-molecular-weight single-stranded donor DNA is recoverable (Piechowska and Fox, 1971; Davidoff-Abelson and Dubnau, 1973a,b). The amount of single-stranded DNA produced is equivalent in mass to the acid-soluble radioactivity present at any given time (Davidoff-Abelson and Dubnau, 1973b; Dubnau and Cirigliano, unpublished observations). The single-strand fragments isolated using current procedures have an average molecular weight of 3 to 5 X 10^6 (Davidoff-Abelson and Dubnau, 1973a). This suggests that 1 to 3 single-strand fragments can be produced from each double-strand fragment of 10 to 20 X 10^6 daltons, if one strand equivalent from each fragment is degraded to yield the acid-soluble material. Lacks (1962) proposed that a membrane-localized exonuclease may degrade one strand of incoming double-stranded DNA, generating a single strand that is simultaneously transported across the membrane barrier of the cell. This model is supported by our observations. Further support comes from the fact that, although the double-strand fragments are external to the cell membrane, the single-strand material is resistant to the action of extracellular DNase (Davidoff-Abelson and Dubnau, 1973b). More recently, using benzoylated-napthoylated DEAE-cellulose columns (Schlegel et al., 1972), we have obtained evidence for the existence of partially single-stranded fragments in deproteinized extracts of cells transformed with [^{3}H]DNA. These are predicted intermediates according to the Lacks transport hypothesis.

FORMATION OF DONOR-RECIPIENT COMPLEX

The single-strand fragments are a precursor of the donor moiety of donor-recipient complex. About 5% of the donor radioactivity bound to the cells 3 min after the addition of transforming DNA is retained following treatment with extracellular DNase. This DNA is entirely single-stranded and moves almost quantitatively (∿75% conversion) into stable association with recipient DNA (Davidoff-Abelson and Dubnau, 1973b).

About 16 recombination-deficient radiation-sensitive mutants
of *B. subtilis* have been studied. These mutations occur in at
least seven genes, five of which play a role in transformation
(Dubnau and Cirigliano, 1974). All of these mutant strains, when
transformed, produce apparently normal double- and single-stranded
fragments from donor DNA. Mutations in three genes (*recA, recD,
recE*), however, prevent the next step in the transformation process,
which is the stable association of donor and recipient DNA (Dubnau
et al., 1973). Nothing is known of the biochemical lesions in
these strains.

The donor-recipient complex has been described by several
investigators working with the *B. subtilis* system, all of whom have
concluded that donor DNA is physically inserted in the recipient
chromosome (Ayad and Barker, 1969; Bodmer and Ganesan, 1964; Dubnau
and Davidoff-Abelson, 1971; Harris and Barr, 1969, Pène and Romig,
1964). Bodmer and Ganesan (1964) showed that the donor moiety in
this structure is single-stranded and is paired with a homologous
recipient strand. This result was confirmed by Dubnau and Davidoff-
Abelson (1971). Perhaps the least understood aspect of genetic
transformation concerns the process by which single-stranded donor
DNA invades the homologous region of the recipient chromosome and
replaces a resident strand. It is attractive to suppose that
specific sequences on the incoming single strands possess affinity
for pairing proteins that facilitate synapsis by binding to these
sequences and to homologous sequences or to structural singulari-
ties on the resident chromosome (Holliday, 1968; Sobell, 1972).
This process may also involve a melting-protein analogous to the
gene *32* protein of phage T4, which is required for recombination
(Tomizawa *et al.*, 1966). Such a protein may increase the probability of donor-recipient DNA interaction by maintaining single-
stranded DNA in a relatively extended configuration. The folded
chromosome model of Worcel and Burgi (1972) is attractive in this
connection, since it provides for a highly compact chromosomal
structure in which all segments are potentially available for pairing with an incoming single-stranded fragment.

Donor radioactivity appears in association with recipient DNA
earlier than this donor-recipient complex develops the capacity to
transform secondary recipients for a donor-specific marker (Dubnau
and Davidoff-Abelson, 1971). This was taken as evidence that the
early donor-recipient complex possesses single-strand interruptions,
which are later repaired. It was shown from physical evidence that
the donor and recipient moieties of this early complex exist in a
noncovalent form of association (Dubnau and Davidoff-Abelson, 1971;
Dubnau and Cirigliano, 1973a). This structure, which is analogous
to the joint molecules described by Tomizawa *et al.* (1966) in bacteriophage T4, may consist of a duplex in which the single-stranded
donor moiety is completely paired to the homologous recipient strand.

Alternatively, it may consist of a branched intermediate such as that proposed by Cassuto and Radding (1971).

The single-strand donor moiety, when freed from the noncovalent donor moiety at pH 13.0, has a molecular weight of 1 to 5 X 10^6, with a broad peak value of 2.5 to 3 X 10^6 (Dubnau and Cirigliano, 1973a). The size of the integrated donor moiety was also determined by using ^{3}H,^{2}H-labeled donor DNA and determining the density displacement of the donor-recipient complex as a function of double-strand molecular weight. This study suggested an average single-strand molecular weight of 2.8 X 10^6 for the donor piece (Dubnau and Cirigliano, 1972c). Thus, the single-strand precursor of the donor-recipient complex, the donor moiety of the noncovalent complex, and the donor moiety of the fully sealed donor-recipient complex are all approximately equivalent in size. This is consistent with the kinetic data described above, which shows that about 75% of the single-strand donor DNA present after 3 min incubation is later found in association with recipient DNA.

INTEGRATION IN RELATION TO DNA SYNTHESIS

Recently we have begun to explore the possible role of DNA polymerases in transformation. *B. subtilis* possesses three known DNA polymerases. Polymerase III (PolIII) is required for DNA replication and is reversibly inhibited *in vitro* and *in vivo* by 6-(*p*-hydroxyphenylazo)uracil (HPU) (Gass and Cozzarelli, 1973; Brown, 1971). PolI, the major DNA polymerase detectable in extracts probably plays a role in repair, while the role of PolII is unknown. We have studied the effect on transforming efficiency of the *polA59* mutation (Searashi and Strauss, 1965). Mutants carrying this lesion are sensitive to UV light and methyl methanesulfonate and have no detectable PolI activity in extracts (Gass and Cozzarelli, 1973). In several experiments comparing BD274 (*trpC2 thr-5 polA59*) with BD170 (*trpC2 thr-5*) it was found that uptake of ^{3}H-labeled *B. subtilis* DNA was indistinguishable in the two strains. The yield of Trp$^+$ and Thr$^+$ transformants in the *polA59* strain was always 50 to 100% of that in the Pol$^+$ strain. Thus, PolI deficiency results in a slight diminution of transforming efficiency, if any. Laipis and Ganesan (1972) have reported that a different mutant, *polA5*, is fully transformable. We have shown that HPU has no discernible effect on the extent and rate of formation of donor-recipient complex in the Pol$^+$ strain BD170 (Dubnau and Cirigliano, 1973b). This was determined from the appearance of donor and recombinant transforming activity measured in extracts of transformed cells as well as from direct physical measurements. Since in these experiments the residual incorporation of [^{3}H]thymidine was about 0.5% of that in the absence of HPU, the results demonstrated that chromosomal replication is not required for the integration of transforming

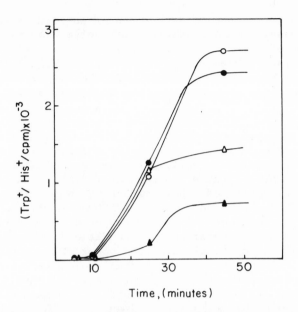

Time, (minutes)

Figure 2.   Recovery of donor transforming activity in Pol[+] and
polA59 competent cells in the presence and absence of HPU. Competent cells of BD170 (*trpC2 thr-5*) and of BD274 (*trpC2 thr-5 polA59*)
were incubated at 37°C with 1 μg/ml ^{3}H-labeled BD204 DNA (*thy hisB2*)
each with and without HPU (400 μM).   Samples were withdrawn at 5,
10, 25, and 45 min and washed twice, and the suspensions were lysed
with lysozyme and SDS, treated with Pronase (1 mg/ml) for 2 hr at
48°C and dialyzed extensively against 0.1X SSC.   Aliquots of each
were withdrawn for radioactive counting and additional aliquots
were used to transform BD55 (*trpC2 hisB2*) for *his* and *trp*.   The
yield of Trp[+] (donor-type) transformants was normalized to the
number of His[+] (recipient-type) transformants obtained and to the
uptake of radioactive donor DNA determined on each sample. Pol[+]
strain without HPU (●); Pol[+] strain with HPU (O); *polA59* strain
without HPU (Δ); *polA59* strain with HPU (▲).

DNA, as had been suggested (Erickson and Braun, 1968; Erickson and
Copeland, 1972, 1973).   Levin and Landman (1973) have reached the
same conclusion.

     The recovery of donor transforming activity from eclipse
(Venema *et al.*, 1965) has also been determined in extracts of the
polA59 strains transformed in the presence and absence of HPU
(Fig. 2).   Recovery of donor transforming activity in the *polA59*
strain proceeds at about half the rate seen in the Pol[+] strain.
HPU has no effect on the Pol[+] strain but has further depressed
recovery in the PolI-deficient strain.   The identical result was

obtained when the appearance of recombinant transforming activity
was measured. This result implies that DNA polymerase is required
for the formation of donor-recipient complex with donor transforming
activity. It further suggests that both PolI and PolIII can fulfill
this requirement. The recovery observed in the *polA59* strain in
the presence of HPU may depend on residual PolI, II, or III activity,
or it may indicate that some integration does not require DNA polymerase.

It is reasonable to postulate that DNA polymerase is required
to carry out repair synthesis during the covalent completion of the
donor-recipient complex. Levin and Landman (1973) estimated that
the residual incorporation of [^{3}H]thymidine by competent cells in
the presence of HPU corresponded to about 5000 to 6000 nucleotides
per chromosome. Since about 10% of the competent cells are transformed for a given marker under optimal conditions, we can assume
that about 10^8 daltons of single-stranded donor DNA are integrated
per transformed cell (assuming a chromosomal molecular weight of
2×10^9). Since each integrated fragment consists of about 2.8×10^6 daltons, we can estimate that the residual incorporation of
[^{3}H]thymidine measured by Levin and Landman allows for an upper
limit of 50 to 100 nucleotides incorporated per integrated fragment.

It is also possible that the exonuclease usually associated
with DNA polymerase is required for the formation of donor-recipient
complex. Although the PolI of *B. subtilis* has been reported to
lack exonuclease activity (Okazaki and Kornberg, 1964), it is possible that this activity was lost in purification. The PolIII of
B. subtilis possesses exonuclease activity sensitive to HPU (Gass
and Cozzarelli, 1973).

SUMMARY

To understand the interaction of parental DNA molecules, which
produces recombinant progeny during transformation, we must describe
the properties of these parental molecules and of the product of
their interaction. In *Bacillus subtilis*, transforming DNA is bound
to the cell surface at one or a few points on each duplex molecule,
possibly at the ends. Donor DNA is then fragmented to yield pieces
with an average size of about 1 to 2×10^7 daltons. These double-
stranded fragments are probably produced by endonucleolytic action
across both strands of the donor DNA. An endonuclease that may perform this role *in vivo* has been identified. The double-stranded
fragments are converted to single strands with molecular weights
of 3 to 5×10^6, and an equivalent mass of acid-soluble, donor-
derived material is released into the culture medium. The single
strands then associate with recipient DNA, first in a noncovalent
and then in a covalent donor-recipient complex. This complex is a

heteroduplex structure, consisting of recipient DNA in which single-stranded donor segments with an average weight of 2.8×10^6 have been inserted. Mutants blocked at several steps in this pathway have been isolated and mapped. They fall into at least five distinct loci, three of which are required for donor-recipient complex formation. Chromosomal replication is not required for the formation of a covalently linked donor-recipient complex. However, some DNA synthesis may be required for this process, since evidence exists that the formation of a covalently linked donor-recipient complex requires DNA polymerase activity.

ACKNOWLEDGMENTS

We thank I. Smith, L. Mindich, B. Scher, and E. Dubnau for valuable discussions, A. Howard for expert secretarial assistance, and N. Cozzarelli for his gift of polymerase-deficient strains.

This work was supported by National Science Foundation Grant GB-18146, Public Health Service Grant AI-10311 from the National Institute of Allergy and Infectious Diseases, and Public Health Service Career Development Award 1-K4-GM8837 from the National Institute of General Medical Sciences.

REFERENCES

Arwert, F. and G. Venema. 1973. Evidence for a non-covalently bonded intermediate in recombination during transformation of *Bacillus subtilis*. In (L. J. Archer, ed.) Bacterial Transformation. p. 203-214. Academic Press, London.

Ayad, S. R. and G. R. Barker. 1969. The integration of donor and recipient deoxyribonucleic acid during transformation of *Bacillus subtilis*. Biochem. J. 113: 167.

Bodmer, W. F. and A. T. Ganesan. 1964. Biochemical and genetic studies of integration and recombination in *Bacillus subtilis* transformation. Genetics 50: 717.

Brown, N. C. 1971. Inhibition of bacterial DNA replication by 6-(*p*-hydroxyphenylazo)-uracil: differential effect on repair and semi-conservative synthesis in *Bacillus subtilis*. J. Mol. Biol. 59: 1.

Cassuto, E. and C. M. Radding. 1971. Mechanism for the action of λ exonuclease in genetic recombination. Nature New Biol. 229: 13.

176

D. DUBNAU AND C. CIRIGLIANO

Davidoff-Abelson, R. and D. Dubnau. 1973a. Conditions affecting the isolation from transformed cells of *Bacillus subtilis* of high-molecular-weight single-stranded deoxyribonucleic acid of donor origin. J. Bacteriol. 116: 146.

Davidoff-Abelson, R. and D. Dubnau. 1973b. Kinetic analysis of the products of donor deoxyribonucleate in transformed cells of *Bacillus subtilis*. J. Bacteriol. 116: 154.

Dubnau, D. and C. Cirigliano. 1972a. Fate of transforming DNA following uptake by competent *Bacillus subtilis*. III. Formation and properties of products isolated from transformed cells which are derived entirely from donor DNA. J. Mol. Biol. 64: 9.

Dubnau, D. and C. Cirigliano. 1972b. Fate of transforming DNA following uptake by competent *Bacillus subtilis*. IV. The endwise attachment and uptake of transforming DNA. J. Mol. Biol. 64: 31.

Dubnau, D. and C. Cirigliano. 1972c. Fate of transforming deoxyribonucleic acid after uptake by competent *Bacillus subtilis*: Size and distribution of the integrated donor segments. J. Bacteriol. 111: 488.

Dubnau, D. and C. Cirigliano. 1973a. Fate of transforming DNA following uptake by competent *Bacillus subtilis*. VI. Non-covalent association of donor and recipient DNA. Mol. Gen. Genet. 120: 101.

Dubnau, D. and C. Cirigliano. 1973b. Fate of transforming deoxyribonucleic acid after uptake by competent *Bacillus subtilis*: Non-requirement of deoxyribonucleic acid replication for uptake and integration of transforming deoxyribonucleic acid. J. Bacteriol. 113: 1512.

Dubnau, D. and C. Cirigliano. 1974. Genetic characterization of recombination-deficient mutants of *Bacillus subtilis*. J. Bacteriol. 117: 488.

Dubnau, D. and R. Davidoff-Abelson. 1971. Fate of transforming DNA following uptake by competent *Bacillus subtilis*. I. Formation and properties of the donor-recipient complex. J. Mol. Biol. 56: 209.

Dubnau, D., R. Davidoff-Abelson, B. Scher and C. Cirigliano. 1973. Fate of transforming deoxyribonucleic acid after uptake by competent *Bacillus subtilis*: Phenotypic characterization of radiation-sensitive recombination-deficient mutants. J. Bacteriol. 114: 273.

Erickson, R. J. and W. Braun. 1968. Apparent dependence of transformation on the stage of deoxyribonucleic acid replication of recipient cells. Bacteriol. Rev. 32: 291.

Erickson, R. J. and J. C. Copeland. 1972. Structure and replication of chromosomes in competent cells of *Bacillus subtilis*. J. Bacteriol. 109: 1075.

Erickson, R. J. and J. C. Copeland. 1973. Congression of unlinked markers and genetic mapping in the transformation of *Bacillus subtilis* 168. Genetics 73: 13.

Gass, K. B. and N. R. Cozzarelli. 1973. Further genetic and enzymological characterization of the three *Bacillus subtilis* DNA polymerases. J. Biol. Chem. 248: 7688.

Harris, W. J. and G. C. Barr. 1969. Some properties of DNA in competent *Bacillus subtilis*. J. Mol. Biol. 39: 245.

Haseltine, F. P. and M. S. Fox. 1971. Bacterial inactivation of transforming deoxyribonucleate. J. Bacteriol. 107: 889.

Holliday, R. 1968. Genetic recombination in fungi. In (W. J. Peacock and R. D. Brock, eds.) Replication and Recombination of Genetic Material. p. 157–174. Australian Acad. Sci., Canberra.

Lacks, S. 1962. Molecular fate of DNA in genetic transformation of *Pneumococcus*. J. Mol. Biol. 5: 119.

Lacks, S. and B. Greenberg. 1973. Competence for deoxyribonucleic acid uptake and deoxyribonuclease action external to cells in the genetic transformation of *Diplococcus pneumoniae*. J. Bacteriol. 114: 152.

Laipis, P. J. and A. T. Ganesan. 1972. A deoxyribonucleic acid polymerase I-deficient mutant of *Bacillus subtilis*. J. Biol. Chem. 247: 5867.

Levin, B. C. and O. E. Landman. 1973. DNA synthesis inhibition by 6-(*p*-hydroxyphenylazo)-uracil in relation to uptake and integration of transforming DNA in *Bacillus subtilis*. In (L. J. Archer, ed.) Bacterial Transformation. p. 217–240. Academic Press, London.

Morrison, D. A. and W. R. Guild. 1973. Breakage prior to entry of donor DNA in *Pneumococcus* transformation. Biochim. Biophys. Acta 299: 545.

Okazaki, T. and A. Kornberg. 1964. Enzymatic synthesis of deoxyribonucleic acid. XV. Purification and properties of a polymerase from *Bacillus subtilis*. J. Biol. Chem. 239: 259.

Pène, J. J. and W. R. Romig. 1964. On the mechanism of genetic recombination in transforming *Bacillus subtilis*. J. Mol. Biol. 9: 236.

Piechowska, M. and M. S. Fox.   1971.   Fate of transforming deoxyribonucleate in *Bacillus subtilis*.   J. Bacteriol. 108: 680.

Scher, B. and D. Dubnau.   1973.   A manganese-stimulated endonuclease
from *Bacillus subtilis*.   Biochem. Biophys. Res. Commun. 55: 595.

Schlegel, R. A., R. E. Pyeritz and C. A. Thomas, Jr.   1972.   Analysis of DNA bearing single-chained terminals by BNC chromatography.
Anal. Biochem. 50: 558.

Searashi, T. and B. Strauss.   1965.   Relation of the repair of
damage induced by a monofunctional alkylating agent to the repair
of damage induced by ultraviolet light in *Bacillus subtilis*.
Biochem. Biophys. Res. Commun. 20: 680.

Sobell, H. M.   1972.   Molecular mechanism for genetic recombination.
Proc. Nat. Acad. Sci. U.S.A. 69: 2483.

Tomizawa, J.-I., N. Anraku and Y. Iwama.   1966.   Molecular mechanisms
of genetic recombination in bacteriophage.   VI. A mutant defective
in the joining of DNA molecules.   J. Mol. Biol. 21: 247.

Venema, G., R. H. Pritchard and T. Venema-Schroder.   1965.   Fate
of transforming deoxyribonucleic acid in *Bacillus subtilis*.   J.
Bacteriol. 89: 1250.

Williams, G. L. and D. M. Green.   1972.   Early extracellular events
in infection of competent *Bacillus subtilis* by DNA of bacteriophage
SP82G.   Proc. Nat. Acad. Sci. U.S.A. 69: 1545.

Worcel, A. and E. Burgi.   1972.   On the structure of the folded
chromosome of *Escherichia coli*.   J. Mol. Biol. 71: 127.

IN VITRO TRANSFORMATION IN TOLUENIZED *BACILLUS SUBTILIS*

Sumi Imada and Noboru Sueoka

Department of Molecular, Cellular and Development

Biology, University of Colorado, Boulder, Colorado 80302

Studies on bacterial transformation have contributed to the understanding of the physical state of transforming DNA in recipient cells. In the early stage of transformation a double-stranded DNA with low transforming activity was found in periplasm of *Bacillus subtilis* (Dubnau and Davidoff-Abelson, 1971). Single-stranded intermediates were found in *Pneumococcus* (Lacks, 1962) and in *B. subtilis* (Piechowska and Fox, 1971; Davidoff-Abelson and Dubnau, 1973a) which were later found as heteroduplex donor-recipient complexes in *Pneumococcus, Haemophilus,* and *B. subtilis* (Lacks, 1962; Fox and Allen, 1964; Notani and Goodgal, 1966; Davidoff-Abelson and Dubnau, 1973b). However, the molecular mechanisms of transformation, which may involve enzyme(s), cellular structure(s), and other factors, still remain obscure. In this paper we report on transformation studies in toluene-treated *B. subtilis*, in which DNA, protein, and RNA synthesis in the presence of proper substrates and ATP has been shown to occur.

MATERIALS AND METHODS

Bacterial Strains

Derivatives of *B. subtilis* 168 strain were used. Donor DNA was purified from *trp*2 *thy* double mutant cells by the method described by Dubnau and Davidoff-Abelson (1971). The *his*B2 *thy* double mutant was used as a toluenized recipient for transformation experiments. Strain *his*B2 *trp*2 was used as a recipient cell to assay biological activity of DNA isolated from a transformed toluene-treated cell. The *his*B2 and *trp*2 markers are linked 50-60% by transformation (Nester *et al.*, 1963).

179

Preparation of Recipient Cells

Maximum competent-stage cells obtained by the method of Cahn
and Fox (1968) were harvested on Millipore filters, washed once
with 0.012 M $MgSO_4$-0.5% glucose in 0.1 M potassium phosphate buffer
(pH 7.0), and resuspended in the same buffer at a concentration
50-fold that of the original culture. The transformation efficiency was between 10^{-3} and 10^{-4}. Toluene treatment was performed
either before or after addition of donor DNA. Treatment of the
cells before transformation with toluene was as described by Matsushita and Sueoka (1971), in which the cells were incubated with
1% of toluene at 25°C for 10 min with gentle shaking and pelleted
by centrifugation. For toluenization after transformation, the
transformation mixture was diluted 5-fold with ice-cold buffer and
maintained at 0°C for 20 min with vigorous shaking four times (5
sec each) in the presence of 5% toluene. Then the cells were
pelleted by centrifugation. Cell survival after this toluene
treatment was 0.001 - 0.01%.

Transformation Procedure

The recipient cell (either toluenized or untreated) was resuspended in a reaction mixture and the transformation was performed at
37°C with 2-10 µg/ml of donor DNA. The complete reaction mixture
contained 12 mM $MgSO_4$, 33 µM dGTP, dATP, dTTP, and dCTP, 2 µM
diphosphopyridine nucleotide, 0.5% glucose, 2 mM dithiothreitol,
and 1.3 mM ATP in 0.07 M potassium phosphate buffer (pH 7.4).

RESULTS AND DISCUSSION

As shown in Table 1, the toluene-treated cells took up tri-
tiated double-stranded donor DNA with an efficiency similar to that
of the untreated cell. When heat-denatured DNA was used, the incorporation efficiency was approximately 30% of that of native DNA in
both toluenized and untreated cells. This suggests that the toluenized cell retains the selectivity for native DNA. The recovery
of the donor-type marker was reproducibly 4- to 5-fold higher in
toluenized cells than in untreated cells in several experiments
(Table 2). Recombinants in the toluenized cell were low compared
with the untreated cell (Table 2), and it is not clear whether they
are true recombinants. Various efforts to raise the recombination
frequency in toluenized cells have been without success. Both
[^{3}H]DNA incorporation and the recovery of the donor marker in
toluenized cells were depressed by omitting ATP from the reaction
mixture. The same effect was observed by adding (β, γ-methylene)
adenosine 5'-triphosphate (an antagonist of ATP) in 6-fold excess
of ATP. This may show that there is an energy-dependent step in
the entry of transforming DNA, as suggested by Strauss (1970).

Table 1. Incorporation of ^{3}H-labeled DNA into recipient cells

Incubation time (min)	Incorporation of radioactivity (cpm)	
	Toluenized cells	Untreated cells
1.5	628	1536
5	1021	1854
10	1666	1826
20	3432	2698
40	3688	3090

Recipient cells, prepared as described in Materials and Methods, were divided in two, and one half was treated with toluene. Both toluenized and untreated cells were resuspended in the complete reaction mixture at a concentration 50-fold that of the original culture and incubated with 10 µg/ml of native [^{3}H]DNA (30,000 cpm/µg) at 37°C. At 1.5, 5, 10, 20, and 40 min incubation, samples were taken into ice-cold buffer [0.1 M potassium phosphate (pH 7.0)-12 mM MgSO$_4$-0.5% glucose-100 µg/ml of calf thymus DNA] with 5-fold dilution, followed by Vortex mixing. Then the cell was washed by centrifugation, and trichloroacetic acid-precipitable radioactivity was counted. Cell numbers in each sample corresponded to 5 ml of original culture.

Omission of other constituents in the reaction mixture had no effect on either the uptake of donor DNA or the recovery of donor transforming activity. These results showed that the toluenized cell took up native transforming DNA, but recombinant formation was ambiguous. This suggests that the transformation process was seriously damaged by toluene treatment at some stage before the formation of recombinant molecules. Absence of physical association between donor DNA and recipient DNA was observed in the toluenized cell by density gradient centrifugation with ^{3}H,[2]H,[15]N-labeled donor DNA. However, when the heavy DNA was used as the donor, after 45 min of incubation at 37°C in a toluenized recipient, the donor transforming activity had a definite shoulder toward a lighter density in a CsCl gradient, although the radioactivity appeared as a single peak at the heavy position. The profiles were reproducible in three different experiments and were essentially the same with

Table 2. Recovery of biological activity in toluenized and untreated cells

Incubation time (min)	Toluenized cells			Untreated cells		
	$\frac{(his^+)-(his^+trp^+)}{trp^+}$	$\frac{his^+trp^+}{trp^+}$	$\frac{his^+trp^+}{his^+}$	$\frac{(his^+)-(his^+trp^+)}{trp^+}$	$\frac{his^+trp^+}{trp^+}$	$\frac{his^+trp^+}{his^+}$
10	1008×10^{-7}	22.4×10^{-7}	0.022	852×10^{-7}	88.2×10^{-7}	0.10
20	2419×10^{-7}	31.0×10^{-7}	0.013	1048×10^{-7}	181.7×10^{-7}	0.15
40	6164×10^{-7}	85.6×10^{-7}	0.014	1594×10^{-7}	315.8×10^{-7}	0.17
60	4399×10^{-7}	80.9×10^{-7}	0.018	1624×10^{-7}	384.7×10^{-7}	0.18

The transformation was carried out as described in the legend of Table 1. The washed cells were resuspended in a solution of 0.15 M NaCl-0.1 M EDTA-0.05 M KCN (pH 7.0) and treated with 0.5 mg/ml of lysozyme at 37°C for 10 min. Then the cells were lysed by adding 0.1% sodium dodecyl sulfate followed by protease treatment (0.5 mg/ml) at 50°C for 1.5 hr. The lysate was phenolized once and the extracted DNA was precipitated by ethanol and redissolved in 1/10 SSC. The DNA was incubated with competent culture of his^-trp^- strain, and the transformants were counted by plating on appropriate plates. The donor (his^+) and recombinant (his^+trp^+) transforming activities are normalized to the level of recipient (trp^+) activity in each sample.

Table 3. Effect of ATP on uptake of donor DNA

Incubation time (min)	Complete medium		Complete medium + ATP	
	Incorporation of radioactivity (cpm)	Recovery of biological activity $\left(\dfrac{his^+}{trp^+}\right)$	Incorporation of radioactivity (cpm)	Recovery of biological activity $\left(\dfrac{his^+}{trp^+}\right)$
0	400	220×10^{-7}	400	399×10^{-7}
10	650	1390×10^{-7}	600	907×10^{-7}
20	1200	3250×10^{-7}	750	1791×10^{-7}
30	1250	4910×10^{-7}	950	2142×10^{-7}
40	1300	4800×10^{-7}	1000	3080×10^{-7}

The transformation was carried out as described in the legend of Table 1, using toluene-treated recipient cells. Uptake of [^{3}H]DNA and recovery of donor transforming activity were measured as described in Tables 1 and 2 in the presence or absence of ATP. Each sample contained cells corresponding to 2 ml of original culture.

or without ATP. The first peak, at the heavy position, had the
majority of radioactivity from the donor DNA, but the specific
activity of transformation was less than 20% that of the original
DNA. This may suggest that this fraction contained an intermediate
reported by Dubnau and Davidoff-Abelson (1971), which was observed
in periplasm as a double-stranded structure with low transforming
activity. The shoulder at intermediate density retained original
transforming activity. The lighter density of this DNA was not
due to a complex with light recipient DNA or to repair DNA synthesis
but probably was caused by complexing with protein or membrane
material. The role of this DNA on bacterial transformation is not
clear. It could be either an intermediate state of donor DNA or a
nonspecific complex.

Thus, there was no evidence that the toluenized cell performed
the transformation event within the membrane. As toluene is known
to attack lipid components of membranes, making cells permeable to
small compounds, there are several possible explanations: (1)
integrity of the membrane was required for transformation, (2)
essential small compound(s) leaked out from toluene-treated cells,
or (3) toluene denatured essential enzyme(s) or structure(s). In
all cases it is possible that the toluene treatment damaged only
the process required for passage of donor DNA through the membrane
and had no effect on the subsequent recombination events. To
clarify this point, the following experiment was done. The recipient cells were exposed to $^3H^2H^{15}N$-labeled donor DNA at 37°C. After
various *in vivo* incubation times (3, 8, 15, 20, and 40 min), samples
were taken and toluenized at 0°C as described in Materials and
Methods. The toluenized cell suspension was divided into two samples; one was kept on ice in 0.05 M KCN (0 min sample) and the other
was incubated in the complete reaction mixture at 30°C for 40 min
(40 min sample). The size and density of the donor DNA of each
sample were examined by sucrose and CsCl gradient centrifugations.
The donor-recipient complex was found in the 0 min sample after 15
min *in vivo* incubation and increased with time of *in vivo* incubation. However, the amount of donor-recipient complex was not
increased by the 40 min *in vitro* incubation in any of the samples.
These results show that the toluene treatment immediately stopped
the transformation events regardless of the state of the donor DNA.

Our study showed that the toluene treatment seriously damaged
the transformation process except for the early event of entrance
of donor DNA into periplasm. In this connection, Sueoka *et al.*
(1973) showed that there was no initiation of new rounds of chromosome replication in toluenized *B. subtilis* cells, where the normal
elongation synthesis was observed. It was pointed out that the
membrane attachment of the replication origin and terminus may be
relevant in regard to this result. It seems reasonable that at
least some of the major reasons for the present results involve
damage of the membrane of recipient cells. The involvement of

membranous material in the bacterial transformation was suggested
also by Nester and Dooley (1973) and Vermeulen and Venema (1974).

ACKNOWLEDGMENTS

This work has been supported by National Institutes of Health
Grant GM20352 and National Science Foundation Grant GB40090X.

REFERENCES

Cahn, F. H. and M. S. Fox. 1968. Fractionation of transformable
bacteria from competent cultures of *Bacillus subtilis* on renografin
gradients. J. Bacteriol. 95: 867.

Davidoff-Abelson, R. and D. Dubnau. 1973a. Conditions affecting
the isolation from transformed cells of *Bacillus subtilis* of high-
molecular-weight single-stranded deoxyribonucleic acid of donor
origin. J. Bacteriol. 116: 146.

Davidoff-Abelson, R. and D. Dubnau. 1973b. Kinetic analysis of
the products of donor deoxyribonucleate in transformed cells of
Bacillus subtilis. J. Bacteriol. 116: 154.

Dubnau, D. and R. Davidoff-Abelson. 1971. Fate of transforming
DNA following uptake by competent *Bacillus subtilis*. I. Formation
and properties of the donor-recipient complex. J. Mol. Biol. 56:
209.

Fox, M. S. and M. K. Allen. 1964. On the mechanism of deoxyribonucleate integration in pneumococcal transformation. Proc. Nat.
Acad. Sci. U.S.A. 52: 412.

Lacks, S. 1962. Molecular fate of DNA in genetic transformation
of pneumococcus. J. Mol. Biol. 5: 119.

Matsushita, T. and N. Sueoka. 1971. Chromosome replication in
toluenized *Bacillus subtilis* cells. Nature New Biol. 232: 111.

Nester, E. W., M. Schafer and J. Lederberg. 1963. Gene linkage
in DNA transfer: a cluster of genes concerned with aromatic biosynthesis in *Bacillus subtilis*. Genetics 48: 529.

Nester, E. W. and D. C. Dooley. 1973. DNA-membrane interactions
in the *B. subtilis* transformation system. In (L. J. Archer, ed.)
Bacterial Transformation. p. 183. Academic Press Inc., New York.

Notani, N. and S. H. Goodgal. 1966. On the nature of recombinants
formed during transformation in *Haemophilus influenzae*. J. Gen.

Physiol. <u>49</u>: 197.

Piechowska, M. and M. S. Fox.   1971.   Fate of transforming deoxyribonucleate in *Bacillus subtilis*.   J. Bacteriol. <u>108</u>: 680.

Strauss, N.   1970.   Early energy-dependent step in the entry of
transforming deoxyribonucleic acid.   J. Bacteriol. <u>101</u>: 35.

Sueoka, N., T. Matsushita, S. Ohi, A. O'Sullivan and K. White.
1973.   In vivo and in vitro chromosome replication in *Bacillus
subtilis*.   In (R. D. Wells and R. B. Inman, eds.) DNA Synthesis
in Vitro.   p. 385.   University Park Press, Baltimore.

Vermeulen, C. A. and G. VENEMA.   1974.   Electron microscope and
autoradiographic study of ultrastructural aspects of competence
and deoxyribonucleic acid absorption in *Bacillus subtilis*: Localization of uptake and of transport of transforming deoxyribonucleic
acid in competent cells.   J. Bacteriol. <u>118</u>: 342.

TRANSFORMATION IN *HAEMOPHILUS INFLUENZAE*

J. Eugene LeClerc[1] and Jane K. Setlow[2]

The University of Tennessee-Oak Ridge Graduate School of

Biomedical Sciences, and Biology Division, Oak Ridge

National Laboratory, Oak Ridge, Tennessee

One of the problems in understanding the mechanism of transformation in *Haemophilus influenzae* has been that no significant amount of single-strand donor DNA has been found following entrance of the transforming DNA into the competent cell (Notani and Goodgal, 1966). Therefore it has been difficult to imagine how specific pairing and integration could occur. We have attempted to investigate (1) the structure of DNA synthesized in competent cells, (2) the structure of transforming DNA after its entrance into the cell, and (3) the interaction between transforming DNA and recipient cell DNA, in the strains listed in Table 1, in order to assess the effects of various mutations on the recombination process.

The results indicate that in strains that permit interaction between transforming DNA and cell DNA, the competent cells contain newly synthesized DNA with single-strand gaps and tails, and that, in all the strains of Table 1, transforming DNA becomes partially single-stranded following uptake into the cell. When the transforming DNA interacts at the site of the single-stranded regions in one strand of the recipient DNA, the strand synthesized before the competence regime begins is broken, except in the strain KW31, which lacks an ATP-dependent nuclease.

Present Addresses:
    [1]Department of Biological Chemistry, Harvard Medical School, Boston, Massachusetts.
    [2]Department of Biology, Brookhaven National Laboratory, Upton, New York.

187

Table 1. Properties of *Haemophilus influenzae* strains

	Relative transformation frequency	Relative phage recombination	References
wild type (strain *Rd*)	1	1	
rec1	10^{-6}	none observable	Setlow *et al.*, 1972
rec2	10^{-7}	none observable	Notani *et al.*, 1972
dna9	1	—	K. L. Beattie and J. E. LeClerc, unpublished data
KW31	0.5-1.0	0.5	Wilcox and Smith, 1974

All the strains when competent take up approximately the same amount of transforming DNA from the medium. All the mutations except that of *rec2* have been transformed into the wild-type strain free of the mutagenized background. Strain *rec2* came from a culture that was not mutagen treated.

Fig. 1 shows sedimentation patterns in alkaline sucrose of DNA from competent and noncompetent wild-type, and also competent *rec2* and *rec1*, cells. The DNA was labeled during two to three cell divisions before the competence regime with [^{14}C]dThd and pulse-labeled at the peak of competence or in exponential growth with [^{3}H]dThd. In the competent wild-type cells, the pulse label is mostly in DNA of single-strand molecular weight about 5×10^7. However, the prelabeled DNA sediments at a position representing a single-strand molecular weight of about 2×10^8. The DNA of exponentially growing wild-type cells also shows no peak comparable to the pulse-label peak in competent cells. Furthermore the DNA of competent *rec2* cells also does not contain comparable breaks in the newly synthesized DNA, although competent *rec1* cells do. Since it was previously shown (Notani *et al.*, 1972) that transforming DNA interacts with recipient DNA in competent wild-type and *rec1* but not in *rec2* cells, we conclude that the single-strand breaks in the DNA of wild-type and *rec1* cells are important for an early step in recombination.

Further evidence for the biological significance of single-strand breaks in competent cells has been obtained by a comparison of transformation frequencies and sedimentation patterns in alkali of DNA from wild-type cells exposed to various amounts of inosine during the competence regime. Miller and Huang (1972) have shown that inosine inhibits the development of competence in *H. influenzae*. Fig. 2 shows that there is a dramatic decrease in transformation with increasing amounts of inosine, and also a decrease in the fraction of pulse-labeled DNA containing single-strand breaks. This experiment indicates that inosine inhibits the formation of the DNA with structural features promoting recombination.

Benzoylated, naphthoylated DEAE-cellulose (BND-cellulose) column chromatography permits the separation of double-stranded DNA containing single-strand regions from completely double-stranded DNA (Iyer and Rupp, 1971). Fig. 3 shows the results of BND-cellulose chromatography on DNA of wild-type cells labeled before competence and pulse-labeled at the peak of competence or in exponential growth. About 75% of the pulse-labeled DNA and 30% of the prelabeled DNA from the competent cells elutes from the column at a position indicating single-strand regions in the DNA. DNA from wild-type exponentially growing cells shows little material in this region, and neither does the DNA from competent *rec2* cells.

Further information on the structure of DNA that elutes from the BND-cellulose columns in a position indicating single-strand regions has been obtained with the use of SI nuclease isolated from *Aspergillus oryzae* (Ando, 1966). This enzyme has no detectable effect on native *H. influenzae* DNA isolated from exponentially

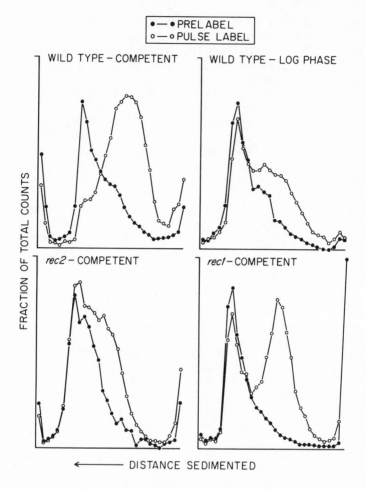

Figure 1.   Alkaline sucrose sedimentation patterns of DNA from cells
made competent in MIV medium (Steinhart and Herriott, 1968) following labeling for 80 to 120 min in Brain Heart Infusion growth medium
(Setlow *et al*., 1968) with [^{14}C]dThd, and pulse-labeled for 10 min
in MIV medium at the peak of competence.   During the 100 min of the
competence regime in nonradioactive MIV medium, the DNA increased
by a factor of 1.8, as measured by the method of Ceriotti (1952).
Exponentially growing wild-type cells were similarly labeled with
[^{14}C]dThd, and pulse-labeled for 10 min.   Cells were lysed following centrifugation and resuspension in 10 mM Tris-HCl (pH 7.6), 1
mM EDTA, by placing 0.1 ml of cell suspension in 0.1 ml 0.5 N NaOH
on top of a 5-20% sucrose gradient at pH 12 containing 0.1 M NaCl.
Sedimentation was in a Beckman SW50.1 rotor in an L350 centrifuge
at 30,000 rpm for 100 min.   Estimation of molecular weights from
sedimentation distance was made according to previously described
methods (Randolph and Setlow, 1972).

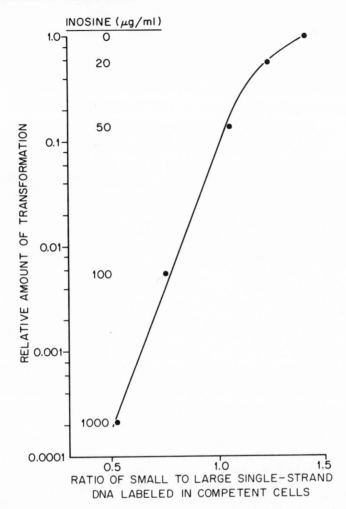

Figure 2. The effect of inosine in the MIV competence medium on
transformation and DNA structure. After cells were submitted to
the competence regime (100 min in MIV medium containing the amounts
of inosine shown), they were either pulse-labeled with [³H]dThd as
described in Fig. 1 or exposed to transforming DNA, and the transformation frequency was assayed as previously described (Setlow *et
al.*, 1968). DNA from the labeled cells was sedimented in alkali as
in Fig. 1. Counts in the high- and intermediate-molecular-weight
fractions from the gradients were added to determine the ratio of
the two types of single-strand material present.

growing or stationary cells but degrades denatured DNA and single-
strand regions in double-stranded DNA (Sutton, 1971). The material
eluted from the columns has been treated with the enzyme. If the

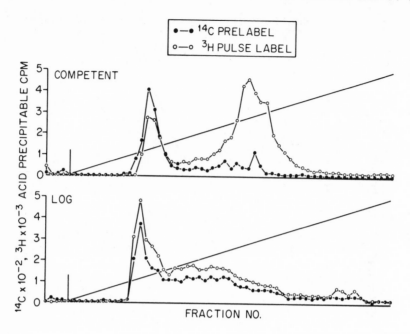

Figure 3.   Benzoylated naphthoylated DEAE–cellulose column chromatography of DNA from competent or exponentially growing wild-type
cells labeled as in Fig. 1 and lysed as previously described (Iyer
and Rupp, 1971).   The gradient was 0-2% caffeine and 0.3-1.0 M
NaCl.

newly replicated DNA (labeled with [^{3}H]dThd) has the structure
shown on the top left of Fig. 4, the SI nuclease should only degrade
the single-strand tails of the ^{3}H-labeled DNA.   If the structure
is as shown on the top right, only the ^{14}C-(pre)labeled strand
should be affected.   What we actually find is that both strands are
affected.   Our interpretation is that the newly replicated DNA in
competent wild-type or *rec*1 cells contains both single-strand tails
and gaps, as shown schematically in the bottom part of Fig. 4.

        The observation of single-strand gaps in the DNA of competent
cells can explain the extra sensitivity to ultraviolet light (UV)
previously seen in competent wild-type but not in competent exci-
sion-defective strains, compared to exponential or stationary-phase
cells (Beattie and Setlow, 1969).   Competent *rec*1 cells are also
more UV-sensitive, but *rec*2 cells show the same UV sensitivity at
competence as in exponential phase (data not shown).   The increased
sensitivity at competence of excision-proficient strains with gaps
in their DNA is reasonable, since a pyrimidine dimer in a single-
strand region would not be expected to be reparable by the excision

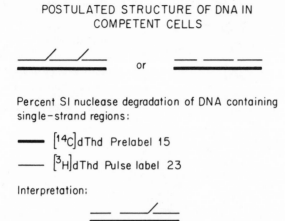

Figure 4. Possible structures of newly replicated DNA in competent wild-type cells (top). DNA from competent cells labeled as in Fig. 1 was subjected to BND-cellulose column chromatography (Fig. 3), and fractions from the righthand peak were collected, dialyzed overnight against 0.01 M NaCl, and exposed to SI nuclease from *Aspergillus oryzae* prepared as described previously (Sutton, 1971). The reaction mixture was essentially as described (Sutton, 1971), except that the final NaCl concentration was 0.2 M. Samples from the mixture of enzyme and DNA were taken at intervals, and the acid-insoluble counts were assayed. The data shown were from samples following maximum degradation (15 min).

---

mechanism (Setlow and Setlow, 1972). A pyrimidine dimer in a single-strand tail might be expected to interfere with subsequent DNA synthesis, since dimers inhibit nucleolytic degradation (Setlow *et al.*, 1964), which would presumably be necessary to remove the tails before normal replication could proceed.

INTERACTION OF TRANSFORMING DNA AND RECIPIENT DNA

Steinhart and Herriott (1968) showed that labeled DNA synthesized before the competence regime in wild-type cells releases its label into the medium as a result of the exposure of competent cells to transforming DNA. As shown schematically in Fig. 5, we have measured this release from cells prelabeled with [^{14}C]dThd and pulse-labeled with [^{3}H]dThd after they have become competent. Assuming that the specific release of label in response to transforming DNA represents displacement of recipient DNA as a result of the interaction between the DNAs, then release will be either from the ^{3}H or the ^{14}C strand, depending upon which strand the transforming DNA enters. The results for wild type, *rec1*, and *rec2* are

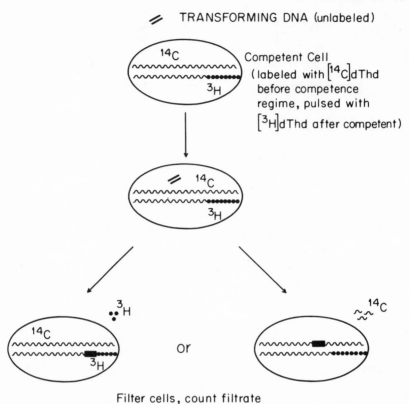

Figure 5.   Schematic diagram of an experiment with results shown in
Fig. 6.   Cells were labeled as in Fig. 1, washed to remove extracellular label, and exposed to a saturating amount of unlabeled
transforming DNA.   After various incubation times, the cells were
put onto 0.45-μm Millipore filters, and the radioactivity in the
filtrate was measured in a scintillation counter.   The total incorporated label was determined as acid-insoluble radioactivity of the
mixture before filtration in order to calculate the fraction of
incorporated label released from the cell DNA into the medium.

seen in Fig. 6, plotted in terms of the fraction of total acid-
insoluble counts at the start of the experiment, after the pulse
of [3H]dThd, against time of incubation of the cells.   In the wild
type there is a slow, nonspecific release of label from cells not
exposed to transforming DNA, and considerably more release of both
labels in response to the transforming DNA.   In the two mutants, the
release is the same with or without the exposure to transforming DNA.
Although the amount of DNA synthesized during the pulse represents
less than 4% of the single-strand genome, in the wild type there is

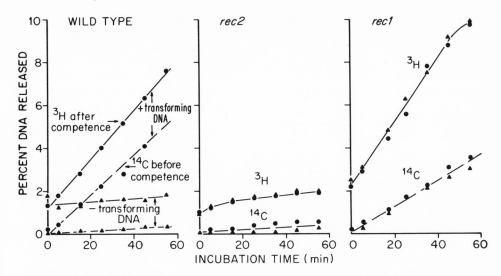

Figure 6. Release of label from DNA of competent cells exposed to
transforming DNA (•) or to M/15 phosphate buffer, pH 7, used as a
diluent for the DNA (▲). Cells were prelabeled with [14C]dThd
(----) and pulse-labeled with [3H]dThd (——) after the competence
regime. Schematic diagram of the experiment is shown in Fig. 5.

a relatively large amount of specific release of ^{3}H label, suggesting
that recombination may occur in the region of the DNA containing
single-strand gaps and tails. The fact that specific release of
both prelabeled and pulse-labeled DNA occurs further suggests that
a single strand of donor DNA can be integrated into either the prelabeled strand or the strand labeled at competence. In *rec2*, in
which there is no association of donor DNA and recipient DNA (Notani
et al., 1972), the release of both labels is similar to those
observed in wild-type cells not exposed to transforming DNA.
However, the release of label from *rec1* cells, whether or not transforming DNA has entered the cell, is considerably greater than the
nonspecific release in wild-type cells, suggesting that there is
degradation at the site of the broken strand synthesized during the
competence regime.

For further information on the interaction of transforming DNA
and cell DNA, experiments shown schematically in Fig. 7 were performed on mutants and wild type cells. Transforming DNA labeled
with 32P was taken up by competent cells, labeled with [3H]dThd
either before or after the competence regime. After various times
of incubation of cells with transforming DNA followed by DNase
treatment, the cells were either lysed on top of an alkaline sucrose
gradient or lysed before neutral sucrose sedimentation. Fig. 8 shows

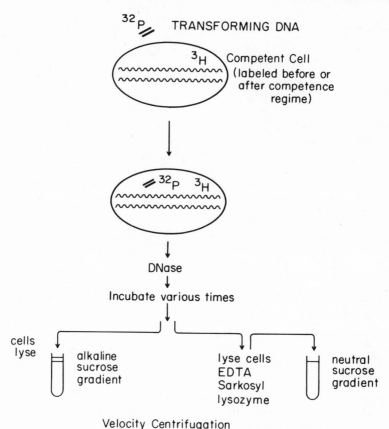

Figure 7.   Schematic diagram of experiments illustrated by Figs. 8,
9, 10, 11, and Table 2.

---

alkaline sucrose profiles for wild type, *rec2*, and *rec1* for two
times of incubation following entrance of transforming DNA into
cells labeled before competence.   In the wild type, breaks are
apparent in the strand labeled before competence as a result of
interaction with transforming DNA, whereas the prelabeled strand
contains little or no material sedimenting at an intermediate position in the gradient when the cells have not been exposed to transforming DNA (Fig. 1).   After 30 min almost all the transforming DNA
label is covalently associated with cell DNA that sediments in
alkaline sucrose as single-strand pieces in the position of pulsed
DNA (Fig. 1).   In competent *rec2*, which contains no DNA with single-
strand regions (Fig. 1), there is no interaction between transforming DNA and cell DNA, and no breakage of the prelabeled cell DNA.
In competent *rec1*, which does contain DNA with tails and gaps, the
interaction between the DNAs is hardly visible at 0 time, but by 30

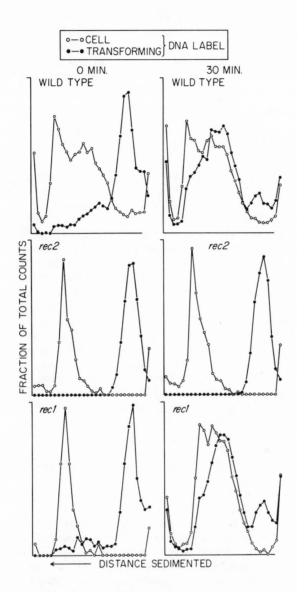

Figure 8. Alkaline sucrose sedimentation patterns of DNA from cells labeled with [3H]dThd for three cell generations before the competence regime and exposed to 32P-labeled transforming DNA after they had become competent. The experimental procedure is outlined in Fig. 7. Sedimentation was carried out as in Fig. 1. Time 0 means after the uptake of transforming DNA and 2 min treatment with 50 μg/ml DNase.

min again some of the prelabeled strands are broken; the transforming DNA has formed covalent bonds with the recipient DNA, and
sediments mostly in an intermediate position, suggesting linkage
with the broken prelabeled strand and/or the strand synthesized
during the competence regime containing single-strand tails and
gaps.

THE ROLE OF DNA SYNTHESIS IN THE INTERACTION OF
TRANSFORMING DNA AND RECIPIENT DNA

Experiments similar to those of Figs. 7 and 8 have been performed with strain $dna9$, a mutant temperature-sensitive for DNA
synthesis. In this strain, incorporation of [^{3}H]dThd shuts off
within 2-3 min when the temperature is raised to 41°C and resumes
at the normal rate when the temperature is shifted back to 36°C,
provided that the time at 41°C has been no more than about 90 min.
After uptake of transforming DNA at 36°C, the cells were incubated
either at the permissive or the restrictive temperature for DNA
synthesis. Alkaline sucrose profiles are shown in Fig. 9, from
which two conclusions may be drawn: (1) Covalent association of
transforming DNA with cell DNA takes place without DNA synthesis.
(2) At the restrictive temperature the transforming DNA goes into
larger-molecular-weight DNA much more rapidly than when DNA synthesis is taking place. Thus, after 30 min at 36°C there is a considerable amount of transforming DNA covalently associated with
recipient DNA of intermediate molecular weight, but at the restrictive temperature almost all the associated transforming DNA is in
high-molecular-weight DNA by 30 min.

NONCOVALENT ASSOCIATION OF TRANSFORMING DNA AND RECIPIENT DNA

A summary of the alkaline and neutral gradient information for
$dna9$ is shown in Fig. 10, in which the percent associated donor DNA
is plotted against time at the permissive or restrictive temperatures. There is more association seen in the neutral gradients
(double-strand) than in the alkaline gradients (single-strand),
especially at early times, suggesting that some of the transforming
DNA is held in place only by hydrogen bonds. At 30 min about 90%
of the associated donor DNA is covalently bonded, as judged by the
ratio of association seen in alkaline and neutral gradients. Similar results were obtained with the wild type and with $rec1$.

EFFECT OF THE $rec1$ MUTATION ON INTERACTION
OF DONOR AND RECIPIENT DNA

We have already shown that competent $rec1$ cells contain DNA
with gaps and tails, and that there is some DNA breakdown in such

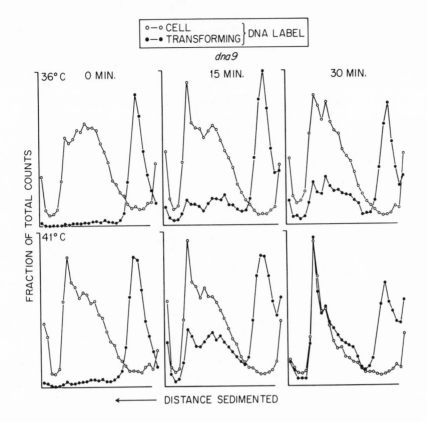

Figure 9. Alkaline sucrose sedimentation patterns of DNA from *dna*9 cells treated as in Fig. 8, except that following uptake of DNA at 36°C the mixture of cells and transforming DNA was exposed to DNase for 2 min either at 36°C or at 41°C. Samples were removed following DNase treatment (time 0), and incubation of the remaining mixtures was continued at these temperatures for further sampling at the times shown.

---

cells, presumably at the sites of the single-strand regions in the DNA (Fig. 6). The double mutant *dna*9*rec*1 has been constructed, and experiments of the type in Fig. 7 have been done with incubation of the double mutant at the permissive (36°C) or restrictive (41°C) temperature for DNA synthesis, following uptake of transforming DNA at 36°C. Table 2 shows some of the results, in comparison with results of similar experiments with the single mutant *dna*9. In neither strain is there appreciable covalent association of donor label at time 0 (see Fig. 9 for *dna*9 at this time). However, in both strains at 30 min there is covalent association of donor label even in the absence of DNA synthesis. This result in *dna*9*rec*1 eliminates the possibility that the association of donor label seen

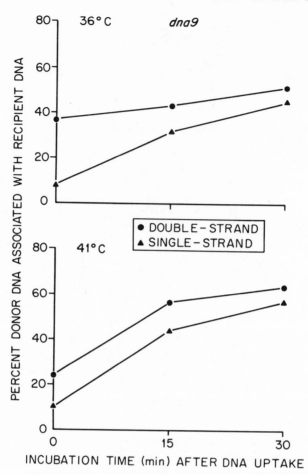

Figure 10. Association of ^{32}P label from transforming DNA with ^{3}H label from cell DNA as a function of time of incubation following uptake of DNA into the cell and 2 min treatment with DNase. Experimental procedure as in Figs. 7 and 9. Sedimentation in alkaline gradients (single-strand) was at 30,000 rpm for 100 min, and in neutral gradients (double-strand) was at 20,000 rpm for 180 min. For determination of the fraction of associated donor label, ^{32}P counts were added together from each of the two parts of the gradients of Fig. 9 and from the corresponding neutral gradients.

---

in the *rec*1 mutant is caused by degradation of transforming DNA followed by resynthesis into recipient DNA. Furthermore, two new phenomena are seen: (1) At neither the permissive nor the restrictive temperature is there appreciable transforming DNA covalently associated with high-molecular-weight DNA in *dna*9*rec*1, unlike the

Table 2. Calculations from sucrose gradient data (30 min incubation)*

| | | Alkaline sucrose | | Neutral sucrose |
| | | % of transforming DNA associated with recipient DNA | | |
Strain	Temp.	Of high molecular weight	Of intermediate molecular weight	M_w (x 10^{-8})
dna9rec1	36°C	4	20	3.5
	41°C	2	20	1.5
dna9	36°C	10	31	3.5
	41°C	31	18	3.8

*Experiments were of the type shown in Fig. 7.

situation in the single mutant $dna9$.   (2) At the restrictive temperature double-strand breaks are formed in the recipient DNA of
the double mutant as a result of the interaction of transforming
DNA.   Such breaks are not seen in the DNA of this strain without
the exposure to transforming DNA.   We conclude that the degradation
that presumably occurs at the site of association of transforming
DNA with recipient DNA in $rec1$, seen from the release data (Fig.
6), prevents the associated transforming DNA from going into high-
molecular-weight recipient DNA, and that this degradation, in the
absence of DNA synthesis, together with the break made in the
strand synthesized before the competence regime, causes the recipient DNA to come apart.

THE ROLE OF THE ATP-DEPENDENT NUCLEASE IN
INTERACTION OF DONOR AND RECIPIENT DNA

Strain KW31 lacks ATP-dependent nuclease (Wilcox and Smith,
1974), which has been extensively studied by Friedman and Smith
(1972, 1973).   This strain behaves like wild type in that the DNA
of competent cells shows sedimentation profiles like those of Fig.
1 for wild type and $rec1$.   Transformation and phage recombination
are only slightly depressed in this strain (Table 1), and association of transforming DNA with recipient DNA, as judged by the
experiment outlined diagrammatically in Fig. 7, is almost as high
as in wild-type cells.   The one striking difference between the
sedimentation profiles of transforming KW31 and wild type concerns
the DNA labeled before the competence regime, which in wild type
shows some material sedimenting at an intermediate position in
alkaline gradients after the introduction of transforming DNA (Fig.
8).   Fig. 11 shows such sedimentation profiles of prelabeled cell
DNA in alkali from KW31 and wild type, after association with
transforming DNA.   In KW31 the DNA is not broken as it is in the
wild type.   This result led us to postulate that in strain KW31
transforming DNA could only be inserted into the gapped strand.
Our evidence that in wild-type cells the non-gapped strand is broken as a result of the interaction of transforming DNA with cell
DNA suggested that it might be possible to have insertion of two
linked markers from transforming DNA into two different strands of
recipient DNA during the same recombination event.   We further predicted that this type of recombination would be impossible in KW31,
because of its inability to break the non-gapped strand.   To
attempt to test these hypothesis, the experiment summarized in
Table 3 was performed.   Cells were exposed to transforming DNA
containing three linked antibiotic-resistance markers (novobiocin,
kanamycin, and streptomycin) and plated without drugs, and colonies
were picked and tested on all combinations of the three antibiotics.
We considered that clones that contained cells resistant to two
different antibiotics, but that did not contain any doubly transformed cells, might reflect an initial transformation event in

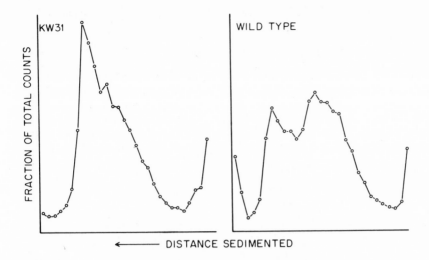

Figure 11. Alkaline sucrose sedimentation patterns of DNA from wild-type or KW31 cells prelabeled with [³H]dThd for three cell generations before the competence regime, exposed to transforming DNA after they had become competent, and then incubated 15 min before lysis on alkaline sucrose gradients. Sedimentation was as in Fig. 1.

----

which two linked markers went into two different strands of recipient DNA. We found four wild-type clones of this kind, but none from KW31. Unfortunately, the statistics of this experiment leave a great deal to be desired, since only about 4,000 clones were isolated and tested. Nevertheless we believe that the results are at least suggestive, and the number of mixed clones found from the wild-type population appears to represent too high a fraction of the transformants to be accounted for in terms of a second transformation event. From the data shown in Table 3 we can by no means exclude the possibility of such mixed clones in KW31.

DISCUSSION AND MODEL

Fig. 12 shows our model of how transformation works in *H. influenzae*. The recipient DNA is shown with single-strand tails and gaps in the newly synthesized strand. We have presented evidence that the *rec2+* gene must be present for the formation of this structure. The transforming DNA, indicated by the heavy lines, is shown with single-stranded ends. We have assumed this structure from experiments in which labeled transforming DNA, which is unaffected by SI nuclease before it enters the cell, becomes 10-15% degradable with this enzyme after it enters the cell, including all

Table 3.   Drug-resistant transformants from nonselected clones*

Drug	Number of clones containing drug-resistant cells		Number of clones also containing K-resistant cells but no double transformants	
	Wild type	KW31	Wild type	KW31
N	24	14	3	0
S	18	27	1	0
K	39	13		
NK	0	3		
KS	2	2		
NS	0	0		
NKS	1	5		

*Competent cells were exposed to DNA containing linked drug markers and were plated nonselectively. Clones were tested individually for the seven possible combinations of markers. Genetic map: N KS.   Abbreviations: N, novobiocin; S, streptomycin; K, kanomycin.

the mutants of Table 1. All we know about the enzyme responsible for the change in structure of the transforming DNA upon entry is that it is not the ATP-dependent nuclease, since the result is the same in KW31, which lacks this enzyme. The single-strand ends of the transforming DNA can pair either with the single-strand tail of the recipient DNA or at the gap, before covalent bonds are formed between the two DNAs. We postulate that rarely, as in the example shown in Fig. 12, is there pairing at both sites. Covalent bonds are first formed between the transforming DNA and the gapped strand of recipient DNA. A break is made by the ATP-dependent nuclease in the recipient strand, which was originally without gaps or tails. It is of interest that a similar endonucleolytic function with a similar substrate has been postulated for the *recBC* nuclease in *Escherichia coli* (A. J. Clark, this volume). In the double mutant *dna9rec1*, in which there is degradation at the site of the breaks in recipient DNA, we presume that it is the break made by the ATP-

MODEL FOR TRANSFORMATION IN *Haemophilus influenzae*

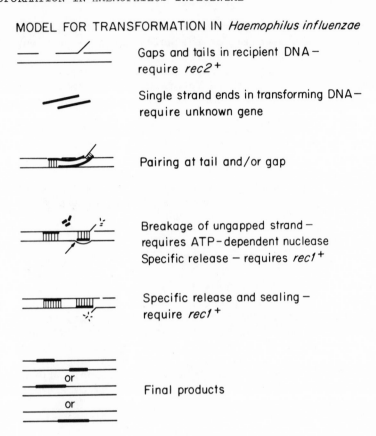

Gaps and tails in recipient DNA — require *rec2*[+]

Single strand ends in transforming DNA — require unknown gene

Pairing at tail and/or gap

Breakage of ungapped strand — requires ATP-dependent nuclease
Specific release — requires *rec1*[+]

Specific release and sealing — require *rec1*[+]

Final products

Figure 12. Model for the postulated mechanism of interaction of transforming DNA (▬▬) and cell DNA (———) in *H. influenzae*.

---

dependent nuclease that, in the absence of DNA synthesis, causes a double-strand break in the recipient DNA.

As the transforming DNA, hydrogen-bonded to the tailed piece of recipient DNA, displaces the originally ungapped strand, pieces of recipient DNA are released from both strands, and there is also degradation of the transforming DNA that will not become integrated. There is little or no such degradation in *rec2* (Notani *et al.*, 1972), suggesting that transforming DNA is degraded as a consequence of its interaction with cell DNA, since *rec2* shows no such interaction. Note that part of the originally gapped recipient strand is further degraded at a site different from where the transforming DNA enters. The release of recipient DNA pieces from the originally ungapped strand, on the other hand, is postulated to result from a direct displacement by the single strand of transforming DNA. We have shown that the *rec1*[+] gene is required for release of recipient

label from both strands as a result of the interaction of the two
DNAs. The beginning of sealing of the holes takes place along with
the specific release. Our data suggest that the original gapped
strand is sealed first, and that there is too much degradation in
the *rec*1 mutant at the site of the interaction to permit sealing of
the transforming DNA into high-molecular-weight DNA. We postulate
that when DNA synthesis is taking place in a *rec*1$^+$ strain, the sealing is retarded because of elongation of the tails and the necessity
for subsequent elimination of recipient DNA to accommodate the
longer tails.

The final product can be either a single strand of transforming
DNA inserted into the Watson or the Crick strand, or the postulated
rare staggered insertion into both strands.

ACKNOWLEDGMENTS

We are grateful to Kent Wilcox for his generous gift of strain
KW31, to M. E. Boling, R. Elespuru, B. LeClerc, L. Munchausen, and
B. Sedgwick for help in the clone isolation experiment, to M. E.
Boling for measuring the UV sensitivity of competent *rec*1 and *rec*2,
and to K. L. Beattie and R. F. Kimball for reviewing the manuscript.
J. E. LeClerc is an Oak Ridge Graduate Fellow under appointment from
Oak Ridge Associated Universities. Oak Ridge National Laboratory
is operated by Union Carbide Corporation for the U. S. Atomic Energy
Commission.

REFERENCES

Ando, T. 1966. A nuclease specific for heat-denatured DNA isolated from a product of *Aspergillus oryzae*. Biochim. Biophys. Acta
114: 158.

Beattie, K. L. and J. K. Setlow. 1969. Killing of *Haemophilus
influenzae* cells by integrated ultraviolet-induced lesions from
transforming deoxyribonucleic acid. J. Bacteriol. 100: 1284.

Ceriotti, G. 1952. A microchemical determination of desoxyribo-
nucleic acid. J. Biol. Chem. 198: 297.

Friedman, E. A. and H. O. Smith. 1972. An adenosine triphosphate-
dependent deoxyribonuclease from *Hemophilus influenzae* Rd. J.
Biol. Chem. 247: 2846.

Friedman, E. A. and H. O. Smith. 1973. Production of possible
recombination intermediates by an ATP-dependent DNase. Nature New
Biol. 241: 54.

Iyer, V. N. and W. D. Rupp. 1971. Usefulness of benzoylated naphthoylated DEAE-cellulose to distinguish and fractionate double-stranded DNA bearing different extents of single-stranded regions. Biochim. Biophys. Acta 228: 117.

Miller, D. H. and P. C. Huang. 1972. Identification of competence-repressing factors during log phase growth of *Haemophilus influenzae*. J. Bacteriol. 109: 560.

Notani, N. K. and S. H. Goodgal. 1966. On the nature of recombinants formed during transformation of *Hemophilus influenzae*. J. Gen. Physiol. 49(6, part 2): 197.

Notani, N. K., J. K. Setlow, V. R. Joshi and D. P. Allison. 1972. Molecular basis for the transformation defects in mutants of *Haemophilus influenzae*. J. Bacteriol. 110: 1171.

Randolph, M. L. and J. K. Setlow. 1972. Mechanism of inactivation of *Haemophilus influenzae* transforming deoxyribonucleic acid by sonic radiation. J. Bacteriol. 111: 186.

Setlow, J. K., M. E. Boling, K. L. Beattie and R. F. Kimball. 1972. A complex of recombination and repair genes in *Haemophilus influenzae*. J. Mol. Biol. 68: 361.

Setlow, J. K., D. C. Brown, M. E. Boling, A. Mattingly and M. P. Gordon. 1968. Repair of deoxyribonucleic acid in *Haemophilus influenzae*. J. Bacteriol. 95: 546.

Setlow, R. B., W. L. Carrier and F. J. Bollum. 1964. Nuclease-resistant sequences in ultraviolet-irradiated deoxyribonucleic acid. Biochim. Biophys. Acta 91: 446.

Setlow, R. B. and J. K. Setlow. 1972. Effects of radiation on polynucleotides. Ann. Rev. Biophys. Bioeng. 1: 293.

Steinhart, W. L. and R. M. Herriott. 1968. Fate of recipient deoxyribonucleic acid during transformation in *Haemophilus influenzae*. J. Bacteriol. 96: 1718

Sutton, W. D. 1971. A crude nuclease preparation suitable for use in DNA reassociation experiments. Biochim. Biophys. Acta 240: 522.

Wilcox, K. W. and H. O. Smith. 1974. Isolation and characterization of mutants of *Haemophilus influenzae* deficient in an ATP-dependent DNase activity. J. Bacteriol. in press.

ON THE ROLE OF RESTRICTION ENZYMES OF *HAEMOPHILUS* IN

TRANSFORMATION AND TRANSFECTION

Rosa Gromkova and Sol H. Goodgal

Department of Microbiology, University of Pennsylvania,

Philadelphia, Pennsylvania 19104

For the past few years we have been studying the biological effects of restriction enzymes in *Haemophilus* (Gromkova and Goodgal, 1972; Goodgal and Gromkova, 1973a; Gromkova *et al.*, 1973; Smith and Wilcox, 1970). It has been relatively easy to demonstrate the action of restriction enzymes on DNA *in vitro*; however, it is not so easy to demonstrate that these enzymes function in the same way in the cell. Although DNA restriction has been regarded as a process apart from the phenomenon of recombination, the ability of restriction enzymes to generate unique segments of DNA with specific ends indicates that these enzymes may play an essential role in the recombination process. The *in vitro* construction of biologically functional bacterial plasmids by the use of restriction endonucleases supports this view (Morrow and Berg, 1972; Mertz and Davis, 1972; Cohen *et al.*, 1973). In the experiments presented below, we have attempted to compare the actions of restriction enzymes of *Haemophilus in vitro* and *in vivo* and to draw some general conclusions about the specific restriction systems involved.

The *Haemophilus* system is a particularly good one for studying the biological role of restriction enzymes, since it contains a rich source of restriction enzymes, is an efficient transformation system, and allows one to study the fate of transforming DNA directly both *in vitro* and *in vivo*. The enzymes we have used in this study are in Table 1. For convenience, we have followed the classification system proposed by Boyer (1971) to distinguish enzymes that require ATP, AdoMet and Mg^{2+} from those that require only Mg^{2+}. We have examined the effects of these enzymes *in vitro* on both bacteriophage and bacterial DNA and compared these activities against the cells' ability to accept or reject bacteriophage and bacterial DNA

209

Table 1.   Endo R enzymes

Type I	Type II
Requires ATP, AdoMet, Mg^{2+}	Requires only Mg^{2+}
HindI	HindIII
HinbI	HpaI
	Hae

in transfection and transformation. The enzyme HindI (Gromkova *et al.*, 1973) is an endonuclease that is obtained from restrictive cells of *H. influenzae* and requires ATP and AdoMet. The effects of this enzyme on modified and unmodified phage and prophage DNAs are shown in Table 2. The enzyme inactivates unmodified phage and prophage DNAs; however, modified phage and prophage DNAs are not affected. These results correlate well with the ability of restrictive cells to restrict unmodified DNA and accept modified phage or

Table 2.   The effect of endo R·HindI on the transfecting efficiency of S2 phage and prophage DNAs

DNA	Enzyme Treatment	Recipient	
		19S	2R
S2.19S	+	0.01[a]	–
19S (S2)	+	0.02	–
S2.2R	+	0.8	–
2R (S2)	+	0.9	–
In vivo			
S2.19S	–	1	0.1
19S (S2)	–	1	0.1
S2.2R	–	1	1
2R (S2)	–	1	1

[a] Transfection efficiency

prophage DNA. A similar enzyme HinbI, extracted from *H. influenzae* type b cells (Goodgal and Gromkova, unpublished results), has a different specificity of restriction (Piekarowicz and Glover, 1972) and shows a similar correlation between inactivation *in vitro* of unmodified DNA and the ability to restrict unmodified DNA *in vivo*. The data suggest, therefore, that restrictive cells reject bacterio-phage DNA by means of specific restriction enzymes.

The effect of type 1 restriction enzymes on transforming activity of bacterial DNA is a little more complicated. The results of one experiment are shown in Table 3. It is clear that the enzyme is capable of attacking transforming DNA *in vitro*; however, its efficiency appears to be relatively low. Indeed, the best way of demonstrating this activity is by its effect on relatively long segments of DNA that carry linked markers. We have shown previously that type 1 enzymes make relatively few breaks in unmodified bac-terial DNA, compared to the endo R type 2 enzymes that produce relatively smaller fragments of DNA. Since the fragments produced are large, transforming activities for single markers are poorly inactivated. On the other hand, linked markers are inactivated in proportion to their relative distance apart on the DNA, as shown by a comparison of the effects of this enzyme on the streptomycin-novobiocin linkage group and on the streptomycin-dalacin linkage pair, representing markers that are considerably further apart. Modified DNA, as expected, is not inactivated by this restriction enzyme. In contrast to the restriction *in vitro* there is no evi-dence for restriction of transforming DNA by restrictive compared

Table 3. The effect of endo R·HindI on modified and unmodified transforming DNA in the presence of ATP and AdoMet

Marker	Modified	Unmodified
str	0.8	0.49
nov	0.94	0.61
dal	1.0	0.71
str-nov	1.0	0.16
str-dal	0.79	0.08

to nonrestrictive recipients. These data suggest that the elements
taken up by the cell and subjected to the cell's restriction systems
are still sufficiently large to be integrated efficiently. On the
other hand, it is possible that the bacteriophage DNA can be restricted but that the bacterial DNA is somehow protected from the
action of the restriction system.

Type 2 restriction enzymes do not require ATP and AdoMet but
only magnesium ions. As noted before, these enzymes produce smaller
segments of DNA than the type 1 enzymes when acting on heterologous
bacteriophage or bacterial DNAs. The first system tested utilized
the endo R·HpaI from *Haemophilus parainfluenzae* and S2 bacteriophage DNA from phage grown in the nonrestrictive *H. influenzae*
strain. In testing for *in vivo* restriction we used *H. parainfluenzae* as the recipient. Table 4 shows that endo R·HpaI can completely
inactivate phage and prophage DNA *in vitro*. The *in vivo* effects
are somewhat more complicated, in that the *H. parainfluenzae* recipient appears to be even less restrictive for transfection than the
nonrestrictive *H. influenzae* recipient. Prophage DNA, on the other
hand, is completely restricted by the *H. parainfluenzae* recipient.
In this respect prophage DNA behaves more like bacterial DNA than
like phage DNA. The mechanism of protection of bacteriophage S2
DNA against the action of endo R·HpaI *in vivo* is not clear. Although
the action of type 2 enzymes on bacterial DNA *in vitro* produces
relatively small fragments of DNA, the sizes of these fragments
vary, leading to the preferential survival of some markers over
others (Table 5). The nal^r and nov^r markers that are on relatively
large segments of DNA have survived treatment by HpaI, whereas the
smaller segments of DNA show relatively reduced activity (Goodgal
and Gromkova, 1973a). In heterospecific transformation between *H.
influenzae* and *H. parainfluenzae,* there is considerable variation in
marker survival. The heterospecifically reduced survival of markers
like those for novobiocin and naladixic acid may be explained by the
presence of other endo restriction enzymes in the recipient.

When treated DNA is tested for transformation heterospecifically
it is found that some markers survive with efficiencies higher than
their efficiencies homospecifically. For example, the erythromycin
marker is capable of transforming *H. influenzae* to a much greater
extent than its homospecific recipient *H. parainfluenzae* (Table 6).
The fact that the erythromycin marker survives in the heterospecific
recipient even though its average molecular weight is of the order
of 10^6 suggests that this segment of DNA has somehow preserved the
sites that are required for recombination in *H. influenzae*.

Although it appears that endo R·HpaI may play a role in exclusion of bacterial DNA heterospecifically, the effects of other type
2 restriction enzymes in other *Haemophilus* species raise additional
questions. If one examines the more closely related species *H. in-*

Table 4. The effect of endo R·HpaI on the transfecting activity of S2 phage and prophage DNAs

DNA	Enzyme Treatment	Recipient	
		H. influenzae 19S	*H. parainfluenzae*
S2.19S	+	<0.01	<0.01
19S (S2)	+	<0.01	<0.01
	In vivo		
S2.19S	−	1	3
19S (S2)	−	1	0.005

Table 5. The effect of endo R·HpaI on the transforming activity of *H. influenzae* DNA

Marker	Enzyme Treatment	Activity in Recipient	
		H. influenzae	*H. parainfluenzae*
str	+	<0.01	−
nal	+	2.	−
dal	+	<0.01	−
nov	+	0.9	−
ery	+	<0.01	−
kan	+	<0.01	−
	In vivo (homo- vs. heterospecific transformation)		
str	−	1	0.006
nal	−	1	0.005
dal	−	1	0.05
nov	−	1	0.0008
ery	−	1	0.1
kan	−	1	0.02

Table 6. Effect of endo R·HindIII on the transforming activity of
H. parainfluenzae DNA

	Recipient
Marker	*H. parainfluenzae*	*H. influenzae*
str	<0.01	<0.01
nov	0.1	0.1
ery	<0.01	1.0
nal	0.1	0.1

fluenzae, *H. aegyptius*, and *H. i. Reid* (Goodgal and Gromkova, 1973b),
it is found that their DNAs are sensitive to heterologous type 2
enzymes *in vitro*. For example, it is found that *H. aegyptius* type
2 restriction enzymes will attack *H. influenzae* or *H. i. Reid* DNA
in vitro, or *H. influenzae* type 2 enzymes will attack *H. aegyptius*
or *H. i. Reid* DNA. Each of these three strains, however, acts as
a very efficient recipient for the DNA of each of the others.
These data suggest that *in vivo* either the endo type 2 restriction
enzymes are nonfunctional or a protective mechanism exists for preventing their action. It therefore appears that type 2 enzymes do
not play a role in exclusion of DNA from closely related species,
although they may act on DNA from species that are more distantly
related.

Evidence for a direct role of restriction enzymes in transformation comes from recent experiments on *com⁻*, a mutant of *H. influenzae*
b that has lost its restriction modification function (presumably
by a mutation in its recognition site) and has become transformation
deficient (Caster *et al.*, 1972). Transfer of the r^+m^+ function into
r^-m^- restores competence capacity. It is possible that restriction
and competence represent closely linked genetic elements; so far
they have not been separated. It is of interest that *H. influenzae*
type c contains no type 1 restriction system and is deficient in
transformation.

In summary it may be noted that *Haemophilus* type 1 restriction
enzymes, those that exclude bacteriophage DNA, are strain specific;
i.e., one finds different enzymes in closely related strains. On
the other hand, *Haemophilus* type 2 restriction enzymes that produce
relatively small fragments of DNA are species specific and exert
their action on heterologous DNA but are controlled in the cell to
prevent activity on the DNA of closely related species. In two

cases, now, there is a correlation between the presence or absence of a type 1 restriction function and the ability of cells to transform.

REFERENCES

Boyer, H. 1971. DNA restriction and modification mechanisms in bacteria. Ann. Rev. Microbiol. 25: 153.

Caster, J. H., E. H. Postel and S. H. Goodgal. 1972. Competence mutants: Isolation of transformation deficient strains of *Haemophilus influenzae*. Nature 227: 515.

Cohen, S. N., A. Chang, H. Boyer and R. B. Helling. 1973. Construction of biologically functional bacterial plasmids *in vitro*. Proc. Nat. Acad. Sci. U.S.A. 70: 3640.

Goodgal, S. H. and R. Gromkova. 1973a. Separation of specific segments of transforming DNA after treatment with endodeoxyribonuclease. Proc. Nat. Acad. Sci. U.S.A. 70: 503.

Goodgal, S. and R. Gromkova. 1973b. The biological specificity of *Haemophilus* endodeoxyribonucleases which attack heterologous DNA. In (L. J. Archer, ed.) Bacterial Transformation. Academic Press, London.

Gromkova, R., J. Bendler and S. H. Goodgal. 1973. Restriction and modification of bacteriophage S2 in *Haemophilus influenzae*. J. Bacteriol. 114: 1151.

Gromkova, R. and S. H. Goodgal. 1972. Action of *Haemophilus* endodeoxyribonuclease on biologically active deoxyribonucleic acid. J. Bacteriol. 109: 987.

Mertz, J. and R. W. Davis. 1972. Cleavage of DNA by R_1 restriction endonuclease generated cohesive ends. Proc. Nat. Acad. Sci. U.S.A. 69: 3370.

Morrow, J. and P. Berg. 1972. Cleavage of simian virus 40 DNA at a unique site by a bacterial restriction enzyme. Proc. Nat. Acad. Sci. U.S.A. 69: 3365.

Piekarowicz, A. and S. W. Glover. 1972. Host specificity of DNA in *Haemophilus influenzae*. The two restriction and modification systems in strain R_a. Mol. Gen. Genet. 116: 11.

Smith, H. O. and K. W. Wilcox. 1970. A restriction enzyme from *Haemophilus influenzae* I. Purification and general properties. J. Mol. Biol. 51: 379.

ROLE OF A DEOXYRIBONUCLEASE IN BACTERIAL TRANSFORMATION

Sanford Lacks

Biology Department, Brookhaven National Laboratory,

Upton, New York 11973

In the genetic transformation of *Diplococcus pneumoniae,* donor
DNA is converted to single strands either during or just after its
uptake by the cell (Lacks, 1962). This conversion may be regarded
as the first step in preparation of the DNA for recombination, since
a single-strand segment of donor DNA is ultimately inserted into
recipient cell DNA (Fox and Allen, 1964). In addition to its role
in the recombination process, this step may be an essential part
of the mechanism for DNA entry.

The appearance of donor DNA degradation products within the
cells during uptake of DNA suggests that a cellular DNase facilitates entry of single strands by degrading the complementary strands
(Lacks, 1962). But the internal degradation products do not correspond quantitatively with the amount of single-strand material
(Morrison and Guild, 1972). Oligonucleotide fragments of donor DNA,
however, accumulate outside the cells in amounts about equal to the
DNA taken up (Morrison and Guild, 1973; Lacks and Greenberg, 1973).
A DNase at the surface of the cell could conceivably draw in one
strand of DNA as it repetitively attached to and hydrolyzed the
opposite strand, the products of which would remain outside the
cell.

Pneumococcal cells contain two major DNases: an endonuclease
that hydrolyzes DNA to oligonucleotides and an exonuclease that
produces mononucleotides (Lacks and Greenberg, 1967). Endonuclease-
deficient (*end*) mutants were selected by a DNase plate assay in
which colonies are grown in agar containing DNA and methyl green
(Lacks, 1970). Around normal colonies, a colorless zone appears
after 30 h incubation, due to degradation of the surrounding DNA.

217

Around *end* mutants at this time the blue color persists. However, after 54 h colorless zones appear, due to the exonuclease, and exonuclease-deficient (*exo*) mutants were selected at this time. The *end,exo* strains originally examined were normally transformable, and donor DNA underwent its usual fate with the cells (Lacks, 1970). One such strain, R6endlexo2, was selected as a point of departure for further mutation that might affect transformability.

TRANSFORMATION-DEFECTIVE MUTANTS

Mutants defective in transformation were selected by two different procedures, called NOZ and NTR. The NOZ procedure was based on the observation that R6endlexo2 colonies still formed small colorless zones in the DNase plate assay after 4 days of incubation. Clones that gave no zones at this time were selected. In the NTR procedure, clones were screened for transformation on agar plates as previously described (Lacks and Greenberg, 1973).

Two classes of defective mutants were obtained. One class, called *noz* because most of its members were selected by the NOZ procedure, shows reduced transformability, generally to ∿0.1% of normal (but in one mutant to ∿10% of normal). Uptake of [^{32}P]DNA into a form resistant to externally added DNase is also very much reduced. However, the *noz* mutants bind considerable amounts of donor DNA to the outside of cells, in a DNase-susceptible form. This binding requires the presence of sugar and the prior activation of the cells by competence factor (Lacks *et al.*, 1974). Another class of mutants, called *ntr*, fail to give any transformants (<0.01% of normal), and neither binds DNA to the outside nor takes it up into the cell. Table 1 lists properties of mutants typical of the two classes. The mutations exert similar effects when transferred to another strain (also *endl,exo2*) as they do in the original mutant strains.

DNase CONTENT OF MUTANTS

Fractionation of DNase activity in extracts of normal strains reveals three enzymes: an endonuclease, an exonuclease, and a less active polymerase-exonuclease (Lacks, 1970). Gently prepared extracts of *endl,exo2* strains contain residual DNases which fractionate similarly to the normal endonuclease and exonuclease (Lacks *et al.*, 1974). Both the normal and residual endonucleases produce oligonucleotides similar in size to the fragments found outside cells after DNA uptake.

Table 2 compares the DNase contents of mutant strains with those of their normally transformable progenitors. Mutants of the

Table 1. Properties of transformation -defective strains

Strain[a]	Selection procedure	Relevant genotype	Transform- ability[b]	Binding[c] of DNA	Uptake[d] of DNA
Mo*end*1*exo*2	–	normal	2.4	6	23
T6*trt*1*hex*4	–	normal	2.1	3	20
R6*end*1*exo*2*ntr*11	NOZ	*noz*-11	0.02	24	2
T6*trt*1*hex*4*noz*11	NOZ	*noz*-11	0.06	16	4
R6*end*1*exo*2*ntr*19	NOZ	*noz*-19	0.007	55	2
T6*trt*1*hex*4*noz*19	NOZ	*noz*-19	0.005	23	2
Mo*end*1*exo*2*ntr*48	–	*noz*-48	0.003	38	2
T6*trt*1*hex*4*ntr*48	NTR	*noz*-48	0.003	35	2
Mo*end*1*exo*2*ntr*37	NTR	*ntr*-37	< 0.0001	0	0
Mo*end*1*exo*2*hex*3*ntr*37	NTR	*ntr*-37	< 0.0001	0	0

[a]Original mutants not indented; derivatives obtained by trans-formation are indented.

[b]Transformants to str^R, after 10 min with DNA and 100 min for phenotypic expression, per 100 CFU present at time of DNA addition.

[c]DNA bound (ng/100 CFU) in a DNase-sensitive form after 10 min with [^{32}P]DNA.

[d]DNA taken up (ng/100 CFU) in a DNase-resistant form after 10 min with [^{32}P]DNA.

ntr class are unchanged in DNase content. *Noz*-type mutants still contain both the residual exonuclease and the polymerase-exonuclease but have lost the residual endonuclease activity. These findings support a role for this enzyme in DNA entry. It may act as a DNA translocase by sequentially degrading one strand to oligonucleotides, which are left outside the cell while the opposite strand is drawn into the cell.

IDENTITY OF THE *noz* AND *end* LOCI

To determine whether the residual endonuclease implicated in DNA entry was a mutant form of the major endonuclease or a distinct enzyme present in *end*+ cells, a genetic analysis was performed by introducing DNA from a strain containing the mutations *end*-1 and *noz*-48 into normal cells (Table 3). All the transformants selected for *noz*-48 were also deficient in endonuclease. Only one of 16 *end* transformants failed to incorporate the *noz* marker as well. This shows that *end*-1 and *noz*-48 are closely linked but not identical

Table 2. DNase content of transformation-defective strains

Relevant genotype	Strain	Transformation frequency ($str^R/10^2$ CFU)	DNase content[a] (units/mg protein)	
			Endo-nuclease	Exonu-cleases
normal	R6	0.9	23.0	53.0
*end*1, *exo*2	Mo*endl*exo2	3.2	1.9	23.2
	T6*trtl*hex4	1.2	3.3	10.2
*end*1, *exo*2, *ntr*	Mo*endl*exo2ntr37	<0.0001	3.2	20.9
*end*1, *exo*2, *noz*	T6*trtl*hex4noz11	0.017	0.0	6.9
	T6*trtl*hex4noz19	0.0004	0.0	3.8
	Mo*endl*exo2ntr48	0.005	0.1	8.4
	T6*trtl*hex4ntr48	0.0004	0.1	4.2

[a]Enzymes fractionated on CM-cellulose and assayed in presence of Mn^{2+}. Mn^{2+} enhances the major exonuclease activity 4-fold with respect to the other DNases, which give the same activity with either Mn^{2+} or Mg^{2+}.

mutations. The common genetic locus of *end* and *noz* indicates that the residual endonuclease is most likely a mutant form of the major endonuclease.

Several newly obtained *end* mutants show reduced transformability and other properties typical of *noz* mutants. The *end* mutation in these cases results in more severe impairment of endonuclease activity than does *end*-1. This experience with *end* mutations provides a useful lesson in attempting to implicate enzymes in other biological processes, such as recombination, for example. Absence of an enzyme activity *in vitro* does not prove that the enzyme is unable to carry out its function *in vivo*. Positive evidence for the role of an enzyme (that is, correlation of absence of an enzyme activity *in vitro* with absence of an *in vivo* function) is more conclusive. This lesson may be pertinent to the controversy on the role of ATP-dependent DNases in recombination.

TWO STEPS IN DNA UPTAKE

Analysis of the properties of the two classes of transformation-defective mutants suggests a mechanism of DNA uptake consisting of two steps. The first step, binding of DNA to the outside of the

Table 3. Linkage of *noz* and *end* mutations

Transformation cross

	Strain	Relevant genotype	Phenotype[a]
DNA donor:	Moend1exo2ntr48	end1,noz48	end⁻,noz⁻
Recipient cells:	T6trt1hex4exo2	end⁺,noz⁺	end⁺,noz⁺

Analysis of progeny

	Number of clones of phenotype[a]			
Selection method	end^-,noz^-	end^-,noz^+	end^+,noz^-	other
No zone, DNase plate assay, 30 h	15	1	0	0
No transformation, agar plate test	7	0	0	1[b]

[a]DNase activity of end^- extracts was 8-15% of end^+. Transformability of noz^- was 0.1-1.0% of noz^+.

[b]Showed high DNase activity and failed to transform (<0.01% of noz^+). May represent a spontaneous *ntr* mutant in the recipient population.

cell, is missing in *ntr* mutants. The second step, entry of DNA, is missing in *noz* mutants. Further details of the two steps are listed in Table 4. [This scheme is based also on the data of others to which reference is made in Lacks *et al.* (1974).] Entry may not require additional energy since the hydrolysis of one strand could provide the energy for transporting its complementary strand into the cell.

The function of a major DNase in pneumococcal cells as a DNA translocase for uptake of DNA in transformation may have general implications. Other enzymes that simply hydrolyze DNA *in vitro* may have other, more significant activities *in vivo*. For example, it is possible that a DNase *in vivo* may transfer one polynucleotide chain to another, rather than to water. Such transferase activity would allow direct recombination of DNA strands without breakage and ligation. It may obviate the need for coincidental breaks in models of genetic recombination.

ACKNOWLEDGMENTS

This work was done in collaboration with Bill Greenberg and Marjorie Neuberger. It was carried out at Brookhaven National Laboratory under the auspices of the U.S. Atomic Energy Commission.

Table 4. Mechanism of DNA uptake in transformation

Step I. Binding	Step II. Entry
1. DNA bound to outside of cell in a form sensitive to DNase and shear	1. DNA within cell, protected from external agents
2. Requires activation by competence factor (inhibited by growth with trypsin)	2. Requires a cellular DNase functioning as a DNA translocase
3. Divalent cations not necessary	3. Requires Mg^{2+} or Mn^{2+}
4. Requires a source of energy (sugar)	4. May not need additional energy
5. Blocked in *ntr* mutants	5. Blocked in *noz* mutants

REFERENCES

Fox, M. S. and M. K. Allen. 1964. On the mechanism of deoxyribonucleate integration in pneumococcal transformation. Proc. Nat. Acad. Sci. U.S.A. 52: 410.

Lacks, S. 1962. Molecular fate of DNA in genetic transformation of pneumococcus. J. Mol. Biol. 5: 119.

Lacks, S. 1970. Mutants of *Diplococcus pneumoniae* that lack deoxyribonuclease and other activities possibly pertinent to genetic transformation. J. Bacteriol. 101: 373.

Lacks, S. and B. Greenberg. 1967. Deoxyribonucleases of pneumococcus. J. Biol. Chem. 242: 3108.

Lacks, S. and B. Greenberg. 1973. Competence for deoxyribonucleic acid uptake and deoxyribonuclease action external to cells in the genetic transformation of *Diplococcus pneumoniae*. J. Bacteriol. 114: 152.

Lacks, S., B. Greenberg and M. Neuberger. 1974. Role of a DNase in a genetic transformation of *Diplococcus pneumoniae*. Proc. Nat. Acad. Sci. U.S.A., in press.

Morrison, D. A. and W. R. Guild. 1972. Transformation and deoxyribonucleic acid size: extent of degradation on entry varies with size of donor. J. Bacteriol. 112: 1157.

Morrison, D. A. and W. R. Guild. 1973. Breakage prior to entry of donor DNA in pneumococcus transformation. Biochim. Biophys. Acta 299: 545.

MARKER EFFECTS IN PNEUMOCOCCAL TRANSFORMATION

Jean-Gérard Tiraby* and Maurice S. Fox

Department of Biology, Massachusetts Institute of Technology, Cambridge, Massachusetts 01239

Genetic markers may be transferred from one pneumococcal strain to another as the result of exposure of competent recipient bacteria to double-stranded DNA isolated from donor bacteria. Several investigators have shown that markers representing single-site mutations can be divided into several classes according to the frequency with which those markers are represented among transformants. These mutations appear to fall into four classes, the distribution of which varies according to the loci analyzed (Lacks, 1966; Sirotnak and Hachtel, 1969; Tiraby and Sicard, 1973a). The two predominant classes of markers are those that yield a high frequency of transformants (HE, for high efficiency of integration) and those that yield a low frequency of transformants (LE, for an efficiency of integration about tenfold lower) (Ephrussi-Taylor *et al.*, 1965; Ephrussi-Taylor and Gray, 1966). When a large number of spontaneous mutations within a given locus are analyzed, two more classes are observed, one corresponding to markers with a very high efficiency of integration (from 1.5- to 2-fold more efficient than HE markers) (VHE) and the other corresponding to markers with an intermediate efficiency (IE). VHE markers are about 20 times more efficient than LE markers. The characteristic integration efficiency of a marker belonging to one of these classes is manifested in transformation of both wild-type bacteria with mutant DNA and mutant bacteria with wild-type DNA.

By following the mode of transmission of the acquired marker to

---

*Present address: Laboratoire de Génétique, Université de Toulouse, 118, Route de Narbonne, 31-Toulouse-France.

daughter cells at successive divisions following DNA uptake,
Ephrussi-Taylor (1966) reported that LE markers segregate transformant progeny one generation earlier than HE markers. Her interpretation was that transformants become homozygous or homoduplex
for LE markers one replication cycle earlier than for HE markers.
Louarn and Sicard (1968) reached the same conclusion by analyzing
the composition of clones produced by bacteria that had experienced
two independent transformation events, including one HE and one LE
marker. The observation that LE markers appear to express their
phenotype earlier than do HE transformants (Ephrussi-Taylor, 1966;
Louarn, 1970) is consistent with this view.

The function (*hex*) responsible for the discrimination between
markers can be altered by mutations (Lacks, 1970; Tiraby *et al.*
1973). With strains termed nondiscriminating (*hex⁻*), all markers
are introduced with the same efficiency as that observed with VHE
markers in the discriminating strain (*hex⁺*) (Tiraby and Sicard,
1973b; Tiraby and Fox, 1973). When a *hex⁻* strain is used as a
recipient, all markers behave like VHE markers in a *hex⁺* strain
(Tiraby and Sicard, 1973b; Claverys and Roger, personal communication).

Genetic transformation of pneumococcus proceeds through the
insertion of single-stranded fragments of donor DNA into the genome
of the recipient bacteria (Fox and Allen, 1964). Thus, after insertion and before replication of the recipient genome, the DNA of the
transformed cells contains regions which are both genetically heterozygous and physically heteroduplex (Guerrini and Fox, 1968;
Gurney and Fox, 1968). The initial steps of integration leading to
the formation of a donor-recipient heteroduplex appears to be identical for both LE and HE markers (Ephrussi-Taylor and Gray, 1966;
Shoemaker and Guild, 1974). It appears, therefore, that the *hex*
function acts on the heteroduplex structure harboring certain base-
pair mismatches. The action of the *hex* function is relatively fast,
since the selective loss of LE transformants is completed within a
few minutes at 37°C (Shoemaker and Guild, 1974). The nature of the
mechanism, which results in the loss of more than 90% of the putative
LE transformants and renders homozygous the fraction of LE markers
that escape destruction, has been investigated. Two basically
different hypotheses can be proposed to account for the characteristics of LE markers.

(1) Transformation involving LE markers results in the formation of a class of base-pair mismatches that suffer efficient lethal
endonucleolytic cleavage unless the integration event has occurred
in advance of the normal replication fork, in which case the marker
is rendered homozygous and escapes cleavage.

(2) Single-strand endonucleolytic cleavage occurs at the site

of those base-pair mismatches represented by LE markers. We assume
that the incision is followed by exonucleolytic digestion.   In
those cases, perhaps half, in which the donor strand is cleaved,
the newly introduced marker is lost. When the cleavage occurs in
the recipient strand, exonucleolytic digestion may proceed to the
terminus of the inserted fragment and produce a lethal event unless
covalent joining of the fragment has occurred. Such lethal events
are presumed to account for the loss of many of the remaining LE
transformants. The LE transformants that survive would include
those in which digestion had failed to reach the terminus of the
inserted fragment and those in which the fragment had become covalently joined prior to digestion of the complementary region. Both
of these classes would experience repair and would thus appear as
homozygous transformants.

    The following observations exclude the first hypothesis and
offer support for the second.

REPLICATION FORK HYPOTHESIS

    Integration of LE markers results in the formation of a class
of mismatched base pairs that are recognized by a specific double-
strand endonuclease whose action is lethal to the transformant.

    The viable LE transformants would be those in which the inte-
gration event occurred sufficiently close to an approaching replication fork so as to be rendered homozygous by replication prior to
action of the endonuclease.   In contrast, the classes of mismatched
base pairs formed by HE markers are not recognized, and therefore
the integration of HE markers is independent of the position of the
replication fork. If the replication indeed allows a fraction of
LE markers to escape destruction by the mismatch-specific enzyme,
this fraction might be expected to decline in the absence of DNA
synthesis.   Independent double-transformation events involving two
unlinked LE markers would, according to this hypothesis, depend on
the presence of more than one replication fork. The incidence of
such events might be expected to be even more sensitive to inhibition of DNA synthesis.

    Inhibition by 6-(p-hydroxyphenylazo)uracil (HPUra), which
blocks semi-conservative DNA synthesis in some gram-positive bacteria (Brown, 1971), permitted examination of these possibilities.
Figure 1 depicts the effect of HPUra on the incorporation of
labeled thymidine and on the viable count of pneumococcus. The
drug stops the synthesis of new DNA almost immediately, as shown
by the cessation of thymidine incorporation, without any significant
loss of viability of the cells. Table 1 shows the result of the
transformation of R6 cells (hex^+) in the presence and absence of

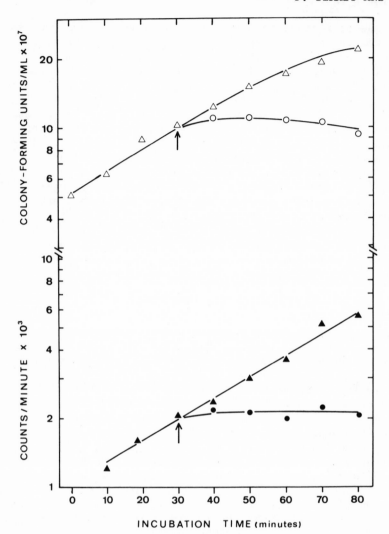

Figure 1. Effect of HPUra on thymidine incorporation and viability
of exponentially growing R6 cells. Thawed precompetent cells of
strain R6 Thy A, Thy B, were diluted at 1/20 in CH medium deprived
of uridine and adenosine but supplemented with 10 μg/ml of cold
thymidine. After 60 min incubation at 37°C, corresponding to time
0 of the figure, 20 μCi of [³H]thymidine were added to the culture.
Thirty minutes later the culture was divided into two equal aliquots,
one receiving 25 μg/ml of HPUra (kindly provided by Neal Brown,
Baltimore). The two cultures were further incubated at 37°C. At
10-min intervals after time 0, the radioactivity incorporated into
a cold trichloroacetic-acid-precipitable form and the number of
colony-forming units were determined.

Table 1. Number of single and double transformants on transformation of HPUra-treated and untreated competent R6 bacteria

Determination	Untreated			HPUra-treated		
	Colony-forming units/ml	Single/*str-r41*	Double/*sulf-str*	Colony-forming units/ml	Single/*str-r41*	Double/*sulf-str*
Total viable cells	1.55×10^8			1.25×10^8		
Single transformants						
str-r41	7.4×10^6	1		9.8×10^5	1	
sulf-d	9.6×10^6	1.3		14×10^5	1.4	
nov-r1	0.75×10^6	0.10		1.20×10^5	0.12	
opt-r2	1.35×10^6	0.18		1.45×10^5	0.15	
rif-r17	0.80×10^6	0.11		0.975×10^5	0.10	
bac-r2	0.875×10^6	0.12		1.75×10^5	0.18	
Double transformants						
sulf-str	780×10^3		—	1.55×10^4		—
nov-opt	2.4×10^3		0.3×10^{-2}	35 (175/5 ml)		0.2×10^{-2}
nov-rif	1.7×10^3		0.2×10^{-2}	40 (160/4 ml)		0.3×10^{-2}
nov-bac	1.75×10^3		0.2×10^{-2}	59 (237/4 ml)		0.4×10^{-2}

A freshly prepared competent culture was divided into two aliquots of 7.5 ml and 2.5 ml. Both cultures were mixed with an equal volume of prewarmed CH medium (30°C), the largest volume containing 50 µg/ml of HPUra. After 10 min incubation at 30°C, DNA was added to both cultures (5 µg/ml). Twenty minutes later deoxyribonuclease was added for 5 min for the untreated culture and 10 min for the HPUra-treated culture, and the cells were sedimented, washed, and resuspended in B medium containing 10% glycerol. The numbers of single and double transformants were determined by the overlay method.

HPUra. The relative yield of LE transformants is not affected by
the inhibition of DNA synthesis during transformation. The relative frequencies of independent double transformants for several
LE-LE pairs also remain unaffected by the inhibition of DNA synthesis.

Preliminary physical experiments were also carried out in
order to investigate the possible intervention of the replicating
fork in the integration of the LE markers. These experiments involve the transfer of competent R6 (hex^+) cells grown in a light
medium to a medium containing nutrients labeled with the heavy
isotopes ^{15}N and ^{13}C and, after incubation for 10 min, the addition
of light transforming DNA. After allowing transformation with
donor DNA carrying both an LE and an HE marker, DNA was extracted
from the transformed population and sedimented to equilibrium in a
cesium chloride gradient. The hypothesis predicts that, in comparison with the HE marker activity, the newly synthesized DNA,
hybrid in density, should be enriched for the LE marker activity,
whereas the light DNA that has not been replicated should be deple-
ted in LE marker activity. Table 2 summarizes the results obtained
from fractions of three gradients in which, following transformation, approximately 5%, 50%, and 75% of the DNA of the recipient
bacteria had replicated in the heavy medium. DNA carrying LE marker
activity does not become hybrid any more rapidly than does DNA
carrying HE activity.

These experimental observations appear to rule out the hypothesis implicating the replication fork in the survival of LE transformants.

LETHAL EVENTS THAT FOLLOW SINGLE-STRAND CLEAVAGE BY AN ENDONUCLEASE RECOGNIZING CERTAIN BASE-PAIR MISMATCHES

Some years ago, Ephrussi-Taylor suggested a model involving an
excision-repair system selective for mismatches and acting on the
donor-recipient heteroduplex harboring LE markers. In order to
explain the 10-fold excess of LE transformants compared to HE transformants, she further assumed preferential excision of the donor
strand. We suggest a modification of this hypothesis, introducing
the notion that lethal events are responsible for the loss of a substantial fraction of potential LE transformants. The features of
this model, outlined in Fig. 2, are the following: in the case of
an LE marker, a mismatch-specific endonuclease acts with equal probability on either strand of the donor-recipient heteroduplex structure. The endonucleolytic cleavage is followed by exonucleolytic
digestion involving removal of on the order of 1000 nucleotides, and
in the absence of lethal events involving disruption of the continuity of the bacterial genome the digested sequence is repaired by new

Table 2. Relative activities of LE and HE donor markers in newly duplicated and unduplicated DNA of newly transformed bacteria

Time of incubation of transformed culture (min)	% of the genome duplicated	Hybrid-density fraction (duplicated DNA)			Light-density fraction (unduplicated DNA)		
		Str-r transformants (HE)	Nov-r transformants (LE)	$\dfrac{Nov\text{-}r}{Str\text{-}r}$	Str-r transformants (HE)	Nov-r transformants (LE)	$\dfrac{Nov\text{-}r}{Str\text{-}r}$
5	1-5	0.51×10^3	82	0.16	7.2×10^3	11×10^2	0.15
30	50	8.5×10^3	14×10^2	0.17	7.8×10^3	12×10^2	0.16
60	75	7.0×10^3	11×10^2	0.16	4.6×10^3	8×10^2	0.18

Competent R6 hex^+ Ery-r bacteria were suspended in ^{13}C, ^{15}N-containing growth medium and exposed to light-DNA-carrying markers Str-r (HE) and Nov-r (LE) for 30 min. DNase was added and incubation was continued. At the times indicated fractions were removed, and the DNA was isolated and fractionated in equilibrium CsCl gradients. Competent R6X hex^- bacteria were used to determine transforming activities of extracts. DNA isolated from the transformed bacteria gave an activity ratio $\dfrac{\text{HE donor } (Str\text{-}r)}{\text{LE donor } (Str\text{-}r)}$ of 2×10^{-3} and an activity ratio of $\dfrac{\text{LE donor } (Nov\text{-}r)}{\text{HE donor } (Str\text{-}r)}$ of 0.19. The duplication of recipient $(Ery\text{-}r)$ of $\dfrac{\text{recipient } (Str\text{-}r)}{(Ery\text{-}r)}$ the genome was estimated on the basis of the relative amount of recipient transforming activity $(Ery\text{-}r)$ appearing at the hybrid density position in the CsCl gradient.

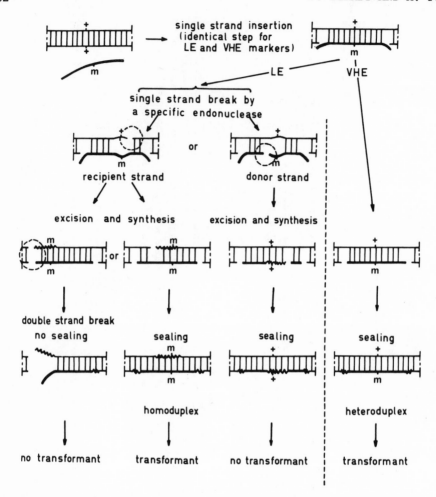

Figure 2.   Caricature of the suggested mechanism of elimination of
LE transformants in *hex*[+] strains.

synthesis, using the complementary strand as a template. Half of
the excision events occur on the donor DNA strand leading to the
loss of donor LE marker. For the remaining half of the LE trans-

Figure 3.   Inactivation of the biological activity of the DNA by
shearing. DNA isolated from the strain R6x carrying the markers
sulf-d (VHE), *Ery*-r2 (HE), *Opt*-r2 (LE), and *Str*-r53 (LE) in 1 M
NaCl, 0.015 M saline citrate was stirred at 40,000 rpm in the Virtis
45 homogenizer at a concentration of 5 µg/ml. The biological activity of sheared DNA was assayed on the *hex*[+] strain R6 and the *hex*[-]
strain R6x *Nov*-r.

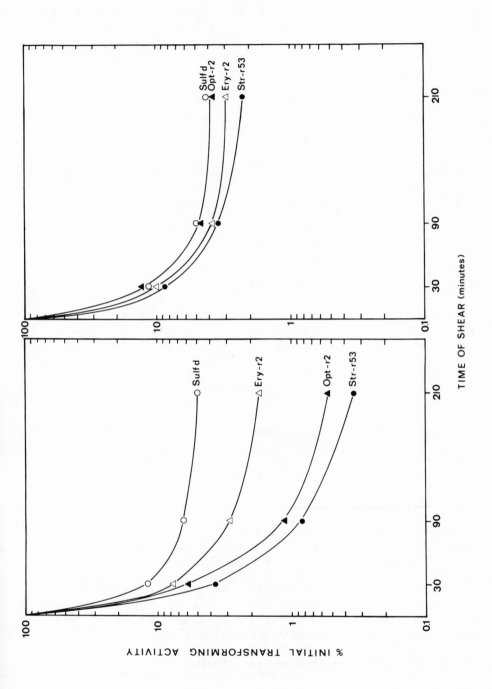

formants, cleavage occurs on the recipient strand and digestion
proceeds toward the terminus of the inserted fragment of donor DNA.
Depending on the position of the LE marker with respect to the ends
of the donor strand and the rate and extent of digestion, the excision may reach an extremity of the donor strand not yet ligated and
thus create a lethal double-strand break of the continuity of the
recipient chromosome. An LE transformant occurs either when the
length of the DNA excised is shorter than the distance separating
the LE marker from the terminus of the donor strand or when covalent
joining of the donor strand has preceded the exonucleolytic digestion.

We have examined the feature of this hypothesis that suggests
that the discrimination between an HE and an LE marker should be
amplified as a result of a reduction of the average length of the
inserted fragment. When transformation is carried out with DNA
whose molecular weight is greater than 10^7, the average mass of
the fragment of DNA integrated is estimated to be 2-3 X 10^6 daltons
(Gurney and Fox, 1968). Reduction of molecular weight by exposure
to shear results in a loss of biological activity for all markers
(Gurney, 1965; Cato and Guild, 1968).

The molecular weight of DNA carrying a VHE marker (*sulf*-d), an
HE marker (*Ery*-r2), and two LE markers (*Opt*-r2 and *Str*-r53) was
reduced by shearing. The surviving activities of the various markers were determined on a discriminating (hex^+) strain and on a
nondiscriminating (hex^-) strain (Fig. 3). The LE markers exhibit a
substantially greater shear sensitivity when tested on the hex^+
strain than does the VHE marker on either strain.

It appears that the probability of survival of an LE transformant in a discriminating strain can be reduced even further by
reducing the average length of DNA separating the marker site from
the terminus of the integrated fragment.

This observation is consistent with the proposal described in
Fig. 2 to account for marker discrimination. The following features seem essential: The presence in discriminating (hex^+) strains
of an endonuclease responsible for single-strand breaks and specific
for both of the possible base-pair mismatches that occur in the
heteroduplex region of LE transformants. An exonuclease expands
the gap that may result in a lethal event when the endonucleolytic
cleavage occurs in the recipient strand, and the digestion expands
to include a terminus of the donor DNA fragment that has not yet
become covalently joined to the recipient DNA.

Those LE transformants that are detected in discriminating
strains result from events in which the excision in the recipient
strand either fails to include an unjoined terminus or expands into
a terminus that has already been covalently joined. Repair

synthesis of these structures would be responsible for homozygosity among the surviving transformants.

ACKNOWLEDGMENTS

This work was supported by grant number AI 05388 from the U.S. Public Health Service. G. T. was supported by fellowships from the Pierre Philippe Foundation and the Foundation for Research in Medicine and Biology.

REFERENCES

Brown, N. C. 1971. Inhibition of bacterial DNA replication by 6-(p-hydroxyphenylazo)-uracil: differential effect on repair and semi-conservative synthesis in *Bacillus subtilis*. J. Mol. Biol. 59: 1.

Cato, A. and W. R. Guild. 1968. Transformation and DNA size. I. Activity of fragments of defined size and a fit to a random double crossover model. J. Mol. Biol. 37: 157.

Ephrussi-Taylor, H. 1966. Genetic recombination in DNA-induced transformation of pneumococcus. IV. The pattern of transmission and phenotypic expression of high and low efficiency donor sites in the ami-A locus. Genetics 54: 211.

Ephrussi-Taylor, H. and T. C. Gray. 1966. Genetic studies of recombining DNA in pneumococcal transformation. J. Gen. Physiol. 49: 211.

Ephrussi-Taylor, H., A. M. Sicard and R. Kamen. 1965. Genetic recombination in DNA-induced transformation of pneumococcus. I. The problem of relative efficiency of transforming factors. Genetics 51: 455.

Fox, M. S. and M. K. Allen. 1964. On the mechanism of deoxyribonucleate integration in pneumococcal transformation. Proc. Nat. Acad. Sci. U.S.A. 52: 412.

Guerrini, F. and M. S. Fox. 1968. Effects of DNA repair in transformation-heterozygotes of pneumococcus. Proc. Nat. Acad. Sci. U.S.A. 59: 1116.

Gurney, T. Jr. 1965. A minimum molecular weight for transforming DNA. Ph.D. Thesis, Yale University.

Gurney, T. Jr. and M. S. Fox. 1968. Physical and genetic hybrids formed in bacterial transformation. J. Mol. Biol. 32: 83.

Lacks, S.   1966.   Integration efficiency and genetic recombination in pneumococcal transformation.   Genetics 53: 207.

Lacks, S.   1970.   Mutants of *Diplococcus pneumoniae* that lack deoxyribonucleases and activities possibly pertinent to genetic transformation.   J. Bacteriol. 101: 373.

Louarn, J. M.   1970.   Etude de la recombinaison genetique chez *Diplococcus pneumoniae*.   Thesis, University of Toulouse, France.

Louarn, J. M. and A. M. Sicard.   1968.   Transmission of genetic information during transformation in *Diplococcus pneumoniae*. Biochem. Biophys. Res. Commun. 30: 683.

Shoemaker, N. B. and W. R. Guild.   1974.   Destruction of low efficiency markers is a slow process occurring at the heteroduplex stage of transformation.   Mol. Gen. Genet. in press.

Sirotnak, F. M. and S. L. Hachtel.   1969.   Increased dihydrofolate reductase synthesis in *Diplococcus pneumoniae* following translatable alteration of the structural gene.   I.   Genotype derivation and recombinational analyses.   Genetics 61: 293.

Tiraby, J.-G., J.-P. Claverys and A. M. Sicard.   1973.   Integration efficiency in DNA induced transformation of pneumococcus.   I.   A method of transformation in solid medium and its use for isolation of transformation-deficient and recombination-modified mutants. Genetics 75: 23.

Tiraby, J.-G. and M. S. Fox.   1973.   Marker discrimination in transformation and mutation of pneumococcus.   Proc. Nat. Acad. Sci. U.S.A. 70: 3541.

Tiraby, J.-G. and A. M. Sicard.   1973a.   Integration efficiencies of spontaneous mutant alleles of amiA locus in pneumococcal transformation.   J. Bacteriol. 116: 1130.

Tiraby, J.-G. and A. M. Sicard.   1973b.   Integration efficiency in DNA-induced transformation of pneumococcus.   II.   Genetic studies of a mutant integrating all the markers with a high efficiency. Genetics 75: 35.

RECOMBINATION IN FUNGI

GENETIC AND BIOCHEMICAL STUDIES OF RECOMBINATION IN *USTILAGO MAYDIS*

R. Holliday, W. K. Holloman, G. R. Banks, P. Unrau and

J. E. Pugh

National Institute for Medical Research, Mill Hill,

London NW7 1AA

Genetic studies of recombination with several species of fungi have led to the accumulation of a large body of information about genetic fine structure and the relationships between reciprocal and nonreciprocal recombination. Molecular models of genetic recombination that appear to be capable of explaining most of the genetic observations have been formulated (Holliday, 1968, 1973; Whitehouse, 1969; Fincham and Holliday, 1970; Leblon and Rossignol, 1973). The models depend on the breakage and reunion of polynucleotide chains, the formation of hybrid or heteroduplex DNA, and the correction of mismatched bases. The following proteins are likely to be required for these processes: deoxyribonucleases, a DNA-binding protein (like the bacteriophage T4 gene 32 product), DNA polymerase, and polynucleotide ligase. Very little information has previously been obtained about proteins or enzymes of this type in fungi that have DNA as their substrate.

We have set out to remedy this situation, using the yeast-like smut fungus *Ustilago maydis*. A genetic system in this organism was developed some years ago, and mutants defective in repair, recombination, and replication have been isolated and partially characterized (see Holliday, 1974). The general aim of the present investigation is to purify and characterize from wild-type cells the enzymes likely to be involved, and then to identify the biochemical defects in the mutants. In this way we hope to begin to unravel the steps involved in recombination, as well as those in the related processes of repair and replication.

239

THE GENETIC SYSTEM IN *USTILAGO*

U. maydis can be grown in haploid or diploid form. Haploids of opposite *a* mating type readily fuse on a special medium containing charcoal to form heterokaryons, and from these diploids can be selected (Day and Agnostakis, 1971). Heterozygous diploids recombine by mitotic crossing-over to expose recessive auxotrophic or other markers, and heteroallelic diploids recombine predominantly by gene conversion to yield prototrophs. Mitotic recombination is strongly stimulated by UV light or ionizing radiation, and it may be the result of a recombination repair process (Holliday, 1971). Crosses can be carried out only by using the natural environment of the fungus, namely its host *Zea mays*. After inoculation of haploids of opposite mating type or vegetative diploid strains, diploid teliospores can be harvested a few days later from the host tissue. The spores undergo meiosis when germinated on agar medium, and the haploid products can be analyzed either by tetrad or random progeny analysis.

THE ISOLATION AND GENETIC CHARACTERIZATION OF MUTANTS

Radiation-Sensitive Mutants

U. maydis was the first eukaryotic organism used to isolate mutants of this type (Holliday, 1965). Although many are available, only a few have been characterized. *rec1* and *rec2* (previously designated *uvs1* and *uvs2*) are recessive mutations sensitive to both UV and ionizing radiation, and some of their effects on recombination have been previously reported (Holliday, 1967). In summary, each blocks radiation-induced mitotic conversion, and in combination they are deficient also in spontaneous conversion. Crosses homozygous for *rec2* yield meiocytes (promycelia), but no haploid meiotic products are formed. This effect should be distinguished from simple sterility, as shown for instance by some auxotrophic strains, which blocks the formation of diploid teliospores in the host. Crosses between *rec1* strains can be made, but as well as the usual haploids, many aneuploid, diploid, or inviable products are formed. Amongst haploids, the recombination frequency is normal. Detailed studies of mitotic recombination have been made with a number of *rec1* diploids, including one of the following genotype:

$$\frac{rec1\text{-}1 \quad inos1\text{-}4 \; nic1\text{-}1 \; nar1\text{-}1 \; ad1\text{-}1 \quad a_2 \quad + \quad b_1}{rec1\text{-}2 \quad inos1\text{-}5 \; nic1\text{-}2 \; nar1\text{-}6 \quad + \quad a_1 \; pan1\text{-}1 \; b_2} \; .$$

With this diploid allelic recombinants can be selected at any of four heteroallelic loci. The *rec1* alleles do not complement, but spontaneous *rec*[+] recombinants can be selected because they are radiation resistant. They provide a control strain isogenic with the original diploid. Its recombination behavior is perfectly normal. The *rec*1 diploid has the effect of increasing the spontaneous recombination frequency at each of the heteroallelic auxotrophic loci, but it almost completely blocks radiation-induced recombination. At least 70% of spontaneous *inos*+ recombinants are no longer heteroallelic for the distal *nic*1 locus. These recombinants have been analyzed further: some are hemizygous and some are homozygous for one or other of the *nic* alleles. In the control *rec*+ strain only 12% of the *inos*+ recombinants are no longer heteroallelic for *nic*1. These results, which will be published in detail elsewhere, indicate that classical nonreciprocal gene conversion does not occur frequently, if at all, in *rec*1 strains. Instead, crossing-over seems to take place at increased frequency but is often associated with the breakage of one of the two interacting chromosomes. This is supported by the finding that diploid *rec*1 strains are always variable for colony size and morphology, whereas *rec*1 haploids are not (Holliday, 1967).

Recently another radiation-sensitive strain has been found to be recombination defective. This has been provisionally designated γs 7, and it is not yet known if the phenotype is due to a single mutation. The reason for this is that in crosses with wild-type strains meiotic division is blocked (in the same way as in *rec*2 X *rec*2 crosses), so that progeny cannot be analyzed. Diploids heterozygous for γs 7 are significantly more sensitive to radiation than control diploids, and in addition they have a very low frequency of spontaneous or induced recombination at heteroallelic loci (Fig. 1). Although mitotic crossing-over occurs at approximately normal frequency, no radiation-sensitive diploids homozygous for γs 7 have been detected among over 5,000 colonies. Possibly they are lethal. Like *rec*1 strains, γs 7 produces inviable cells during growth. Its dominance for some phenotypic characteristics suggests that it might be a regulatory mutation, and this is borne out by the discovery that it has an increased level of DNase III, an enzyme described below. Preliminary evidence indicates that there are some complex interactions with other radiation-sensitive strains that affect both repair and recombination.

Some radiation-sensitive strains are known to have normal recombination, for instance *uvs*3 and pyrimidine-requiring mutants. The latter are repair deficient, whatever step in pyrimidine biosynthesis is blocked. It is known that the pool of thymidine triphosphate is abnormally low in these mutants, and it is possible that the enzyme responsible for repair replication cannot operate normally (Moore, 1974a, b).

Deoxyribonuclease-Deficient Mutants

Badman (1972) isolated a number of mutants deficient in DNases

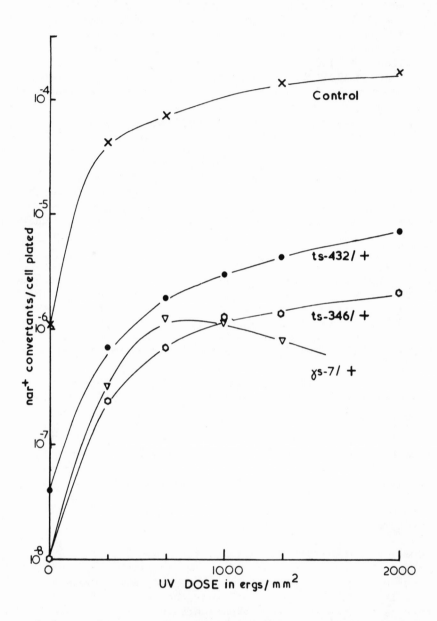

Figure 1.   Recombination in *nar*1-1/*nar*1-6 heteroallelic diploids
heterozygous for γs 7, *tsd*346, or *tsd*432, and a control diploid.
Recombinants are scored on nitrate minimal medium. (*nar* strains
lack nitrate reductase and cannot grow on this medium.)

by a two-step procedure. First, strains that lacked an extra-cellular enzyme (*nuc*1, phenotype e⁻) were obtained, and these were then used to isolate mutants deficient also in an intracellular enzyme activity (*nuc*1 *nuc*2, phenotype e⁻i⁻). Diploids homozygous for *nuc*1 and *nuc*2 mutations are not radiation sensitive, but they are recombination deficient. Both spontaneous and induced conver-sion was shown to be blocked at the *nar*1 locus (Badman, 1972), and subsequently the same effect was seen at heteroallelic *nic*1 and *inos*1 loci. In attempting to discover whether both mutants or only *nuc*2 was involved in the control of recombination, difficulty was experienced in scoring the e⁻ and i⁻ phenotypes by the same DNA plate test that was used to isolate the mutants in the first place. Instead, progeny have been classified for their ability or inability to recombine at heteroallelic loci. The type of analysis carried out is shown in Fig. 2. From Cross M207, 14 progeny of the appro-priate genotype were tested; 11 showed normal recombination at the 3 heteroallelic loci, whereas 3 had a 50- to 100-fold reduction in frequency. Representative data are summarized in Table 1.

In the other crosses between *nuc*1 *nuc*2 strains and wild type, it has also been shown that significantly less than half the prog-eny have a *rec*⁻ phenotype. The segregation ratio shown in Table 2 suggests that two genes control the ability to recombine, and in the absence of evidence to the contrary, we assume that these are the original *nuc*1 and *nuc*2 mutations. The puzzling observation is that although the recombination phenotype segregates so clearly, we

Cross M207

nar 1-1 nic 1-2 inos 1-5 ad 1-1 rec 1-1 a₂b₂ x nar 1-1 pan 1-1 nuc 1-1 nuc 2-1 a₁b₁
        (rec⁺)   (rec⁻)

            nar⁻ nic⁻ inos⁻ pan⁻ progeny tested in diploids:-

    nar 1-1 nic 1-2 inos 1-5 pan 1-1   +   ?   ?   a₁b₁
    _____

    nar 1-6 nic 1-1 inos 1-4   +   ad 1-1 nuc 1-1 nuc 2-1 a₂b₂

Figure 2. The procedure for isolating diploids heteroallelic for three loci. One parent of the cross is deficient in intracellular and extracellular DNases and is known to be recombination deficient (Badman, 1972). The other parent is recombination proficient, even though it carries *rec*1-1 (see text). Random meiotic progeny with the four requirements indicated, lacking *rec*1-1, were crossed to a *nuc*1-1 *nuc*2-1 (*rec*⁻) tester strain to construct triply heteroallelic diploids. Of 14 progeny, 3 were blocked in recombination at all three loci and 11 were normal. Plate tests for DNase activity were ambiguous, but it is presumed that the *rec*⁻ diploids are homozygous for *nuc*1-1 and *nuc*2-1.

Table 1. Spontaneous and ultraviolet-induced recombination at
heteroallelic loci in diploids isolated by the procedure shown
in Fig. 2. Cells were plated on supplemented nitrate minimal
medium lacking ammonium ions, nicotinic acid, or inositol.

| Pheno-type | Recombination frequencies per 10^8 cells plated | | | | | |
| | nar^+ | | nic^+ | | $inos^+$ | |
	C	UV	C	UV	C	UV
rec^+	279	37,500	375	16,800	48	3,240
rec^-	0.2	20	<0.1	<0.5	<0.1	11

UV = 1,400 ergs, >80% survival. C = spontaneous control.

Table 2. The segregation of recombination proficiency from various
crosses between strains deficient in intra- and extracellular DNase
and in wild type. In each case *nar*1-1 (or *nar*1-6) haploid progeny
were scored by making heteroallelic diploids with tester *nar*1-6
(or *nar*1-1) strains which were *nuc*1 *nuc*2. The use of *nuc*+ tester
strains established that the components of *rec*⁻ diploids were indeed
heteroallelic: Ultraviolet-induced allelic recombination was measured by a spot test.

| Cross | Recombination phenotype of progeny | |
	rec^+	rec^-
M200 (*nuc*1-1 *nuc*2-1 X + +)	12	4
M204 (*nuc*1-1 *nuc*2-1 X + +)	12	6
M207 (*nuc*1-1 *nuc*2-1 X + +)	10	3
M219 (*nuc*1-1 *nuc*2-2 X + +)	14	3
	48	16

have not always found that the same is true of DNase activity, as
measured in crude extracts and plate tests. The pair of mutant
alleles that give the clearest results are *nuc1-1* and *nuc2-2*.
From crosses in which these are segregating, we have been able to
correlate DNase I activity with the ability to recombine (Holloman
and Holliday, 1973). Although the results with *nuc* strains clearly
implicate DNase I in genetic recombination, we are inclined to think
·that the mutants may be altered in regulatory functions rather than
in the structural genes for enzymes. Further genetic and biochemical analysis is in progress.

Mutants Temperature Sensitive for DNA Synthesis

Amongst a large number of mutants unable to grow at the re-̯
strictive temperature of 32°C, several that are blocked in DNA synthesis have been identified (Unrau and Holliday, 1970). Amongst
these, one, *pol1-1*, has been found to have a reduced level of DNA
polymerase, and the evidence strongly suggests that the mutation
is in the structural gene for the enzyme (Jeggo *et al.*, 1973).
pol1-1 is not radiation sensitive or recombination deficient.
Interestingly enough, teliospores homozygous for *pol1* germinate and
produce haploid products at the restrictive temperature. If these
are rescued at 22°C and scored, it is found that the crossover frequency is fairly normal. The results indicate that the *pol1* gene
product is required only in vegetative growth, not meiosis. *pol1*
strains may therefore be particularly useful in identifying any DNA
polymerases that may be specific for meiocytes. (The DNA polymerase
responsible for most of the activity in extracts from wild-type
vegetative cells has been purified 5,000-fold and characterized,
but these results will not be described, as there is no evidence
as yet that the enzyme is implicated in recombination).

Recently, a search for alleles of *pol1* yielded two further temperature-sensitive mutants defective in DNA synthesis with unusual
properties. These mutants, provisionally designated *ts*346 and
*ts*432, have identical phenotypes and are probably alleles, but they
are not linked to *pol1*. Diploids heterozygous for either mutant
do not grow at 32°C. Moreover, the mutants are also dominant
with regard to their effect on recombination at 22°C. Diploids
heterozygous for *ts*346 or 432, which are heteroallelic for *nar1*,
recombine at 1-5% of the normal rate either spontaneously or after
ultraviolet light treatment, as shown in Fig. 1. On the other
hand, these diploids proceed through meiosis at 32°C and *nar*[+] recombinants are produced at normal frequency. These mutants, like
nuc strains, are not radiation sensitive. Their dominance in vegetative diploids suggests that they are regulatory mutations controlling perhaps the protein required for both mitotic recombination
and replication. This suggested that the "gene 32" DNA-binding

protein described below might be affected, but no evidence for
this has been obtained.

BIOCHEMICAL STUDIES

Deoxyribonucleases

Three enzymes, provisionally designated DNases I, II, and III,
have been detected in broken cell extracts of wild-type *U. maydis*.
DNases I and II, which are separable by column chromatography, are
highly specific for single-stranded DNA and are responsible for
most of the hydrolysis observed when denatured DNA is treated with
portions of crude extracts.   Crude extract values of specific activities are approximate measures of the level of DNase 1, since it
is present in about three times the amount of DNase II.   Table 3
shows the levels of activity in a number of *Ustilago* strains,
including those selected for low deoxyribonuclease activity as
discussed above.   A mutant lacking extracellular DNase activity,
*nuc*1-1, was found to have normal levels of intracellular activity,
and fractionation of DNases I and II by column chromatography
revealed that the proportions of the two activities were unchanged
from that of the wild type.   Thus the *nuc*1-1 locus exerts no
apparent effect on the activity or composition of the intracellular
DNase activity.   However, crude extract values of *nuc*1-1 *nuc*2-2
double mutants consistently were observed to contain low levels of
DNase activity, ranging from 5 to 25% of the wild type.   The residual activity fractionated with behavior identical with and in
approximately the same proportions as DNases I and II from wild-
type cells, yet the absolute amounts of both were reduced.   This
result indicates that there is not a simple relationship between
*nuc*2 and one or the other of the DNases.   However, it is not ruled
out that DNase I and DNase II are different forms of the same
enzyme, coded by a single gene.

In crosses involving the *nuc*1-1 and *nuc*2-2 alleles, we have
been able to show that the ability to recombine (as tested by con-
structing heteroallelic diploids) and the low level of DNase activity segregate together (Holloman and Holliday, 1973).   This esta-
blishes the relationship between the two defects, but at this point
we are still unsure of the basis of the relationship, particularly
as the ability to recombine is controlled by two loci (see above).

Of the two enzymes, we have been concerned for the most part
with the detailed examination of only DNase I (Holloman and Holliday, 1973; Holloman, 1973) and have purified it 8,600-fold to homogeneity.   The enzyme is quite active on RNA as well as on denatured
DNA, and hydrolyzes native DNA at a low but significant rate (1-2%
of the rate of denatured DNA).

Table 3. Levels of deoxyribonuclease activities
in crude extracts of wild-type and various mutant
strains

Strain	Specific activity (units*/mg)	
	DNase I	DNase III
Wild type	316[+]	0.92[+]
*nuc*1-1	376	—
*nuc*1-1 *nuc*2-2	59[+]	0.80
γs 7	324	2.58[+]
*rec*1	296	1.82
*rec*2	276	1.2
*uvs*3	271	0.65
*pol*1-1	257	—

* One unit converts 1 nmole of [^{3}H]thymidylate
residues in [^{3}H]DNA to an acid-soluble form.

+ Average of several determinations

Addition of divalent cation is not required for activity, but
addition of EDTA severely inhibits activity. However, complete
enzymatic activity can be restored by simultaneous addition of an
excess of Co or Zn ion, suggesting the enzyme has a bound metal ion.

Acid-soluble products are liberated immediately upon addition
of the DNase to denatured *Escherichia coli* DNA at a rapid initial
rate until about 50% of the DNA has been solubilized. The reaction
then slows to a second, slower phase. Prolonged incubations, addition of high levels of enzyme, or incubation at high temperature
can result in almost complete conversion of the DNA to acid-soluble
products. When the size of the products of digestion was examined
by chromatography of partial digests on DEAE-cellulose columns run
in 7 M urea, oligonucleotides of a range of sizes were noted

throughout the course of digestion. The absence of a preponderance
of mononucleotides in the early phase of digestion suggested that
the primary mode of digestion of the enzyme was endonucleolytic.
However, mononucleotide was found to be a major proportion of the
material in a limit digest.

Denatured T7 DNA was an excellent substrate for the enzyme.
Partial T7 DNA digests were examined by sedimentation in neutral
sucrose gradients. These results indicate that large pieces accumulate and are progressively converted to smaller and smaller oligomers. The enzyme is capable also of causing single-strand nicks
in native DNA, as determined by sedimentation of a T7 DNA digest
on an alkaline sucrose gradient. If the substrate has previously
been irradiated with UV, much greater activity can be demonstrated,
as shown in Fig. 3.

Examination of the size of the products of digestion suggested
that the enzyme acted in an endonucleolytic fashion. However,
single-stranded circular DNA from φX174 was resistant to digestion
by the enzyme unless the circular DNA was first opened by brief
treatment with a low level of pancreatic DNase. Furthermore, the
sedimentation behavior of φX174 DNA on alkaline sucrose gradients
remained unchanged after treatment with a high level of the *Ustilago*
nuclease. Like φX174 DNA, circular duplex DNA from polyoma virus
was found to be refractory to the nicking action of DNase I when
examined in alkaline sucrose gradients. These results suggested
that free DNA ends were required for activity.

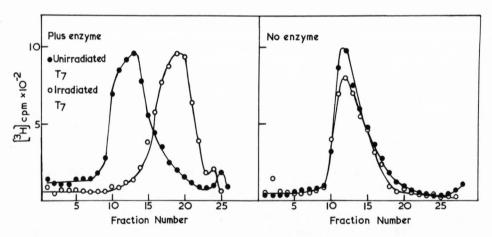

Figure 3.   Sedimentation in alkaline sucrose of native T7 DNA irradiated with 1,000 ergs/mm^2 ultraviolet and untreated T7 DNA after
incubation with a purified preparation of DNase 1. *Left*: parallel
gradients using the two substrates are superimposed. *Right*:
sedimentation of the substrates without enzyme treatment.

Denatured thymus DNA labeled at either the 5´ terminus with ^{32}P or at the 3´ terminus with ^{3}H was exposed at saturating levels to the *Ustilago* nuclease in an attempt to determine the direction of enzymatic attack from DNA ends. The results indicated that the label from either end was initially made acid soluble faster than total nucleotide. This indicates that the enzyme may degrade DNA from either end.

The enzyme fulfills at least a minimal role for a recombination nuclease in that it can degrade single-stranded portions of DNA and nick duplex DNA. The inability to hydrolyze DNA without ends may well be highly significant, as it is obviously essential for a recombination enzyme to avoid cleaving intact chromosomes at random. Its action on UV-irradiated DNA suggests that it may recognize structural distortions, such as mismatched base pairs, but this has yet to be tested.

Very little activity converting native DNA to an acid-soluble form can be detected in cell extracts prepared by crushing cells in low-ionic-strength buffer with or without detergent. We have found, on the other hand, that significant activity can be solubilized if cells are crushed in a buffer containing 2 M salt. This activity, which we term DNase III, was observed to be stimulated several-fold by ATP. This finding was particularly exciting since a number of bacterial enzymes involved in recombination and restriction require nucleoside triphosphates for activity. The investigation, which will be reported in detail elsewhere, was based again upon the commonly used assay which measures degradation of DNA by its conversion to an acid-soluble form. However, it was only when an analysis was made of the products of digestion that it became clear that the conversion of DNA to an acid-soluble form was due not to hydrolysis of DNA into small oligomers but to formation of an unusual acid-soluble DNA-enzyme complex.

Purification 1,600-fold has been achieved. The enzyme is unusual in that it is cold labile. Exposure to 0°C causes a precipitous drop in activity, which is largely reversible by incubation at 37°C for a short time.

Addition of increasing amounts of enzyme to assay mixtures can result in conversion of 60-80% of the substrate DNA to an acid-soluble form. The increase in the amount of DNA rendered acid soluble is not linear, however, but sigmoidal. K^+ and to a lesser degree NH_4^+ are partially effective in abolishing the lag in the enzyme concentration curve.

As mentioned, a number of bacterial DNases require as cofactors or are stimulated by nucleoside triphosphates. At low protein concentrations activity of the *Ustilago* enzyme is stimulated 2- to

3-fold by triphosphates. Diphosphates are also effective, but not
monophosphates or inorganic pyrophosphate. Degradation of DNA by
the ATP-stimulated bacterial DNases is accompanied by hydrolysis
of the ATP. Enhancement of the activity by the ATP analogs β,γ-
methylene-ATP and α,β-methylene-ATP suggests, on the contrary, that
ATP is not hydrolyzed in this case. This point was investigated in
more detail with the use of appropriately labeled isotopes. However,
no hydrolysis could be detected by any of a number of means. Furthermore, chromatographic experiments on Sephadex indicated that
neither the enzyme nor the DNA product was adenylylated nor phos-
phorylated.

     Molecular-weight determination led to an anomaly. The enzyme
was excluded by 6% agarose gels completely, regardless of ionic
strength, pH, presence of detergents, or temperature of the column.
The enzyme displayed a strikingly different behavior when analyzed
by sedimentation. This is probably due to the shape of the enzyme
rather than an aggregation-dissociation phenomenon. It was subsequently found that about 60% of the enzyme by weight was carbohy-
drate.

     Conversion of DNA to an acid-soluble form by less pure frac-
tions is time dependent. In contrast, the reaction by the purified
enzyme preparation ceases within 5 min. Additional DNA is made acid
soluble with addition of more enzyme, but no further solubilization
is observed if more DNA is added.

     Reaction products were examined by chromatography on Sephadex.
DNA rendered 80% acid soluble by the enzyme was passed onto a column
previously calibrated with undigested DNA and DNA digested to 49%
acid solubility with pancreatic DNase. Figure 4A shows that all the
radioactivity applied to the column emerged at the exclusion limit
-- clearly inconsistent with the degree of acid solubility. An
explanation is strong binding of DNA oligomers to the enzyme, forms
a complex large enough to be excluded by the gel. Alternatively,
physical interaction of the enzyme with the DNA alters the acid
solubility of the DNA without reducing it to small oligomers.

     Treatment of the DNA from the excluded fraction in two ways
served to distinguish between the alternatives. In one experiment,
an aliquot of the DNA was treated with acid. The DNA was still 80%
soluble. The supernatant was reapplied to the column. As shown in
Fig. 4B, acid treatment does not liberate small oligomers and the
acid-soluble radioactivity is still excluded, arguing strongly that
the action of the enzyme on DNA is not to reduce it to small oligomers but to alter its properties so that it becomes acid soluble.
To reiterate, conversion to an acid-soluble form is an artifact
resulting from binding of the enzyme to the DNA to form a complex
that is itself acid soluble. Alkali treatment of the DNA has the
effect of slightly reducing the size, indicating that the DNA might

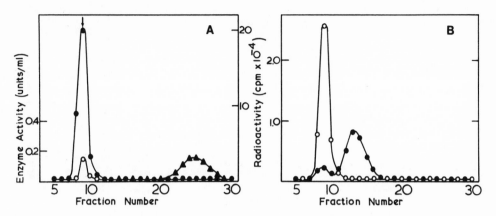

Figure 4.   Analysis of reaction products by gel filtration.
(A)   The reaction mixture (1.5 ml) contained 0.1 M sodium acetate
(pH 5.8), 0.01 M MgCl$_2$, 380 nmoles [^{32}P]DNA, and 60 units of *Ustilago* DNase III.   After 10 min of incubation at 37°C an aliquot
(0.15 ml) was removed and the acid-soluble radioactivity was determined.   A few drops of glycerol were added to the remaining mixture,
and the entire sample was applied to the top of a Sephadex G-200
column (1.8 cm^2 X 20 cm) equilibrated at 4°C with 0.05 M Tris.Cl
0.25 M NaCl.   The column was run at 10 ml per hr, and fractions of
1.85 ml were collected.   Radioactivity (●—●) was determined from
1-ml aliquots of each fraction by scintillation counting in 10 ml
of dioxane counting fluid.   Enzyme activity (o—o) was monitored
with [^{3}H]DNA by the standard assay procedure.   The column was previously calibrated with undigested [^{32}P]DNA, indicated by the arrow,
and with DNA digested to 49% acid solubility with pancreatic DNase
(▲—▲).   (B)   Fractions 8 and 9 from the column in (A) were pooled.
To an aliquot of 0.7 ml of this pooled peak were added 0.2 ml of 2
mg/ml carrier DNA and 0.1 ml of 50% trichloroacetic acid.   The mixture was cooled in ice and then centrifuged.   A few drops of glycerol
were added to the supernatant, the mixture was applied to the top of
the Sephadex column, and the radioactivity was determined in each
fraction (o—o).   To another 0.7-ml aliquot of the pooled peak from
the column in A were added 0.2 ml H$_2$O and 0.1 ml 2 N NaOH.   After
incubation of the mixture for 10 min at room temperature, it was
applied to the Sephadex column as before and the radioactivity was
determined (●—●).

be hydrolyzed to a small extent.   This is illustrated further by sedimentation analysis of digested T7 DNA on alkaline sucrose gradients.
Large oligomers of 600 nucleotides in length accumulate (Fig. 5).

Binding of the enzyme to DNA can be measured in a more conven-
tional way through the use of a membrane filter binding assay
(Figure 6).   Again a sigmoidal curve is obtained, which parallels

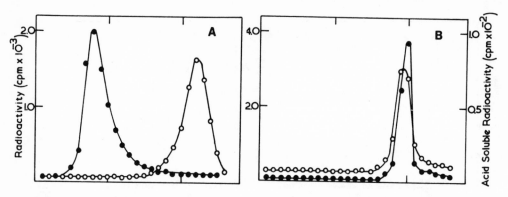

Figure 5. Sucrose gradient centrifugation of T7 DNA after treatment with the *Ustilago* enzyme. A reaction mixture (0.15 ml) containing 0.1 M sodium acetate (pH 5.8), 0.01 M $MgCl_2$, 5.4 nmoles
[^{3}H]DNA from T7, and 10 units of *Ustilago* enzyme was incubated at
37°. After 18 hr NaOH and EDTA were added and the mixture was
layered on top of an alkaline sucrose gradient as described in the
legend to Fig. 3. Centrifugation was for 210 min at 50,000 rpm.
The digested sample (o—o) is compared with an undigested control
(●—●) from a parallel gradient.

the curve obtained with the acid-solubility assay. These curves
may be indicative of cooperative binding, but other interpretations
are possible. However, the DNA saturation curve shown in Fig. 6
is most easily explained in terms of cooperative or nonrandom
binding. A plateau level of the DNA-enzyme complex is reached at
high DNA concentrations and this suggests some DNA molecules are
totally complexed while others are free. Favorable interaction
between neighboring bound enzyme molecules or conformational changes
in the DNA induced by bound enzyme molecules favoring the binding of
other molecules could lead to the selective binding suggested by the
saturation curve.

The structural relationship between the enzyme and DNA is by no
means clear. It does seem likely that a rather basic property of
the DNA is altered through interaction with the enzyme, so that the
polymer remains soluble under acid conditions. It is well known
that a profound change occurs in the structure of DNA in acid solution in which the rigid duplex structure is collapsed, and it is

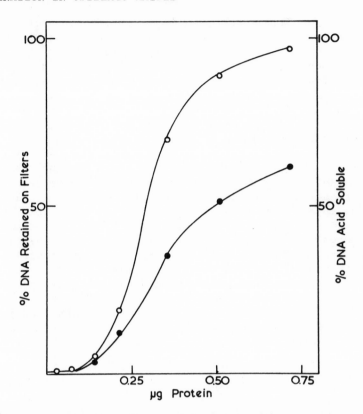

Figure 6. Enzyme concentration curve with the membrane filter
assay. Two identical sets of reaction mixtures (0.15 ml each) containing 0.1 M sodium acetate (pH 5.8), 0.01 M $MgCl_2$, 5.4 nmoles T7
[^{3}H]DNA, and the indicated amounts of *Ustilago* enzyme were incubated at 37°C for 10 min. The acid-soluble radioactivity was
determined in one set (o—o). Reaction mixtures in the other set
were passed through nitrocellulose filters as described in the
legend to Figure 7 (•—•).

popularly believed that under these conditions the DNA is denatured.
However, a large body of evidence based on light scattering, vis-
cometry, and sedimentation analysis indicates to the contrary that
strand separation does not occur. In agreement with a number of
other workers (Dore *et al*., 1972; Cavalieri and Rosenberg, 1957;
Thomas and Doty, 1956; Rice and Doty, 1957; Sturtevant *et al*.,
1958), we find that the buoyant density of DNA after acid treatment
is unchanged from native DNA, indicating that strand separation does
not occur. Aside from protonation of some of the bases, the collapsed structure assumed by DNA in acid may be similar in some
regards to the condensed form of DNA resulting from treatment with
alcohols (Lang, 1969; Geiduschek and Holtzer, 1958), water-soluble

polymers as shown by Lerman (1971), and possibly to the form of DNA
in condensed chromosomes. In this regard it is interesting to note
that acid treatment of isolated interphase nuclei induces the
appearance of prophase-like structures in the nuclei (Ris and
Mirsky, 1949; Philpot and Stanier, 1957). If the acid-mediated
collapse of DNA to the condensed form bears some resemblance to
chromosome condensation, the presence of a molecule in the cell that
might interfere with this process suggests that such a molecule
might be involved in regulation of the process.

In an attempt to establish the physiological role of the enzyme,
a number of mutants defective in functions that may involve DNA
metabolism were screened for the presence of the enzyme (Table 3).
In none of the mutants examined was the enzyme in low levels, but
the radiation-sensitive mutant γs 7 was found to have 3-4 times more
enzyme than normal. *rec*1 also has a significantly increased level.
These mutants are equally sensitive to ultraviolet and ionizing
radiation; both are recombination deficient, have abnormal meiosis,
and produce many nonviable cells during growth; but only γs 7 is
dominant for some of these characteristics. These mutants are
being used to test the hypothesis that DNase III is involved in
chromosome condensation, by the examination of the structure of
nuclei *in vivo* by light and electron microscopy.

DNA-Binding Protein

A DNA-binding protein with properties very similar to those of
the T4 gene protein (Alberts and Frey, 1970) has been purified to
apparent homogeneity from vegetative cells of *Ustilago*. Purification is effected by removal of nucleic acids from cell-free extracts, followed by chromatography on a single-stranded DNA-
cellulose column and then on carboxymethylcellulose. The protein
is eluted from the former by 1.6 M sodium chloride. The single
protein band observed after polyacrylamide gel electrophoresis in
the presence of sodium dodecyl sulfate possesses a mobility that
corresponds to a molecular weight of about 20,000. This is also
the figure for the molecular weight of the binding activity determined by glycerol gradient sedimentation.

The protein is assayed by its ability to bind labeled single-
stranded T7 DNA to nitrocellulose filters (Tsai and Green, 1973)
(Fig. 7).

When the binding activity is plotted versus protein concentration, a sigmoidal curve results. Since the protein by itself binds
to the filters and the degree of washing fails to perturb the
sigmoidal nature of the curve, we believe that this is good evidence
for cooperative binding of the protein to single-stranded DNA. No

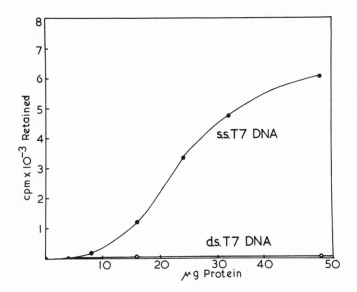

Figure 7. Dependence of the binding activity on protein concentration. Binding protein (0-50 μg as indicated) was incubated at 20°C
for 10 min with 5 μg heat-denatured (●—●) or native (o—o) T7
[^{3}H]DNA in 20 mM Tris·HCl (pH 8.0), 1 mM EDTA, 2 mM 2-mercapto-
ethanol, 50 mM NaCl, and 5% glycerol. The mixture was filtered at
5 ml/min through a nitrocellulose filter (Schleicher and Schull,
BA85) that had been boiled and presoaked in the above buffer. The
filter was washed with 9 ml of this buffer that also contained 1%
dimethyl sulfoxide, dried, and counted in a toluene-based scintillation fluid.

binding to double-stranded DNA can be detected.

The melting temperature of the alternating copolymer poly(dA-
dT) in the presence of the protein, but in the absence of magnesium
ions, was found to be 10.7°C (Fig. 8). This is not an equilibrium
value, since hysteresis was observed on reversing the melting cycle.
In the presence of magnesium ions, a value of 12.5°C was found when
the temperature was increased or decreased. In the absence of the
protein, the melting temperatures under identical conditions were
54 and 62°C, respectively. These results suggest that the protein
decreases the melting temperature by almost 50°C and that magnesium
ions increase the rate of renaturation.

To demonstrate the renaturation of T7 DNA, use was made of the
different buoyant densities of single- and double-stranded DNAs.
Alkali-denatured T7 DNA was incubated with the protein in a buffer
containing 11 mM magnesium chloride. After destruction of any
protein-DNA complexes by sodium dodecyl sulfate, the buoyant density

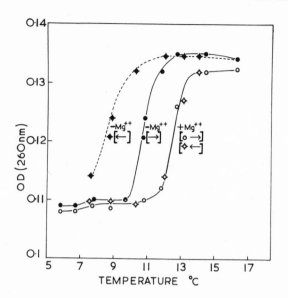

Figure 8.   Denaturation and renaturation of poly(dA–dT) in the
presence of the binding protein.   The reaction mixtures (1.0 ml).
contained poly(dA–dT) (0.125 OD_{260} units) and binding protein (corresponding to a 2-fold saturation of the DNA) in 10 mM KPO_4 (pH
7.5), 33 mM KCl, 0.3 mM EDTA, 1 mM 2-mercaptoethanol, and 5% glycerol at 4°C, with (o—o), ⟡ – ⟡) and without (●—●, ✦ ✦) 10 mM
$MgCl_2$.   The mixtures were placed in cuvettes (1 X 0.2 cm) in a
cooled, thermostatted cuvette holder of a Zeiss PMQII spectropho-
tometer.   The temperature was increased 1°C every 20 min, when the
optical density at 260 nm was determined.   To reverse the cycle,
the temperature was decreased at the same rate as the increase.

of the DNA was determined by analytical centrifugation in a cesium
chloride gradient (Fig. 9).

     When a subsaturating level of protein was used, the DNA band
was rather wide, with a mean buoyant density between those for
single- and double-stranded T7 DNAs.   With a saturating level of
protein, the buoyant density of almost all of the DNA was characteristic of fully native T7 DNA.   Therefore, the protein catalyzes
the reassociation of single strands of T7 DNA.

     The interaction between the protein and the *Ustilago* DNA poly-
merase is now under investigation, but some preliminary results are
known (Fig. 10).

     The protein stimulates 4- to 5-fold the synthesis of DNA by
the polymerase, using denatured calf thymus DNA as template at

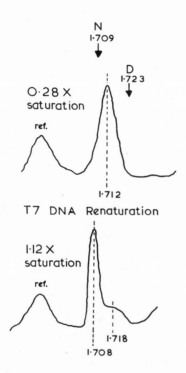

Figure 9. Renaturation of single-stranded T7 DNA in the presence
of the binding protein. The reaction mixtures (0.55 ml) contained
5 µg alkali-denatured, binding protein (at the binding saturation
levels indicated) in 2 mM Tris·HCl (pH 8.0), 1 mM 2-mercaptoethanol,
0.1 mM EDTA, 120 mM KCl, and 10 mM $MgCl_2$. After incubation at 37°C
for 30 min, 100 µg sodium dodecyl sulfate was added, and an aliquot
of each was diluted and CsCl was added (to 1.26 g per ml). The
solution was centrifuged to equilibrium in a Beckman Model E
analytical ultracentrifuge at 44,000 rpm for 20 hr.

approximately a 1:1 DNA:protein ratio. Inhibition, however, is
observed when double-stranded calf thymus DNA that has been nicked
by DNase I is the template. No effect on DNA synthesis using *E.
coli* DNA polymerase I was observed.

We have calculated from the binding activity versus protein
concentration that one molecule of protein binds to about 9 nucleotides. This is a reasonable figure in view of the fact that one
molecule of *E. coli* unwinding protein of molecular weight 22,000
binds to 8 nucleotides (Sigal *et al.*, 1972). There are some 2-5 X
10^5 molecules per *Ustilago* cell. Making rough assumptions about
the topology of DNA replication based on the data of Petes *et al.*
(1973) for yeast replication, 200-400 molecules of protein should

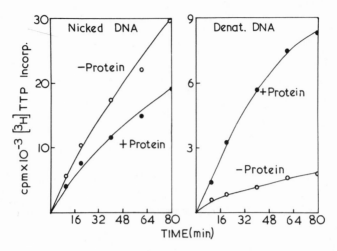

Figure 10.   Stimulation of the DNA polymerase activity by the
binding protein.   The reaction mixtures (0.3 ml) contained 66 mM
Tris·HCl (pH 7.5), 33.3 μM each dATP, dGTP, and dCTP, 3.33 μM
[^{3}H]dTTP, 8 mM MgCl$_2$, 133 mM KCl, DNA polymerase, and 60 μg DNase-
I-nicked or heat-denatured calf thymus DNA with (•—•) or without
(o—o) 40 μg binding protein.   After incubation at 32°C for the
times indicated, the mixtures were assayed for incorporation of
[^{3}H]dTTP into acid-insoluble DNA.

be available for each replication fork, a figure close to those for
T4 and fd phages and *E. coli* (Alberts and Frey, 1970; Alberts *et al.*,
1972; Oey and Knippers, 1972; Sigal *et al.*, 1972).

　　DNA-binding proteins have been detected in meiocytes of several
eukaryotic species, but not in their mitotic cells (Hotta and Stern,
1971a, b), and it was suggested that the proteins were involved in
pairing and crossing-over between homologous chromosomes during
meiosis.   Our results show that a DNA-binding protein with properties very similar to the "Alberts" protein exists in mitotic cells
of *Ustilago*.   Such a protein has recently been isolated from calf
thymus tissue (Herrick and Alberts, 1973).   We now hope to determine
whether the same or different DNA-binding proteins are present in
meiotic cells of *Ustilago*.   We have preliminary evidence that these
cells contain two DNA polymerase enzymes not present in mitotic
cells (Banks, 1973).

　　The levels of the binding protein in the mutants *pol*1-1,
*tsd*432, and *rec*1-1 have been determined.   All three contain normal
levels.

CONCLUSIONS

U. maydis has proved to be useful for experimental investigation of repair, recombination, and replication. It was the first eukaryotic organism successfully used to isolate radiation-sensitive, deoxyribonuclease-deficient, and DNA-polymerase-deficient mutants. Significant progress in the purification and characterization of enzymes and proteins interacting with DNA has also been made.

We do not think the results obtained so far provide evidence for or against particular models of recombination, and it would therefore be premature to discuss details of possible mechanisms. Nevertheless, some general conclusions can be drawn on the basis of existing experimental results. (1) Some radiation-sensitive mutants are defective also in recombination, whereas others are not. Also, some recombination-deficient strains are not radiation sensitive. This suggests that the two processes have some biochemical steps in common but depend on quite distinct pathways or enzymes. (2) Some recombination- and/or repair-deficient mutants are known to be dominant rather than recessive. In one case, γs 7, this is associated with overproduction of an enzyme, DNase III, suggesting that the genetic lesion affects a regulatory function. (3) Mutants can be obtained that are defective in mitotic gene conversion but not crossing over, indicating that at least one biochemical process is not common to both. One possibility is that the length of heteroduplex DNA is very much reduced in these mutants. This would still allow reciprocal exchange but would decrease the opportunity for conversion. Another is that the correction of mismatched bases is eliminated. (4) One class of mutants blocked in gene conversion were isolated as DNase deficient. DNase I is implicated in this process. (5) Temperature-sensitive mutants exist that block mitotic division but not meiosis; others occur that affect mitotic but not meiotic gene conversion. A DNA polymerase, accounting for most of the activity in mitotic cells, is required for vegetative growth but not for recombination or meiosis. (6) There is a glycoprotein DNase III, that binds to DNA and changes its physical properties. There are some grounds for believing that it may be involved in the control of chromosome condensation. A mutant, γs 7, with an excess of this protein, is deranged in several genetic functions. (7) A DNA-binding protein similar to that required for recombination and replication in bacteriophage T4 occurs in mitotic eukaryotic cells. This is contrary to the reports by Hotta and Stern (1971a, b) that a protein of this type is to be found only in meiocytes.

ACKNOWLEDGMENTS

We wish to thank B. J. Maurer, T. L. Olive, and A. Spanos for

their skilled assistance. We are also grateful to Dr. D. H.
Williamson for the ultracentrifugation analysis shown in Figure 9.

REFERENCES

Alberts, B. M. and L. Frey. 1970. T4 bacteriophage gene 32: a
structural protein in the replication and recombination of DNA.
Nature 227: 1313.

Alberts, B. M., L. Frey and H. Delius. 1972. Isolation and
characterisation of gene 5 protein of filamentous bacterial viruses.
J. Mol. Biol. 68: 139.

Badman, R. 1972. Deoxyribonuclease-deficient mutants of *Ustilago
maydis* with altered recombination frequencies. Genet. Res. 20:
213.

Banks, G. R. 1973. A search in fungi for some proteins possibly
involved in recombination of deoxyribonucleic acid. Biochem. Soc.
Trans. 1: 245.

Cavalieri, L. F. and B. H. Rosenberg. 1957. Studies on the structure of nucleic acids. XI. The roles of heat and acid in deoxyribonucleic acid denaturation. J. Amer. Chem. Soc. 79: 5352.

Day, P. R. and S. L. Agnostakis. 1971. Corn smut dikaryon in
culture. Nature New Biol. 231: 19.

Dore, E., G. Fronteli and E. Gratton. 1972. Physico-chemical
description of a condensed form of DNA. Biopolymers 11: 443.

Fincham, J. R. S. and R. Holliday. 1970. An explanation of fine
structure map expansion in terms of excision repair. Molec. Gen.
Genet. 109: 309.

Geiduschek, E. P. and A. Holtzer. 1958. Application of light
scattering to biological systems: deoxyribonucleic acid and the
muscle proteins. Advan. Biol. Med. Phys. 6: 431.

Herrick, G. and B. Alberts. 1973. A nucleic acid helix unwinding
protein from calf thymus. Fed. Proc. 32: 497 (abstract).

Holliday, R. 1965. Radiation sensitive mutants of *Ustilago maydis*.
Mutat. Res. 2: 557.

Holliday, R. 1967. Altered recombination frequencies in radiation
sensitive strains of *Ustilago*. Mutat. Res. 4: 275.

Holliday, R. 1968. Genetic recombination in fungi. In (W. J. Peacock and R. D. Brock, eds.) Replication and Recombination of Genetic Material. p. 157. Australian Academy of Science, Canberra.

Holliday, R. 1971. Biochemical measure of the time and frequency of radiation-induced allelic recombination in *Ustilago*. Nature New Biol. 232: 233.

Holliday, R. 1974. Molecular aspects of genetic exchange and gene conversion. Genetics in press.

Holliday, R. 1974. The genetics of *Ustilago maydis*. In (R. C. King, ed.) Handbook of Genetics. Plenum Press, New York in press.

Holloman, W. K. 1973. Studies on a nuclease from *Ustilago maydis*. II. Substrate specificity and mode of action of the enzyme. J. Biol. Chem. 248: 8114.

Holloman, W. K. and R. Holliday. 1973. Studies on a nuclease from *Ustilago maydis*. I. Purification, properties, and implication in recombination of the enzyme. J. Biol. Chem. 248: 8107.

Hotta, Y. and H. Stern. 1971a. A DNA-binding protein in meiotic cells of *Lilium*. Develop. Biol. 26: 87.

Hotta, Y. and H. Stern. 1971b. Meiotic protein in spermatocytes of mammals. Nature New Biol. 234: 83.

Jeggo, P. A., P. Unrau, G. R. Banks and R. Holliday. 1973. A temperature sensitive DNA polymerase mutant of *Ustilago maydis*. Nature New Biol. 242: 14.

Lang, D. 1969. Collapse of single DNA molecules in ethanol. J. Mol. Biol. 46: 209.

Leblon, G. and J. L. Rossignol. 1973. Mechanism of gene conversion in *Ascobolus immersus*. III. The interaction of heteroalleles in the conversion process. Molec. Gen. Genet. 122: 165.

Lerman, L. S. 1971. A transition to a compact form of DNA in polymer solutions. Proc. Nat. Acad. Sci. U.S.A. 68: 1886.

Moore, P. D. 1974a. Genetic Repair in Pyrimidine Mutants of *Ustilago maydis*. Ph.D. Thesis. C.N.A.A.

Moore, P. D. 1974b. Evidence for an inducible repair mechanism in pyrimidine mutants of *Ustilago maydis*. Heredity in press (abstract).

Oey, J. L. and R. Knippers. 1972. Properties of the isolated gene 5 protein of bacteriophage fd. J. Mol. Biol. 68: 125.

Petes, T. D., C. S. Newlon, B. Byer and W. L. Faugman. 1973. Yeast chromosomal DNA: size, structure and replication. Cold Spring Harbor Symp. Quant. Biol. 38: 9.

Philpot, J. St. L. and J. E. Stanier. 1957. Comparison of interphase and prophase in isolated rat liver nuclei. Nature 179: 102.

Rice, S. A. and P. Doty. 1957. The thermal denaturation of deoxyribose nucleic acid. J. Amer. Chem. Soc. 79: 3937.

Ris, H. and A. E. Mirsky. 1949. The state of the chromosomes in the interphase nucleus. J. Gen. Physiol. 32: 489.

Sigal, N., H. Delius, T. Kornberg, M. L. Gefter and B. A. Alberts. 1972. A DNA unwinding protein isolated from *Escherichia coli*: its interaction with DNA and with DNA polymerase. Proc. Nat. Acad. Sci. U.S.A. 69: 3537.

Sturtevant, J. M., S. A. Rice and E. P. Geiduschek. 1958. The stability of the helical DNA molecule in solution. Disc. Faraday Soc. 25: 138.

Thomas, C. A. and P. Doty. 1956. The mild acidic degradation of deoxyribose nucleic acid. J. Amer. Chem. Soc. 78: 1854.

Tsai, R. L. and H. Green. 1973. Studies on a mammalian cell protein (P8) with affinity for DNA *in vitro*. J. Mol. Biol. 73: 307.

Unrau, P. and R. Holliday. 1970. A search for temperature-sensitive mutants of *Ustilago maydis* blocked in DNA synthesis. Genet. Res. 15: 157.

Whitehouse, H. L. K. 1969. Towards an Understanding of the Mechanism of Heredity. 2nd ed. Arnold, London.

GENETICAL INTERFERENCE AND GENE CONVERSION

Robert K. Mortimer and Seymour Fogel

Division of Medical Physics and Donner Laboratory, and

Department of Genetics, University of California,

Berkeley, California 94720

Gene conversion is a phenomenon associated with a high frequency of crossing-over of flanking markers (Mitchell, 1955; Case and Giles, 1964; Fogel and Hurst, 1967). Within a sample of 907 conversion events at four loci in the yeast *Saccharomyces cerevisiae*, 445 were associated with exchange of bracketing markers (Hurst *et al.*, 1972). The finding that approximately 50% of the conversions were associated with crossing-over applied even when the bracketing alleles were in the same gene as the converted alleles. These results imply a direct relationship between gene conversion and crossing-over. A variety of different models have been proposed to explain recombination as a sequence of molecular events that may result in conversion alone, postmeiotic segregation, or either of these events associated with reciprocal recombination of outside markers (for review see Radding, 1973). A corollary of these models is that a reciprocal recombination event implies the occurrence of a conversion event somewhere between the recombined markers (Fogel and Mortimer, 1969; Paszewski, 1970). However, most and possibly all current models do not address themselves to the question of chiasma interference or the distribution of conversions and/or recombinations in adjacent genetic intervals. For most eukaryotes, with a few notable exceptions, it is well established that a reciprocal recombination event in one interval reduces the probability of occurrence of an additional event in an adjacent interval (*i.e.* positive chiasma interference). Moreover, chiasma interference is very high for regions close to each other and decreases with increasing separation of intervals.

For the two alternatives, conversion alone and conversion
associated with flanking marker exchange, any unitary mechanism of
genetic exchange might be expected to generate equivalent effects
on crossing-over in adjacent intervals. Similarly, if all crossovers result from a common sequence of molecular events that also
generate a region of gene conversion or postmeiotic segregation,
we might expect that conversions of neighboring genes would interfere with each other.

Relevant to the above considerations are Stadler's results
based on a sample of *Neurospora* spores, which were assumed to represent conversional events (Stadler, 1959). He found positive chiasma
interference only for those conversion events that were associated
with exchange of outside markers. However, for those conversion
events that retained the parental array of outside markers, recombination in the adjacent region occurred at control frequencies.
Stadler's findings were based on selected prototrophic spores from
a heteroallelic cross. These spores were assumed to have arisen
from conversion events, though some could also have resulted from
a reciprocal event between the alleles. Additionally, 1+:3- conversions and coconversions were undetected by this selective approach.
For certain allele combinations, coconversions may represent a high
percentage of all conversion events. Thus, the use of selected
samples adds to the possibility of bias. Further, additional biases
may be associated with selective advantages of certain parental or
recombinant genotypes. For these reasons, it seemed worthwhile to
reexamine the relationships between the two classes of conversion
events and their effects on additional crossovers in another biological system and under conditions that avoid some or all of the
above limitations.

We have reexamined data from unselected tetrads of the yeast
S. cerevisiae for one of the hybrids reported in our previous conversion studies (Fogel *et al.*, 1971). This hybrid was marked so
that both recombination of markers flanking the conversion event
and recombination in adjacent intervals could be ascertained and
therefore both chiasma and chromatid interference could be estimated. In addition we have reanalyzed results from selected tetrads
bearing a prototrophic spore. These data are from three crosses
heteroallelic at the *his1* locus on chromosome V (Fogel and Hurst,
1967), which were also suitably marked for interference analysis.

In this paper we demonstrate that conversional events of all
types, if they are associated with a crossover, cause chiasma but
not chromatid interference. However, if the conversion event retains the parental marker array, positive chiasma interference is
not found. Additionally, total conversional events in neighboring
genes were found to occur independently. These findings are considered in relations to various notions on genetic recombination.

CONVERSIONS IN *arg4*

The hybrid X2961 was selected because (a) it was suitably marked for interference analysis, and (b) data from a sufficiently large
sample of unselected tetrads were available. The genotype of X2961
is

	I	II	III	IV	V	VI			
a	0	*pet1*	19	+	17	*thr1*	*cup*	+	*leu1*
α		+	+	16	+	+	*CUP1*	*trp1*	+

+	+	*met1*	*ade2-1*	.
his5	*lys5*	+	*ade2-l*	

The numbers 19, 16, 17 refer to alleles of the *arg4* locus located
on chromosome VIII (Hawthorne and Mortimer, 1960). In this cross,
the approximate map distances (in centimorgans, cM) between markers
on chromosome VIII are

centromere VIII - 4.5 - *pet1* - 3.3 - *arg4-19* - 0.3 - *arg4-16* -

- 0.2 - *arg4-17* - 18 - *thr1* - 29 - *CUP1*

Centromere segregation was scored using *trp1* and *leu1* (Hawthorne
and Mortimer, 1960).

In Table 1 we present the control data for hybrid X2961. The
tetrads are classified according to the number of exchanges in the
centromere - CUP1 interval (tetrad rank) and the distributions of
single and multiple exchanges. The double-exchange tetrads (rank
2) are further classified according to the numbers of strands involved in the two exchanges (*i.e.* 2-, 3-, and 4-strand double exchanges). Omitted in this analysis are those tetrads in which any
of the genes on chromosome VIII failed to segregate in a 2:2 fashion.
Such tetrads represent approximately 1/6 of the total sample, and
notably these tetrads would display the usual high correlation of
recombination on chromosome VIII. Map distances are influenced
both by the conversion-associated exchanges and by the conversion
event alone in the absence of exchange. More appropriately, map
distances between two markers A and B should be estimated by the
relation

$$X = \frac{100 \times 2(T + 6NPD) + C_A + C_B}{4 \ (Total \ tetrads)},$$

where C_A and C_B are the numbers of conversions of A + B, respectively.

The existence of chiasma interference in the data of Table 1
is revealed by the distributions of tetrad ranks. The observed numbers of asci with 0, 1, 2, 3, and 4 exchanges are 333, 1406, 367, 14,
and 3, respectively (average number of exchanges = 1.03). If the ex-

Table 1. Distribution of exchanges on chromosome VIII (control
asci - X2961)

	pet1	19	16	17	*thr1*		*CUP1*	
0 I	II	III	IV	V		VI		

Tetrad rank	Region	No. of asci	Poisson dist. $\overline{n} = 1.03$	Strand relations of double exchanges		
				2st	3st	4st
0		333	754			
1	I	95				
	II	69				
	III	12				
	IV	7				
	V	489				
	VI	737				
		1406	778			
2	I-II	7		1	3	3
	I-V	11		4	5	2
	I-VI	82		20	41	21
	II-III	3		2	1	0
	II-V	3		1	2	0
	II-VI	34		10	18	6
	III-IV	1		1	0	0
	III-VI	2		1	0	1
	V-VI	224		59	121	44
		367	399	99	191	77
3	I-II-III	1				
	I-II-V	4				
	I-II-VI	4				
	I-V-VI	3				
	II-V-VI	1				
	IV-V-VI	1				
		14	147			
4	I-II-V-VI	3	42			
		2123				

changes on chromosome VIII were independent, they would have been
distributed according to the Poisson distribution as follows: 0,
754; 1, 778; 2, 399; 3, 147; 4, 42.   The observed distribution of
tetrad ranks clearly indicates chiasma interference. The coincidence
values for any pair of regions can be calculated from the data in
Table 1.   For example, for the intervals II and V, which straddle
$arg4$, 11 doubles were observed and 44.7 were expected ($C = 0.29$).
For intervals II and VI, which are more widely separated, the coincidence value is 0.63 (42 observed, 66.3 expected).   Furthermore, the
double exchanges exhibit no chromatid interference.   The numbers of
2-, 3-, and 4-strand double crossovers observed were 99, 191, and
77, which does not differ significantly from the expected 1:2:1
distribution.

The various numbers of asci representing conversional events
in $arg4$ as well as recombination events in adjacent regions are
presented in Table 2.   The symbols C_0 (or ——) and C_x (or —x—)
denote conversional events with parental and recombined flanking
marker arrays, respectively.   The symbol R (or x), indicates a
reciprocal recombination event.   The classes of events that contain
two or more exchanges are apportioned in column 4 with respect to
the numbers of chromatids involved in the adjacent exchanges, $i.e.$
2-strand, 3-strand, or 4-strand double exchanges.

The data from Table 2 are presented in summary form in Table
3.   For each category of conversional events, $i.e.$ single-, double-,
or triple-allele conversions, a different combination of flanking
markers was examined to assess whether an exchange was associated
with the conversion.   This is indicated in column 2.   In column 3
are listed the corresponding regions in the $centromere - thr1$ interval that could be examined for additional exchanges.   This interval includes $arg4$ and hence contains regions close to this locus.
In contrast, the $thr1 - CUP1$ interval is distal to and further removed from $arg4$.   The results summarized in Table 3 demonstrate
that of the 91 $arg4$ conversions of the C_0 category, there were 33
with exchanges in $c-thr1$ and 44 with exchanges in $thr1-CUP1$.   If
crossing-over in the adjacent intervals was occurring at the control frequencies (Table 1), the expected numbers of exchanges in
these two regions would be 23.3 and 46.4, respectively.   In effect
then, crossing-over occurs at approximately control frequencies in
marked intervals adjacent to those harboring a conversion event of
the C_0 type (coincidence values = 1.42 and 0.95).   For the 105 asci
with $arg4$ conversions that were exchanged for their flanking markers, C_x, only 10 had additional exchanges in the $centromere-thr1$
interval, and 30 displayed additional exchanges in the more distal
$thr1-CUP1$ region.   The number of additional exchanges that would
have occurred if no interference existed would have been 20.1 and
53.6, respectively (coincidence values = 0.49 and 0.56).   For the
28 asci with a reciprocal event between adjacent $arg4$ alleles, the

Table 2. Conversions in *arg*4 and additional recombinations
in adjacent regions (Diploid X2961; 2566 unselected asci)

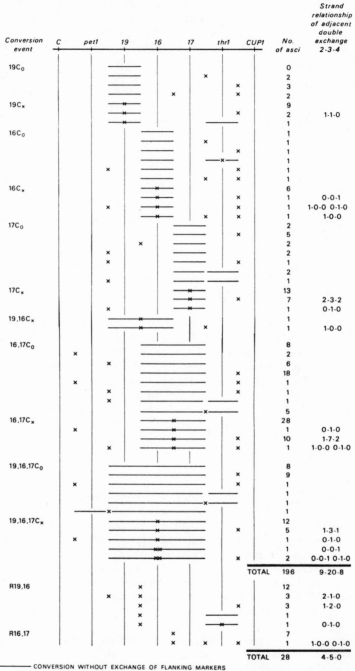

CONVERSION WITHOUT EXCHANGE OF FLANKING MARKERS
CONVERSION WITH EXCHANGE OF FLANKING MARKERS
×   RECIPROCAL EXCHANGE

Table 3. Summary of conversions in *arg4* and additional recombinations in adjacent regions (X2961, 2566 asci)

```
        pet1    19    16    17    18   thr1      CUP1
0 ----------------------------------------------------
       4.5   3.3   0.3   0.2           29
```

Alleles Converted	Flanking Markers	Additional Regions in c–thr	Map length of additional regions	C_O			C_X or R		
				No. of asci	Additional Exchange c–thr	thr–CUP	No. of asci	Additional Exchange c–thr	thr–CUP
19	pet1-16	c–pet, 16-17, 17-thr	22.7	7	4 *3.2*	5	12	0 *5.4*	2
16	19-17	c–pet, pet-19,17-thr	25.8	6	4 *3.7*	3	9	2 *2.3*	3
17	16-thr1	c–pet, pet-19, 19-16	8.1	15	6 *2.4*	6	21	1 *3.4*	7
19-16	pet1-17	c–pet, 17-thr	22.5	0	0	0	2	1 *.9*	0
16-17	19-thr1	c–pet, pet-19	7.8	42	16 *11.4*	20	40	2 *6.2*	11
19-16-17	pet1-thr1	c–pet	4.5	21	3 *2.6*	10	21	4 *1.9*	7
		Total observed		91	33	44	105	10	30
		Expected			*23.3*	*46.4*		*20.1*	*53.6*
		Coincidence			1.42	.95		0.49	0.56
Reciprocal Exchanges	19-16	c–pet, pet-19, 17-thr					20	3	4
	16-17	c–pet, pet-19, 19-16 thr					8	1	1
		Total observed					28	4	5
		Expected						*14.6*	*14.3*
		Coincidence						0.27	0.35

Italicized entries refer to expected numbers of exchanges, calculated from control exchange frequencies and corrected for cases of conversion of outside markers.

corresponding numbers of asci with additional exchanges in these
two intervals were 4 and 5, respectively. Assuming no interference,
the expected numbers in these two intervals would be 14.6 and 14.3
(coincidence values = 0.27 and 0.35).

A clear difference is apparent. If conversion is associated
with exchange of flanking genes, recombination in adjacent regions
is considerably reduced in comparison with meioses in which conversion occurred without exchange. A similar manifestation of
interference is seen for the asci in which a reciprocal event had
occurred between the alleles. The interference effect associated
with C_x events is less pronounced for the more distal *thr1-CUP1*
interval. These findings are consistent with the conclusions based
on selected prototrophic spores from *Neurospora* (Stadler, 1959).

Also from Table 2, it is apparent that the exchanges associated with approximately half of the conversion events do not show
chromatid interference relative to additional exchanges. Of 37
tetrads containing a conversion-associated exchange and an additional exchange, there were 9 2-strand, 20 3-strand, and 8 4-strand
double exchange -- a result consistent with the absence of chromatid interference. A similar lack of chromatid interference was
seen in the asci that segregated normally for markers on chromosome
VIII (Table 1).

CONVERSION IN *his1*

Summarized in Table 4 are the results from selected prototrophic tetrads derived from three hybrids heteroallelic at *his1* (Fogel and Hurst, 1967). The conversions have been classified as in
the analysis of X2961 (Table 3). As was found for events in the
arg4 locus, conversions in *his1* that were not recombined for flanking markers failed to generate interference for additional exchanges
in adjacent regions (coincidence = 3.3, 1.07, and 0.85). However,
conversions that were associated with exchange as well as reciprocal exchanges between the alleles exerted positive chiasma interference (C = 0.96, 0.09, and 0.67). This interference effect is
most pronounced for the *2 - arg6* interval and is considerably reduced for exchanges in *arg6 - trp2*. The anomolous results for the
hom3 - 1 region possibly reflect selective advantages associated
with the wild-type allele of *hom3*.

COINCIDENT CONVERSIONS OF ADJACENT GENES

In X2961, both *arg4* and *thr1* were converting at an approximately 10% frequency. The sample was sufficiently large to establish
whether or not conversion events, *i.e.* with or without recombination, interfered with each other. Of 2566 asci, there were 196

Table 4. Summary of conversions in *his1* and additional recombinations in adjacent regions

```
ura3  0 _____ hom3 _____ 1  2  arg 6 _____ trp2
               2.5          11          20
```

Alleles Converted	Flanking Markers	Additional Regions	C_o				C_x or R			
			No. of Asci	Additional Exchange			No. of Asci	Additional Exchange		
				hom-1	2-arg	arg-trp		hom-1	2-arg	arg-trp
1	*hom3-2*	2-arg6, arg6-trp2	415	-	97	146	220	-	5	55
					90.5	*170*			*47.9*	*90.2*
2	*1-arg6*	*hom3-1*, arg6-trp2	40	6	-	13	68	0	-	23
				1.8		*16.4*		*3.1*		*27.9*
Reciprocal Exchange	1-2	*hom3-1, 2-arg6, arg6-trp2*					91	7	1	19
								4.2	*19.8*	*37.3*
Total observed			455	6	97	159	379	7	6	97
Expected				*1.8*	*90.5*	*186.4*		*7.3*	*67.7*	*155.4*
Coincidence				3.3	1.07	0.85		.96	.09	.62

Italicized entries refer to expected numbers of exchanges calculated from control exchange frequencies.

conversions of one or more alleles in *arg4* and 159 in *thr1*. If
conversions had occurred independently, the expected number of asci,
with coincident conversions of these two genes would be 12.1.   In
this sample, 13 coincident conversions were observed (Table 2).
Thus, conversion events in adjacent regions do not appear to interfere with each other.

These findings are supported by data for *his2* and *SUP6* located 9 cM apart on chromosome VI (Hurst, Fogel, and Mortimer, 1972
and unpublished).   Both genes convert at a relatively high frequency.   In a sample of 2702 unselected asci segregating for both genes,
there were 381 conversions of *his2* and 301 conversions of *SUP6*.
There were 40 asci in which both genes were converted.   Of these,
32 were asymmetrical, ruling out the possibility that they arose by
single coconversional events.   The remaining 8 asci were symmetrical
and could represent coconversions of the two genes or independent
conversions that resulted in a symmetrical distribution.   The probability of symmetrical conversions (only parental genotype spores)
that would arise by chance from independent conversions is 1/8.
Thus, most if not all of the 40 coincident conversions can be accounted for by separate events.   If conversions at *his2* and *SUP6*
had occurred independently, 42.3 coincident conversions would have
been expected.   Again, it appears that conversion events in adjacent
genes in *Saccharomyces* do not interfere with each other.   A similar
conclusion was derived from a study of simultaneous conversions in
linked genes of *Ascobolus immersus* (Paszewski, 1967).

DISCUSSION

The data presented in this paper, which were derived from both
unselected and selected tetrads in yeast, permit the following conclusions:

1.   The two classes of conversion events, *i.e.* with or without
exchange, differ with respect to their effects on crossing-over in
adjacent regions.   Only conversions recombined for their flanking
markers depress crossing-over in adjacent intervals.   This supports
previously reported results (for review see Stadler, 1973) for *Neurospora* (Stadler, 1959) and *Ascobolus* (Baranowska, 1970; Stadler *et
al.*, 1970).

2.   The exchanges associated with conversion and the additional
exchanges do not exhibit chromatid interference.

3.   Reciprocal exchanges between the alleles are equivalent to
conversions associated with exchange with respect to both chiasma
and chromatid interference.

4.   Conversions of markers in adjacent intervals occur independently.

For the most part, molecular recombination models focus on accounting for both gene conversion and associated outside marker exchange in a single DNA segment. The sequences of events that lead to conversion alone or conversion with exchange usually differ only in the final steps that resolve the continuity of the DNA strands. Clearly, however, the two classes of conversion events are dissimilar in their effects on additional exchanges in neighboring genetic regions, and this dissimilarity is not readily accomodated by any of the current models. For example, with the model presented by Holliday (1964), one would need to propose that resolution by breakage and rejoining of the two strands that were broken initially would not cause interference, whereas rejoining of the other two strands would cause interference. It would appear that some additional features must be incorporated into the existing recombination models to account for the results presented above.

In this context, we make the following, somewhat speculative, proposals:

1.   All recombinogenic events have a common molecular basis. All such events result in a converted segment of chromosome that may or may not be associated with outside marker recombination.

2.   These recombinogenic events are distributed along the chromosome in an independent fashion; *i.e.*, the occurrence of an event at one site neither decreases nor increases the likelihood of an event at a neighboring site.

3.   The types of adjacent events, however, are not independent. If the first event results in conversion with an associated crossover, the next event is more likely to be a conversion without crossover.

This proposal accounts both for the chiasma interference observed for conversion events with crossing-over (and the lack of chiasma interference for conversion events not associated with crossing-over) and for the independent occurrence of total conversion events at neighboring genes. Classical chiasma interference is then not a reflection of altered probabilities concerning the fundamental recombinogenic event but is instead a consequence of constraints on the types of adjacent events. The model also predicts that the intensity of chiasma interference would decrease with increasing separation of intervals.

With respect to lack of chromatid interference, conversion-associated exchanges as well as reciprocal intragenic exchanges are equivalent to exchanges detected only on the basis of reciprocal marker exchange. This supports the proposal that all reciprocal recombination is associated with conversion.

None of the molecular models of recombination provide for chiasma interference. If the above proposal is to be incorporated into these models, some signal between adjacent recombinogenic events must exist to constrain that they are usually of opposite types. Because chiasma interference does not extend across the centromere, we presume that the signal postulated above is not propagated across this chromosomal element.

ACKNOWLEDGMENTS

This work was supported by the United State Atomic Energy Commission (R.K.M.) and GM-17317, U.S. Public Health Service (S.F.).

REFERENCES

Baranowska, A. 1970. Intragenic recombination pattern within the 164 locus of *Ascobolus immersus* in the presence of outside markers. Genet. Res. 16: 185.

Case, M. E. and N. H. Giles. 1964. Allelic recombination in Neurospora: Tetrad analysis of a three-point cross within the *pan-2* locus. Genetics 49: 529.

Fogel, S. and D. D. Hurst. 1967. Meiotic gene conversion in yeast tetrads and the theory of recombination. Genetics 57: 455.

Fogel, S. and R. K. Mortimer. 1969. Informational transfer in meiotic gene conversion. Proc. Nat. Acad. Sci. U.S.A. 62: 96.

Fogel, S., D. D. Hurst and R. K. Mortimer. 1971. Gene conversion in unselected tetrads from multipoint crosses. In (G. Kimber and F. P. Rédei, eds.) Stadler Genetics Symposia, Vols. 1 and 2, pp. 89-110. University of Missouri Agriculture Experiment Station, Columbia, Mo.

Hawthorne, D. C. and R. K. Mortimer. 1960. Chromsome mapping in *Saccharomyces:* centromere-linked genes. Genetics 45: 1085.

Holliday, R. 1964. A mechanism for gene conversion in fungi. Genet. Res. 5: 282.

Hurst, D. D., S. Fogel and R. K. Mortimer. 1972. Conversion-associated recombination in yeast. Proc. Nat. Acad. Sci. U.S.A. 69: 101.

Mitchell, M. B.   1955.   Aberrant recombination of pyridoxine mutants
of Neurospora.   Proc. Nat. Acad. Sci. U.S.A. 41: 935.

Paszewski, A.   1967.   A study on simultaneous conversions in linked
genes in *Ascobolus immersus*.   Genet. Res. 10: 121.

Paszewski, A.   1970.   Gene Conversion: Observations on the DNA
hybrid models.   Genet. Res. 15: 55.

Radding, C. M.   1973.   Molecular mechanisms in genetic recombination.
Ann. Rev. Genet. 7: 87.

Stadler, D. R.   1959.   The relationship of gene conversion to crossing-over in Neurospora.   Proc. Nat. Acad. Sci. U.S.A. 45: 1625.

Stadler, D. R.   1973.   The mechanism of intragenic recombination.
Ann. Rev. Genet. 7: 113.

Stadler, D. R., A. M. Towe and J. L. Rossignol.   1970.   Intragenic
recombination of ascospore color mutants in *Ascobolus* and its relationship to the segregation of outside markers.   Genetics 66: 429.

THE RELATIONSHIP BETWEEN GENETIC RECOMBINATION AND COMMITMENT TO CHROMOSOMAL SEGREGATION AT MEIOSIS

Rochelle E. Esposito, Diane J. Plotkin and Michael S. Esposito

Erman Biology Center, Department of Biology, University of Chicago, Chicago, Illinois 60637

INTRODUCTION

When meiocytes are removed from a meiosis-inducing environment at an early stage of development they can revert to mitotic division. At later developmental stages, however, they exhibit an irreversible commitment to the completion of meiosis and lose the ability to return to mitosis (Stern and Hotta, 1969; Ganesan *et al.*, 1958; Simchen *et al.*, 1972).

The events that lead to intragenic recombination during meiosis in yeast occur before cells become committed to the completion of meiosis (Sherman and Roman, 1963). When diploid cells of a suitable genotype are removed from a sporulation-inducing medium, a dramatic increase in the frequency of intragenic recombinants is observed among cells that revert to mitosis and remain diploid.

The present study provides evidence that cells stimulated to enter a meiotic cycle, which are capable of returning to mitosis, can exhibit intergenic recombination at frequencies characteristic of meiosis.

EXPERIMENTAL DESIGN AND RESULTS

A diploid strain, Z193, having the following genotype* was used in these studies:

---

* See following page

```
II                      lys2-1                              HIS7
—o————————————————————————————————————————————————————————————
            80          lys2-2              104               his7

III         a                       trp5-R   leu1  VII        ade6
—o——————————————————————————————————————————————o—————————————
     24     α                       trp5-20  16 LEU1  2    30  ADE6

ura1            XI                         XV                 ade2
—o——————————......o——                ——————o——————————————————
URA1                                               68        ade2
```

---

* Map distances are taken from Mortimer and Hawthorne (1973).
Ura1 was located on chromosome XI by trisomic analysis. The symbols are as follows: *a* and α, mating type alleles; *ade2*, adenine
requiring; *his7*, histidine requiring; *leu1*, leucine requiring; *lys2*,
lysine requiring; *trp5*, tryptophan requiring; *ura1*, uracil requiring.
Roman numerals indicate the chromosome number.

Z193 is heteroallelic at the *lys2* locus on chromosome II and
the *trp5* locus on chromosome VII. In addition, it is heterozygous
for *leu1* located 2 map units from the centromere of chromosome VII,
heterozygous for *ade6* 30 map units from the centromere of chromosome VII, and heterozygous for several other loci as indicated.
Z193 is a homothallic strain. Its meiotic products self-diploidize
upon germination to produce diploid cells homozygous for all markers
except the mating-type locus, which becomes heterozygous during the
diploidization process (Hawthorne, 1963).

The experiments were performed as follows: Z193 was introduced into a medium that induces meiosis and ascospore formation
(for methods see Esposito and Esposito, 1974; Fast, 1973). At
intervals cells were removed and plated on synthetic complete medium
to assay viability, and on lysineless and tryptophanless media to
select prototrophic intragenic recombinants at these loci. The
selected recombinant clones were then analyzed to determine the proportion that originated from cells which reverted to mitotic division (*i.e.* from cells uncommitted to meiotic segregation) and those
that originated from cells which completed the meiotic divisions and
formed meiotic products (*i.e.* from cells committed to meiosis). The
selected prototrophs were also examined to determine whether intergenic recombination had occurred and the extent of this recombination.

Figure 1 shows the recovery of lysine and tryptophan prototrophs from cells plated during sporulation. Prototrophs in excess

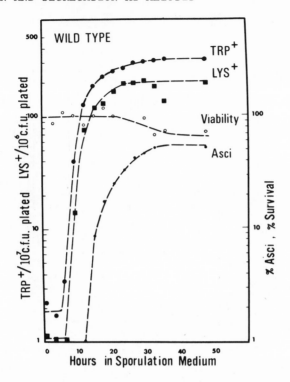

Figure 1.   Intragenic recombination at the *lys2* and *trp5* loci following exposure of diploid Z193 to sporulation medium.   Prototroph
values are given per colony-forming unit (c.f.u.) plated.   Cells
were pregrown in glucose nutrient medium prior to transfer to
sporulation medium (from Esposito and Esposito, 1974).

of the starting background were recovered after 6 hr of incubation
in sporulation medium.   The maximum yield of prototrophs was obtained by 30 hr of sporulation.   Ascus formation began at approximately 12 hr and proceeded to a final level of 50% asci.

     Prototrophs are formed primarily by gene conversion (Fogel and
Mortimer, 1969).   They are recovered among cells that resume mitotic
cell division or complete meiosis and diploidization following
plating.   The procedure used to analyze intergenic recombination
and commitment to meiosis among the prototrophs is summarized in
Fig. 2.   The analysis of lysine prototrophs is used as an example
of the general method employed.   The progeny of prototrophic cells
uncommitted to meiosis are (i) heterozygous at the locus where conversion occurred (*e.g. LYS2/lys2-2*), (ii) heterozygous for markers
closely linked to their centromeres (*e.g. LEU1/leu1*), and (iii)
heterozygous or homozygous for markers at some distance from their

Genetic Recombination and Commitment to Meiosis in a Homothallic Diploid

lys2-1   trp5-20   LEU1   ADE6
lys2-1   trp5-20   LEU1   ADE6

lys2-2   trp5-R   leu1   ade6
lys2-2   trp5-R   leu1   ade6

gene conversion
at lys2

reciprocal exchange
ade6 – centromere

LYS2   trp5-20   LEU1   ADE6
lys2-1   trp5-20   LEU1   ade6

lys2-2   trp5-R   leu1   ADE6
lys2-2   trp5-R   leu1   ade6

Mitosis

Meiosis I, II,
Diploidization of Gametes

(1) LYS2   trp5-20   LEU1   ADE6
    lys2-2   trp5-R   leu1   ade6

(2) LYS2   trp5-20   LEU1   ADE6
    lys2-2   trp5-R   leu1   ADE6

(3) LYS2   trp5-20   LEU1   ade6
    lys2-2   trp5-R   leu1   ade6

(1) LYS2   trp5-20   LEU1   ADE6
    LYS2   trp5-20   LEU1   ADE6

(2) LYS2   trp5-20   LEU1   ade6
    LYS2   trp5-20   LEU1   ade6

(3) LYS2   trp5-R   leu1   ADE6
    LYS2   trp5-R   leu1   ADE6

(4) LYS2   trp5-R   leu1   ade6
    LYS2   trp5-R   leu1   ade6

centromeres depending upon whether gene-centromere recombination
has occurred. When there is no recombination between a gene and
its centromere the marker remains heterozygous. When recombination
occurs, as between $ade6$ and its centromere (Fig. 2), then half of
the equational segregations yield heterozygotes ($ADE6/ade6$) and
half yield homozygotes ($ADE6/ADE6$ and $ade6/ade6$). Prototrophic
clones derived from cells that underwent meiosis and diploidization
are (i) homozygous at the locus where conversion occurred ($LYS2/$
$LYS2$), (ii) homozygous for markers closely linked to their centromeres, and (iii) homozygous for markers located some distance from
their centromeres.

     In summary, the progeny of uncommitted cells are heterozygous
at all loci except when recombination between a gene and its centromere renders the cell homozygous for that gene, while the progeny
of committed cells are homozygous at all loci except the mating-type
locus.

     Dissection and tetrad analysis of prototrophs recovered at 9
hr revealed that 98% of the lysine prototrophs and 96% of the
tryptophan prototrophs recovered at this time represent cells uncommitted to meiosis. Gene-centromere recombination among lysine
and tryptophan prototrophs not yet committed to meiotic segregation
is shown in Table 1. The value in parentheses below each marker is
the percent gene-centromere recombination expected if exchange
occurs at the meiotic level. Among both lysine and tryptophan prototrophs uncommitted to meiosis, the frequency of gene-centromere
recombination is orders of magnitude greater than normally encountered in mitotic cell populations, and it is approximately equal
to the meiotic value in certain intervals. Recombination at frequencies less than the meiotic values in such cells can have two
interpretations. Recombination may never achieve the meiotic value
for a given region or may do so with different rates in different
areas of the genome. A study of the kinetics of recombination in
the $leu1$ - $ade6$ interval was undertaken to determine whether intergenic recombination could exceed the values observed among prototrophs harvested at 9 hr of sporulation (details of procedures and
more extensive results will be published elsewhere).

Figure 2. Analysis of lysine prototrophs. Following gene conversion at the $lys2$ locus, cells revert to mitosis or complete meiosis and diploidization. Twice the percent of $leu1$ auxotrophs in a
sample of lysine prototrophs is used to estimate the fraction of
cells committed to meiosis at the time of plating. The frequency
of $ade6$ homozygotes among lysine prototrophs heteroallelic at the
$trp5$ locus is used to measure recombination in the $leu1$ - $ade6$
interval among cells uncommitted to meiosis. Recombination in the
$leu1$ - $ade6$ interval in diploidized meiotic products was monitored
among leucine auxotrophs homoallelic at the $trp5$ locus.

Table 1. Gene-centromere recombination among prototrophs uncommitted to meiosis in diploid Z193a

Prototrophic class	Number tested	Percent gene-centromere recombination					
		$\frac{ade6}{(30}$	$\frac{leu1}{(2)}$	$\frac{trp5}{(18)}$	$\frac{lys2}{(33)}$	$\frac{his7}{(33)}$	$\frac{ura1}{(33)}$
LYS[+]	99	14.7	2.1	7.0	—	16.7	23.4
TRP[+]	62	14.0	0.0	—	8.8	18.1	29.3

a Prototrophs examined were obtained from samples plated on lysine-less or tryptophanless medium after 9 hr of incubation in sporulation medium.

The kinetics of intragenic recombination and sporulation as well as other parameters measured are shown in Fig. 3. Lysine and tryptophan prototrophs in excess of the starting background were detected at 5 hr. The maximum yield of prototrophs at both loci was observed by 22 hr. Commitment of the lysine prototrophs to meiosis was first detected at 7 hr. Approximately 90% of these prototrophs were finally recovered as meiotic products. Ascospore production was detected beginning at 12 hr and increased to a final level of 70% asci at 22 hr. The data shown in the upper portion

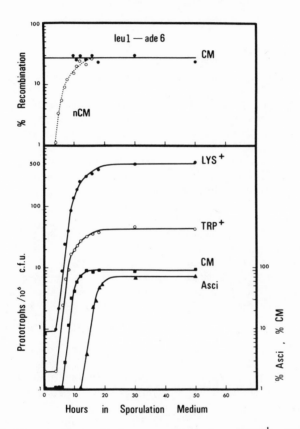

Figure 3. *Bottom:* Intragenic recombination (LYS$^+$, TRP$^+$), commitment to meiosis among lysine prototrophs (CM), and ascus production in Z193. The fraction of LYS$^+$ committed to meiosis is equal to twice the percent of leucine auxotrophs in the sample (*cf.* Fig. 2). Cells were pregrown in acetate nutrient medium prior to transfer to sporulation medium to improve the synchrony and extent of sporulation. *Top:* Kinetics of recombination in the *leu*1 - *ade*6 interval among lysine prototrophs committed to meiotic disjunction (●—●, CM) and cells not committed to meiotic disjunction (o--o, nCM).

of the figure indicate that recombination in the *leu*1 - *ade*6
interval among lysine prototrophs committed to meiotic disjunction
is at the final meiotic value regardless of the time of recovery
of committed prototrophs. Thus, recombination in this interval
among cells which complete meiosis occurs at the same frequency
irrespective of whether cells complete meiosis on selective growth
medium or in sporulation medium. Recombination in the *leu*1 - *ade*6
interval among cells uncommitted to meiosis, however, is initially
less than the meiotic value and with time proceeds to the meiotic
value. Studies in progress indicate that recombination in the centromere - *trp*5 interval is also at first below the meiotic value
and then achieves the meiotic value among cells uncommitted to
meiotic disjunction.

CONCLUSIONS

These data demonstrate that cells stimulated to enter meiosis
exhibit levels of intergenic recombination characteristic of
meiotic products before the cells become irreversibly committed to
a meiotic disjunction of chromosomes. Therefore, it appears that
(i) commitment to recombination precedes the decision to undergo
the meiotic divisions, and (ii) the events of homologous chromosome
pairing and recombination at levels typical of meiosis do not ensure
a meiotic disjunction of centromeres.

ACKNOWLEDGMENT

This research has been supported by NSF Grant GB-27688 and the
Wallace C. and Clara Abbott Memorial Fund of the University of
Chicago. D. J. Plotkin is a predoctoral trainee of the NIH Child
Health and Human Development Training Grant No. HD-174.

REFERENCES

Esposito, R. E. and M. S. Esposito. 1974. Genetic recombination
before commitment to meiosis in Saccharomyces. Proc. Nat. Acad.
Sci. U.S.A. in press.

Fast, D. 1973. Sporulation synchrony of *Saccharomyces cerevisiae*
grown in various carbon sources. J. Bacteriol. 116: 925.

Fogel, S. and Mortimer, R. K. 1969. Informational transfer in
meiotic gene conversion. Proc. Nat. Acad. Sci. U.S.A. 62: 96.

Ganesan, A. T., H. Holter and C. Roberts. 1958. Some observations
on sporulation in Saccharomyces. C. R. Trav. Lab. Carlsberg Ser.
Physiol. 31: 1.

Hawthorne, D. 1963. Directed mutation of the mating type allele as an explanation of homothallism in yeast (Abstr.). Proc. XI Int. Congr. Genet. 1: 34.

Mortimer, R. K. and D. C. Hawthorne. 1973. Genetic mapping in *Saccharomyces*. IV. Mapping of temperature-sensitive genes and use of disomic strains in localizing genes. Genetics 74: 33.

Sherman, F. and H. Roman. 1963. Evidence for two types of allelic recombination in yeast. Genetics 48: 255.

Simchen, G., R. Pinon and Y. Salts. 1972. Sporulation in *Saccharomyces cerevisiae*: Premeiotic DNA synthesis, readiness and commitment. Exp. Cell Res. 75: 207.

Stern, H. and Y. Hotta. 1969. DNA synthesis in relation to chromosome pairing and chiasma formation. Genetics (Suppl.) 61: 27.

PROPERTIES OF GENE CONVERSION OF DELETIONS IN *SACCHAROMYCES*

CEREVISIAE

Gerald R. Fink*

Department of Genetics Development and Physiology,

Cornell University, Ithaca, New York

Studies of large numbers of unselected asci in *Saccharomyces cerevisiae* have shown that gene conversion for heterozygous sites occurs frequently (Fogel and Mortimer, 1969; Hurst *et al.*, 1972). The conversion event is identified by 3+ : 1 m or 3m : 1+ ratios instead of the expected 2+ : 2m. A number of empirical generalizations have emerged from the conversion studies of Fogel, Hurst, and Mortimer. They are (1) *parity* — conversions of the type 3+ : 1m are equal to the type 3m : 1+; (2) *fidelity* — new alleles are not produced by gene conversion; (3) *coconversion* — when two sites within a gene are heterozygous, the alleles convert together as well as separately; (4) *absence of marker effects* — the conversion frequency for a given heterozygous site is constant, unrelated to its position in the map, and not influenced by other alleles within the gene; and (5) *conversion-associated recombination* — the frequency of reciprocal recombination for genes bracketing a site at which gene conversion has occurred is about 50%.

These five conclusions have been derived from studies on the conversion of point mutations of the missense and nonsense types. Little information is available concerning the affects of gross chromosome aberrations on gene conversion. Recently, we have described a procedure for the selection of deletions of the *his4* region in *Saccharomyces* (Fink and Styles, 1974). This region is one of the most intensively studied gene-enzyme systems in yeast (Shaffer *et al.*, 1972). Analysis of unselected asci from crosses

---

* Supported by NIH grant GM 15408

heterozygous for deletions show that gene conversion of deletions occurs. There are many similarities between the conversion of point mutations and the conversion of deletions. One difference is that the presence of a deletion can influence the conversion frequency of another site in the gene.

RESULTS

The deletions of the *his4* region are shown in Fig. 1. The compositions of the various diploids analyzed for gene conversion are depicted in Fig. 2. The number of tetrads analyzed and the composition of each tetrad are shown in Table 1.

Parity

The equality of conversion types 3+ : 1 m and 3m : 1+ in crosses heterozygous for certain of our deletions (26 and 29) indicates that parity can be a property of gene conversion of deletions as well as point mutations. However, deletion *his4-15* shows an excess of 3+ : 1 m conversions. This inequality in conversion types may be unrelated to deletions, as can be seen in the lack of parity for the point mutation *his4-290*.

Fidelity

No new mutations were produced by gene conversion of deletions. The end points of every deletion in the 3m : 1+ asci were tested by recombination and shown to be identical to those of the parent deletion. In addition, when the point mutation *his4-290* was converted, recombination and complementation analysis indicated that the emerging *his4C* alleles were not different from *his4C-290*.

Figure 1. Deletion map of the *his4* region. The heavy solid line represents the yeast chromosome in the *his4* region. Each number on that line stands for an independently isolated mutation. The letters designate the different functional segments within *his4*. Sets of mutations that fail to recombine with one another are grouped vertically. All circled numbers represent nonsense mutations. Those with stripes are amber (UAG) and those without are ochre (UAA). Mutations below the heavy horizontal line are deletions. The positions of the mutational sites above the line were determined by deletion mapping. Distances between the sites are arbitrary.

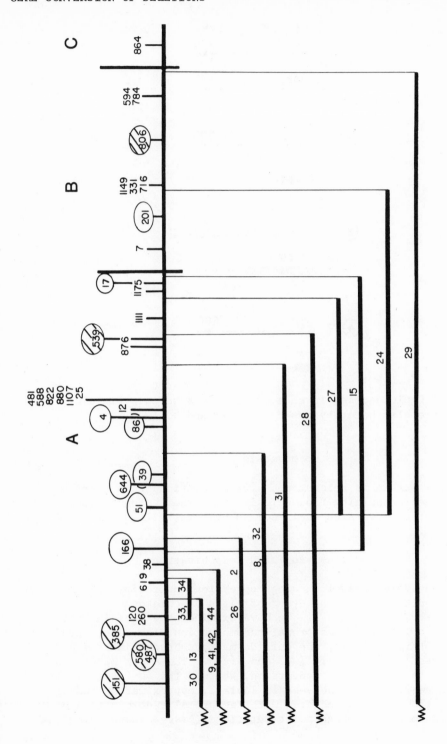

Figure 1. Deletions of the *his4* region.

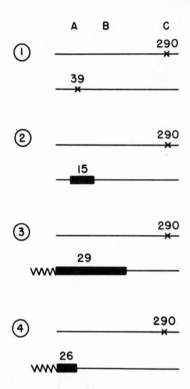

Figure 2. Diploids used in gene conversion studies. Diploids 1, 2, and 3 are also heterozygous for *leu2-1* and *ade2-1*.

Coconversions

When a strain is heterozygous for a deletion and a point muta-tion, the asci resulting from meiosis often show coconversion. The two types of coconversion asci seem to be equally frequent.

Conversion-Associated Recombination

The analysis of asci showing conversion and reciprocal recom-bination indicates that the order of sites on chromosome III is centromere-*leu2-his4A-his4C*. We have examined the asci in Table 1 for the association of reciprocal recombination with gene conver-sion. For this analysis, the outside markers bracketing the con-version event at *his4A* were *leu2* and *his4C*. The *his4C* marker is very close to the site of conversion, whereas the *leu2* site is 16 map units away. As can be seen in Table 2, approximately 50% of the conversions were associated with reciprocal recombination of the outside markers. Both point mutations (*his4-39*) and deletions

Table 1. Meiotic events at the *his4* region (frequency of gene conversion for the diploids shown in Fig. 2)

Diploid	No. of tetrads	Conversion				Coconversion		R[a]
						+→C A→+	C→+ +→A	
		+→C	C→+	+→A	A→+	A→+	+→A	
his4-39/200	404	11	3	10	16	2	5	2
15/290	401	8	7	2	11	3	4	0
29/290	433	4	2	5	3	0	1	1
26/290	131	3	0	4	4	0	0	1

[a] Number of asci showing reciprocal recombination

at *his4* show this high frequency of conversion-associated reciprocal recombination.

Marker Effects

Deletions, unlike point mutations, can show marker effects. As shown in Table 3, the frequency of conversion of *his4-290* is lowered by the presence of deletion *his4-29*. Deletion *his4-15* does not seem to alter the conversion frequency of *his4-290*.

Table 2. Reciprocal recombination associated with gene conversion

Diploid	Type of conversion	
	A→+	+→A
	Fraction reciprocally recombined	
his4-39/290	13/16	4/10
15/290	6/11	0/2
29/290	1/4	3/4
Total	20/31	7/16

Fraction of deletion conversions
with a crossover = 10/21

Table 3.   Conversion frequencies for *his4* mutations

	% Conversions			
Diploid	A		C	
his4-39/290	8.2	$\dfrac{33}{404}$	5.2	$\dfrac{21}{404}$
15/290	5.0	$\dfrac{20}{401}$	5.4	$\dfrac{22}{401}$
29/290	2.0	$\dfrac{9}{433}$	1.6	$\dfrac{7}{433}$

The *his4A* alleles are *his4-39*, *his4-15*, and *his4-29*, respectively; the *his4C* allele is *his4-290* in all three crosses.   The conversion of *his4-290* is significantly lower in the third cross than in the first two.   Using the method of Brandt and Snedecor (Snedecor, 1940), the probability (P) is less than 0.01, indicating significant heterogeneity.

DISCUSSION

Studies on gene conversion of deletions should provide important information concerning the mechanism of recombination in yeast. Our studies have already shown that gene conversion of deletions is similar to gene conversion of point mutations.   One difference is that the presence of a deletion in a gene can influence the conversion frequency of another site within the gene.   Deletion *his4-29* lowers the conversion frequency of the distal site *his4-290*.   This depression is likely to result from aberrant pairing of the heterozygous deletion, as shown by the following result.   Analysis of 244 tetrads from a strain in which deletion *his4-29* was homozygous and the distal *his4* site *his4C-290* was heterozygous (*29/29-290*) gave 6 asci of the type 3+ : 1(*290*) and 6 of the type 1+ : 3(*290*).   In other words, the conversion frequency of *his4-290* (4.9%) returns to normal when the deletion is homozygous.   Clearly, further study of new deletions through the ends of *his4* should provide information on the factors influencing gene conversion.

One note of caution should be added.   Tetrad analysis is really necessary to prove that conversion frequencies are a heritable property of the allele under observation.   This means crossing ascospores from tetrads (several) in which the allele has been segregating 2:2 and showing that the conversion frequency of all His⁻ spores is identical, segregating 2:2 along with the *his⁻* allele.   This type of experiment involves an enormous amount of labor.   To date no one has reported the results of such a study.

REFERENCES

Fink, G. R. and C. Styles. 1974. Gene conversion of deletions in the *his4* region of yeast. Genetics in press.

Hurst, D., S. Fogel and R. K. Mortimer. 1972. Conversion associated recombination in yeast. Proc. Nat. Acad. Sci. U.S.A. **69**: 101.

Fogel, S. and R. K. Mortimer. 1969. Informational transfer in meiotic gene conversion. Proc. Nat. Acad. Sci. U.S.A. **69**: 96.

Snedecor, G. 1940. In <u>Statistical</u> <u>Methods</u>. p. 207. Iowa State College Press, Iowa.

Shaffer, B., S. Edelstein and G. R. Fink. 1972. *His4* a gene complex of *Saccharomyces cerevisiae*. Brookhaven Symp. Biol. **23**: 250.

LACK OF CORRESPONDENCE BETWEEN GENETIC AND PHYSICAL DISTANCES

IN THE ISO-1-CYTOCHROME *c* GENE OF YEAST

Carol W. Moore and Fred Sherman

Department of Radiation Biology and Biophysics, School

of Medicine and Dentistry, and Department of Biology,

University of Rochester, New York 14642

It is necessary to study intragenic recombination at a locus for which the primary sequence analysis of the gene product is available if one wishes an unequivocal check on the positions of the mutant sites in the structural gene, as well as to uncover factors other than distance that might affect frequencies of genetic exchanges. The iso-1-cytochrome *c* gene of the bakers' yeast *Saccharomyces cerevisiae*, therefore, is particularly suitable. Nucleotide sequences of numerous mutant codons have been identified from alterations in functional iso-1-cytochromes *c* produced by intragenic revertants, but all too often an order of *cyc*1 mutational sites establishable from mapping frequencies is not compatible with corresponding alterations in the sequence of amino-acid residues.

We have undertaken an extensive investigation designed to examine how rates of recombination are affected by the nature of mutant base pairs and by adjacent nucleotide sequences. In this paper we report the disparity between physical distances, which are deduced from altered proteins, and map distances, which are based on the rates of X-ray-induced recombination for pairwise crosses of the four defined *cyc*1 mutants, *cyc*1-13, *cyc*1-76, *cyc*1-179, and *cyc*1-239. Our findings indicate that the X-ray mapping procedure is unreliable for measuring physical distances; they also demonstrate that recombinational processes are influenced by particular nucleotide sequences.

MATERIALS AND METHODS

Mutant Codons

The mutational lesions of three of the four mutants, *cyc*1-13, *cyc*1-179, and *cyc*1-239 lie within the region of the gene which corresponds to the dispensable amino-terminal portion of iso-1-cytochrome *c* (Sherman and Stewart, 1973; Stewart and Sherman, 1974). The *cyc*1-13 mutant contains one of the isoleucine codons AUU, AUC, or AUA, instead of the normal AUG initiation codon (Stewart *et al.*, 1971). The *cyc*1-179 mutant contains the UAG (amber) codon corresponding to amino-acid residue position 9 (Stewart and Sherman, 1972). The frameshift mutant *cyc*1-239 has a deletion of a single G·C base pair at the third position of the lysine 4 codon (see Stewart and Sherman, 1974). The fourth mutant, *cyc*1-76, contains an amber codon corresponding to amino-acid position 71 in the total sequence of 108 residues (Stewart and Sherman, 1973).

Strains

Three haploid strains, *cyc*1-13, *cyc*1-76, and *cyc*1-179, were directly derived from D311-3A by mutation (Sherman *et al.*, 1974). The *cyc*1-239 mutant was isolated as a recombinant from a frameshift revertant; therefore, it is not isogenic to the other three *cyc*1 haploid strains. Crosses of all pairwise combinations of the four *cyc*1 alleles were made using the three isogenic haploid strains as well as 11 haploid strains derived from meiotic pedigrees. From 3 to 8 different diploids were constructed for each heteroallelic combination. The potential variability due to the influence of genetic background should be uncovered in the analyses of the 38 resulting heteroallelic and homoallelic diploids.

Media and Selection of Recombinants

Procedures for selecting recombinants and revertants on lactate medium and assaying viability and cell number on glycerol medium have been described by Sherman *et al.* (1974).

Procedure for X-Irradiation

In all experiments fresh cells from liquid-grown cultures were X-irradiated at 2, 4, and 6 krad on the surface of solid lactate and glycerol media in open plastic petri dishes. A Machlett OEG-60-7 X-ray tube, powered by a custom-made X-ray generator (Picker Corp.) was operated at 50 kVp and 25 mA; the dose rate at the surface of the plates was determined to be 28 krads/min by a Model 555 Radcon

II ratemeter with a 555-100 LA Probe (Victoreen Instrument Division).

RESULTS

X-irradiation of all of the 38 heteroallelic and homoallelic strains constructed for this study resulted in the induction of prototrophs with a frequency linearly proportional to dose, except for the homoallelic cyc1-239/cyc1-239 diploid, which rarely gave rise to prototrophs. These linear rates of X-ray-induced prototrophs are expressed in X-ray mapping milliunits, defined as prototrophs per 10^{11} survivors per roentgen. The values for each strain (Table 1) usually varied less than 20% from one experiment to another. It can be seen that values obtained with heteroallelic strains generally were two to three orders of magnitude higher than those for the homoallelic strains. The increases of the heteroallelic values above the corresponding homoallelic values can be assumed to measure primarily interallelic recombination.

Values from independent crosses involving the same cyc1 pair were quite comparable, in spite of the fact that parental haploid strains were not necessarily isogenic. The fact that comparable frequencies were obtained in only partially related strains indicates that these values are properties of the heteroallelic pairs and are not strongly modified by undefined genes. However, some of the two- to threefold variation among strains of the same cyc1 genotype may be strain dependent. For example, CM-12, CM-15, and CM-54 were constructed using the same cyc1-179 and three different cyc1-13 parents; these three diploid strains exhibited twofold higher frequencies than CM-1, CM-14, and CM-98, which share in common another cyc1-179 parent. Also, CM-128 and CM-131 were constructed using the same cyc1-76 strain and two cyc1-13 strains, and their recombination frequencies were similar to each other but were more than double those of CM-135, CM-136, and CM-137, which were constructed from different sets of cyc1-76 and cyc1-13 strains.

The mutational sites of the mutants cyc1-13, cyc1-239, and cyc1-179 delimit two adjacent intervals of 13 base pairs at the beginning of the gene (Fig. 1). Thus, if frequencies of genetic exchanges directly correlate with distances separating altered nucleotides, the two segments should be comparable. The mean frequency for the eight cyc1-13/cyc1-239 diploids was 2200 X-ray mapping milliunits, in marked contrast with only 84 milliunits for the six cyc1-239/cyc1-179 heteroallelic strains. This 26-fold discrepancy in recombination frequencies for two segments of equal physical length is drawn to scale in Fig. 1, along with the relative frequency for the entire cyc1-13—cyc1-179 segment, which is 25 base pairs long and corresponds to 340 milliunits of recombination. The latter

Table 1. X-ray-induced rates of recombination and reversion for

Cross	Strain no.	Rate ± s.d.
*cyc*1-13 X *cyc*1-239	CM-4	2060 ± 61
	CM-18	2450 ± 120
	CM-19	2080 ± 160
	CM-22	2250 ± 99
	CM-57	1800 ± 240
	CM-97	1610 ± 36
	CM-103	2170 ± 82
	CM-104	3180 ± 22
	Mean	2200
*cyc*1-239 X *cyc*1-179	CM-60	47 ± 5
	CM-99	125 ± 9
	CM-100	80 ± 7
	CM-105	115 ± 2
	CM-106	72 ± 7
	CM-107	62 ± 8
	Mean	84
*cyc*1-13 X *cyc*1-179	CM-1	218 ± 41
	CM-12	326 ± 26
	CM-14	257 ± 29
	CM-15	587 ± 74
	CM-54	503 ± 31
	CM-98	207 ± 16
	CM-101	280 ± 24
	Mean	340
*cyc*1-179 X *cyc*-76	CM-127	1510 ± 210
	CM-130	1110 ± 71
	CM-134	1090 ± 73
	Mean	1237

Units are X-ray mapping milliunits: prototrophs/10^{11}survivors/

heteroallelic and homoallelic *cyc*1 strains

Cross	Strain no.	Rate ± s.d.
*cyc*1-239 X *cyc*1-76	CM-118	4010 ± 610
	CM-126	2920 ± 86
	CM-138	1600 ± 120
	CM-139	3000 ± 120
	Mean	2882
*cyc*1-13 X *cyc*1-76	CM-128	3980 ± 100
	CM-131	4080 ± 240
	CM-135	1550 ± 300
	CM-136	2200 ± 120
	CM-137	1380 ± 240
	Mean	2638
*cyc*1-13 X *cyc*1-13	CM-6	3.3 ± 1.9
	CM-102	1.5 ± 0.9
	Mean	2.4
*cyc*1-239 X *cyc*1-239	CM-21	0 ± 0
*cyc*1-179 X *cyc*1-179	CM-3	6.1 ± 1.8
*cyc*1-76 X *cyc*1-76	CM-133	9.7 ± 2.6

roentgen.

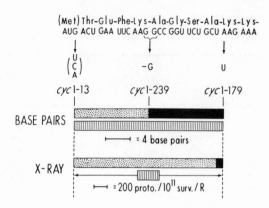

Figure 1. The mutational location and alteration in the messenger
RNA sequence of each of the three mutants, *cyc*1-13, *cyc*1-239 and
*cyc*1-179, and the mean rates of X-ray-induced recombination for the
three possible heteroallelic crosses (see Table 1). Shown on the
top of the figure are the normal amino-acid sequence of the amino-
terminal region of iso-1-cytochrome *c* and the corresponding sequence
of the mRNA (Stewart and Sherman, 1974). The relative rates are
drawn to scale and are represented as follows: stippled bar,
*cyc*1-13 X *cyc*1-239; black bar, *cyc*1-239 X *cyc*1-179; vertically
lined bar, *cyc*1-13 X *cyc*1-179.

is clearly inconsistent with values for either of the two 13 base-
pair segments, by criteria for either additivity or, more important,
known physical distance.

     The fourth mutant, *cyc*1-76, contains an amber codon correspond-
ing to amino-acid position 71. Relative to *cyc*1-76, therefore, the
mutational lesions of *cyc*1-13, *cyc*1-239, and *cyc*1-179 are all separated by approximately the same physical distance. Indeed, the
induced rates of recombination in *cyc*1-76/*cyc*1-13 and *cyc*1-76/*cyc*1-
239 diploids were very similar, but these rates corresponding to the
long intervals were comparable to those for the *cyc*1-13—*cyc*1-239
interval, which includes only 13 base pairs (Fig. 2). Also inconsistent, *cyc*1-179/*cyc*1-76 diploids, which on the basis of physical
distances separating the mutational sites should be similar to
*cyc*1-13/*cyc*1-76 and *cyc*1-239/*cyc*1-76 diploids, measure, on the average, only one half these two heteroallelic classes and, moreover,
measure only one-half the *cyc*1-13/*cyc*1-239 strains whose mutational
sites define an interval of 13 base pairs.

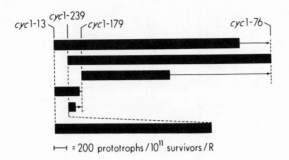

Figure 2. Diagram comparing the physical distances separating the four mutants cyc1-13, cyc1-239, cyc1-179, and cyc1-76, and the genetic distances based on rates of X-ray-induced recombination for the six heteroallelic crosses.

DISCUSSION

Considering the recombinational data presented in this report, it is clear that X-ray-induced rates of prototroph production fail to reflect either the correct order of the mutational sites or relative physical distances separating them. The use of cyc1 mutants with defined nucleotide changes permits the calculation of recombination rates as a function of the number of base pairs separating the mutant sites. Such normalized recombination rates (Table 2) reveal the gross disparity in the rates for the heteroallelic combination, cyc1-13—cyc1-239, which in comparison to rates for the other five heteroallelic pairs are 13 to 72 times greater. This extensive disproportion between genetic and physical distances presumably is due to the combination of nucleotide sequences in the cyc1-13/cyc1-239 diploids; neither cyc1-13 nor cyc1-239, in combination with the other mutants, cyc1-76 and cyc1-179, gives rise to disproportionately high rates of recombination.

There also appear to be disproportionalities among the other five heteroallelic combinations, but to a lower extent. While the ranges of values from strains having the same heteroallelic pairs obscure the comparisons of strains having different heteroallelic pairs, less ambiguous comparisons can be made with isogenic series of crosses. The three haploid strains cyc1-13, cyc1-76, and cyc1-179, directly derived from D311-3A (see Materials and Methods), should be closely related. Normalized values from the series of crosses of these three isogenic haploids to various cyc1 mutants are presented in Table 2. The normalized values from these three series of isogenic crosses not only establish the marked disproportionality of the cyc1-13—cyc1-239 combination but also indicate that there are differences between cyc1-239—cyc1-179 and cyc1-239—cyc1-76 combinations, and possibly between cyc1-13—cyc1-179 and cyc1-13

Table 2. Number of base pairs per X-ray mapping unit for each heteroallelic combination

Cross	cyc1-13 X cyc1-239	cyc1-239 X cyc1-179	cyc1-13 X cyc1-179	cyc1-179 X cyc1-76	cyc1-239 X cyc1-76	cyc1-13 X cyc1-76
Number of base pairs	13	13	25	186	199	211
Base pairs per X-ray mapping unit						
Isogenic strains: X cyc1-13			89			53
X cyc1-239	8.1	113			50	
X cyc1-239	4.1	104			68	
All strains: Range	4.1 to 8.1	105 to 277	43 to 121	123 to 171	50 to 124	52 to 153
Mean	5.9	155	73.5	150	69	80

*cyc*1-76 combinations. In addition, there is little or no overlap
of the values of the groups of *cyc*1-179/*cyc*1-76 strains in comparison to either the groups of *cyc*1-13/*cyc*1-179 or *cyc*1-239/*cyc*1-76
strains, suggesting disproportional rates of recombination. While
it is unreliable to conclude from these results whether the normalized rates for any two different heteroallelic combinations are
truly equivalent, some appear to be at least very similar, such as
the *cyc*1-239/*cyc*1-179 diploids compared to either the *cyc*1-13/*cyc*1-
179 or *cyc*1-13/*cyc*1-76 diploids.

Linear rates of recombination derived by treatments with ionizing radiation have been used to construct genetic maps, first for
the *trp*5 and *arg*4 loci (Manney and Mortimer, 1964) and later, for
the *his*4 (Fink, 1966), *ade*8 (Esposito, 1968), *leu*1 (Nakai and Mortimer, 1967), *cyc*1 (Parker and Sherman, 1969), *ilv*1 (Thuriaux *et*
al., 1971), *asp*1 (Jones, 1973) and *his*1 (Korch and Snow, 1973) loci.
Although nonadditivity between sites was often encountered and many
sites could not be unambiguously ordered, several investigators
assumed that the rates were proportional to the physical distances
between the two sites of a heteroallelic pair. However, it is clear
for the defined *cyc*1 mutants examined in this study that the propor-
tionality fails to hold. The disparity between genetic and physical
distances is dependent not only on disproportionality intrinsic to
different heteroallelic pairs but also to the variability observed
with different strains containing the same heteroallelic pair.
Nevertheless, approximate correspondences may fortuitously appear,
as was apparently the case for the first X-ray map of the *cyc*1 gene
reported by Parker and Sherman (1969) and the related amino-acid
changes in iso-1-cytochrome *c* (Sherman *et al.*, 1970). However, the
amino-acid replacements in the revertants from *cyc*1-8 and *cyc*1-15
(see Putterman *et al.*, 1974) did not correspond to the mutational
lesions in the gene, and the sites were incorrectly assigned. A
genetic map of *cyc*1 alleles, including *cyc*1-8 and *cyc*1-15, was constructed recently by deletion mapping (Sherman *et al.*, unpublished
results), which gives unambiguous order in contrast to X-ray mapping
of two-point crosses. Thus we are forced to emphasize the early
view that "one should be reluctant to equate X-ray-mapping units
with lengths of DNA or protein" (Sherman *et al.*, 1970; Sherman and
Stewart, 1971). This view has been substantiated from the lack of
complete agreement between X-ray mapping and deletion mapping of the
*his*4 locus (Fink and Styles, 1974).

The relationships between recombination rates and physical
distances in yeast are being examined with other mapping procedures,
including the use of spontaneous rates of mitotic and meiotic recombination (Moore and Sherman, in preparation). So far we have not
uncovered any reliable method for measuring physical distances from
recombination rates of two-point crosses.

The lack of correspondence between physical and genetic distances has been established either directly or indirectly in numerous prokaryotic and other eukaryotic systems. Genetic distances inferred from frequencies of recombination often are not additive, and the order of the mutational sites does not necessarily correspond to the order determined by deletion mapping. In fact, in the extensive study of conjugation crosses by Norkin (1970), where mutant sites in the *lac*Z gene of *Escherichia coli* were ordered unambiguously by deletion mapping, distances separating allelic markers were shown to be of negligible importance in recombination between them. Then recently, Stadler and Kariya (1973) described the high recombination behavior of certain tryptophan synthetase mutants of *E. coli* whose nucleotide sequence changes associated with mutant codons were identified from protein analyses of the gene product. There has been no simple explanation for the disproportionalities of recombination frequencies reported in these studies with *E. coli*, nor in other studies with prokaryotes (see review by Stadler, 1973). On the other hand, Leblon (1972a, b) concluded from their studies of spore-color alleles in *Ascobolus immersus* that frameshift mutants act differently in recombination. In contrast, there is no evidence from the studies of *trp*A mutants of *E. coli* (Stadler and Kariya, 1973) or from our studies of *cyc*1 mutants that frameshift mutants necessarily affect recombination differently than base-pair substitution mutants. From our studies, it appears as if combinations of certain nucleotide sequences in some way influence the rate of recombination, and that disproportionalities cannot be explained by the nucleotide sequence of the mutant codons alone. It is our hope that extension of the study with additional defined *cyc*1 mutants at different sites may reveal these sequences.

ACKNOWLEDGMENTS

This investigation was supported in part by U. S. Public Health Service Research Grant GM12702 and in part by the U. S. Atomic Energy Commission at the University of Rochester Atomic Energy Project, Rochester, New York; it has been designated USAEC Report no. UR-3490-542.

REFERENCES

Esposito, M. S. 1968. X-ray and meiotic fine structure mapping of the adenine-8 locus in *Saccharomyces cerevisiae*. Genetics 58: 507.

Fink, G. R. 1966. A cluster of genes controlling three enzymes in histidine biosynthesis in *Saccharomyces cerevisiae*. Genetics 53: 445.

Fink, G. R. and C. A. Styles. 1974. Gene conversion of deletions in the *his4* region of yeast. Genetics in press.

Jones, G. E. 1973. A fine-structure map of the yeast L-asparaginase gene. Molec. Gen. Genet. 121: 9.

Korch, C. T. and R. Snow. 1973. Allelic complementation in the first gene for histidine biosynthesis in *Saccharomyces cerevisiae*. I. Characteristics of mutants and genetic mapping of alleles. Genetics 74: 287.

Leblon, G. 1972a. Mechanism of gene conversion in *Ascobolus immersus*. I. Existence of a correlation between the origin of mutants induced by different mutagens and their conversion spectrum. Molec. Gen. Genet. 115: 36.

Leblon, G. 1972b. Mechanism of gene conversion in *Ascobolus immersus*. II. The relationships between the genetic alterations in b_1 or b_2 mutants and their conversion spectrum. Molec. Gen. Genet. 116: 322.

Manney, T. R. and R. K. Mortimer. 1964. Allelic mapping in yeast by X-ray induced mitotic reversion. Science 143: 581.

Nakai, S. and R. K. Mortimer. 1967. Induction of different classes of genetic effects in yeast using heavy ions. Radiat Res. 7 (Suppl.): 172.

Norkin, L. C. 1970. Marker-specific effects in genetic recombination. J. Mol. Biol. 51: 633.

Parker, J. H. and F. Sherman. 1969. Fine-structure mapping and mutational studies of gene controlling yeast cytochrome c. Genetics 62: 9.

Putterman, G. J., E. Margoliash and F. Sherman. 1974. Identification of missense mutants by amino acid replacements in iso-1-cytochrome c from yeast. J. Biol. Chem. 235 in press.

Sherman, F., J. W. Stewart, J. H. Parker, G. J. Putterman, B. B. L. Agrawal and E. Margoliash. 1970. The relationship of gene structure and protein structure of iso-1-cytochrome c from yeast. Symp. Soc. Exp. Biol. 24: 85.

Sherman, F. and J. W. Stewart. 1971. Genetics and biosynthesis of cytochrome c. Ann. Rev. Genet. 5: 257.

Sherman, F. and J. W. Stewart. 1973. Mutations at the end of the iso-1-cytochrome c gene of yeast. In (J. K. Pollak and J. W. Lee,

eds.) The Biochemistry of Gene Expression in Higher Organisms.
p. 56. Australian and New Zealand Book Co., Sydney.

Sherman, F., J. W. Stewart, M. Jackson, R. A. Gilmore and J. H.
Parker. 1974. Mutants of yeast defective in iso-1-cytochrome c.
Genetics in press.

Stadler, D. 1973. The mechanism of intragenic recombination.
Ann. Rev. Genet. 7: 113.

Stadler, D. and B. Kariya. 1973. Marker effects in the genetic
transduction of tryptophan mutants of $E.$ $coli$. Genetics 75: 423.

Stewart, J., F. Sherman, N. A. Shipman and M. Jackson. 1971.
Identification and mutational relocation of the AUG codon initiating
translation of iso-1-cytochrome c in yeast. J. Biol. Chem. 246:
7429.

Stewart, J. and F. Sherman. 1972. Demonstration of UAG as a nonsense codon in bakers' yeast by amino-acid replacements in iso-1-
cytochrome c. J. Mol. Biol. 68: 429.

Stewart, J. W. and F. Sherman. 1973. Confirmation of UAG as a nonsense codon in bakers' yeast by amino acid replacements of glutamic
acid 71 in iso-1-cytochrome c. J. Mol. Biol. 78: 169.

Stewart, J. W. and F. Sherman. 1974. Yeast frameshift mutations
identified by sequence changes in iso-1-cytochrome c. In (M. W.
Miller, ed.) Molecular and Environmental Aspects of Mutagenesis.
C. C. Thomas, Springfield, Illinois, in press.

Thuriaux, P., M. Minet, M. M. A. Ten Berge and F. K. Zimmerman.
1971. Genetic fine structure and function of mutants at the $ilv1$-
gene locus of $Saccharomyces$ $cerevisiae$. Molec. Gen. Genet. 112: 60.

RECOMBINATION OF MITOCHONDRIAL GENES IN YEAST

Bernard Dujon

Centre de Génétique Moléculaire du C.N.R.S.

91190, Gif-sur-Yvette, France

INTRODUCTION

Mitochondrial mutations conferring resistance to specific antibiotics have been isolated in the yeast *Saccharomyces cerevisiae*. These mutations are located in the mitochondrial DNA (mtDNA) molecule (Nagley and Linnane, 1972; Faye *et al.*, 1973; Deutsch *et al.*, 1974). Mitochondrial recombination in yeast is interesting to consider in a symposium on mechanisms in recombination for several reasons: (1) mitochondrial genetics is a population genetics similar in certain aspects to bacteriophage genetics, (2) the elementary acts of recombination are of the nonreciprocal type, and (3) the occurrence of repetitive sequences in mtDNA of ρ^- mutants offers a tool to study recombination in segments of repeated genes. Recently, extensive studies on multifactorial mitochondrial crosses have been published (Kleese *et al.*, 1972; Suda and Uchida, 1972; Avner *et al.*, 1973; Wolf *et al.*, 1973; Howell *et al.*, 1973; Rank, 1973 and Netter *et al.*, 1974), using a standard cross procedure described by Coen *et al.* (1970), in which a random sample of a population issued from many zygotes after some 20 cell divisions is analyzed. From these studies features of exchanges of mitochondrial genetic material appeared, permitting Dujon *et al.* (1973) to develop a model for recombination of mitochondrial genes which integrates all the present experimental facts. This model is composed of two parts, the first part dealing with the process of pairing between mtDNA molecules and the second dealing with the mechanism of recombination between paired mtDNA molecules. This article will be essentially focused on the second part with a short summary of the first one.

307

FEATURES OF GENETIC EXCHANGES IN MITOCHONDRIA

Genetic features of multifactorial crosses are (1) a high
positive coincidence for both close and distant markers; *i.e.*,
there are at least twice as many double recombinants as expected
from the product of frequencies of single recombinants; (2) an
upper limit of frequency of recombinants of around 20 to 25% for
pairs of genetically unlinked markers; (3) a variable input fraction from one cross to another depending on nuclear genetic backgrounds and physiological conditions; (4) a coordinated output of
all the alleles issued from the same parent depending on variations
of input. All these features are in favor of the idea that mitochondrial genomes constitute a panmictic pool of molecules characterized by a variable input fraction and undergoing several mating
rounds that are random in time. Therefore, mitochondrial genetics
is similar in this aspect to the bacteriophage genetics described
by Visconti and Delbrück (1953), which is the genetics of a dynamic
population of molecules. The genetic composition of this population
evolves as a function of the average number of mating rounds. It
should be stressed that since frequencies of recombinants are functions of both the probabilities of genetic exchanges and the average
number of mating rounds, an independent estimate of this latter
parameter is necessary to determine the former. These calculations
permit speculations on the mechanisms involved in recombination.

ELEMENTARY ACTS OF RECOMBINATION BETWEEN mtDNA MOLECULES

Distinction has to be made between the products of a single
elementary act of recombination and the products of several rounds
of matings and several acts of recombination among the total population of molecules. A situation in which two reciprocal recombinants appear with equal frequencies in the population can be
explained either by a reciprocal elementary act of recombination
or by a nonreciprocal elementary act. In the latter case each
elementary act produces only one type of recombinants, and statistically the two reciprocal types are produced with equal frequencies.
The main difference between these two mechanisms is that the first
one produces two recombined molecules while the second one produces
one parental concomitantly with one recombined molecule per each
elementary act. The second mechanism therefore requires twice as
many mating rounds to produce the same number of recombinant molecules as the first mechanism. On the contrary, a situation in which
two reciprocal recombinants appear at the population level with
drastically unequal frequencies is in favor of a nonreciprocal
elementary act of recombination. Furthermore, the nonreciprocal
elementary act has to occur in the population of molecules always
in the same direction.

The main argument favoring the nonreciprocity of elementary

acts of recombination in mitochondria comes from the discovery of
a specific locus (ω) of the mitochondrial genome which governs
polarity of recombination (Bolotin *et al.*, 1971). The ω locus is
closely linked to the segment of ribosomal genes (see Fig. 1).
Two allelic forms of ω have been found among wild-type yeast strains
studied so far (Coen *et al.*, 1974). This determines the existence
of two types of crosses. On one hand crosses between an ω^+ and an
ω^- strain exhibit a significant polarity of recombination in the
ribosomal segment of mtDNA (heterosexual or polar crosses). On the
other hand crosses between two strains carrying the same ω allele
(ω^+ X ω^+ or ω^- X ω^-) never show any significant polarity of recombination for the ribosomal segment (homosexual or nonpolar crosses).
In polar crosses the value of the polarity of recombination between
two markers depends on the distance between the marker the most
proximal to ω and the ω locus. Indeed, the closer a marker is to
ω, the higher is the polarity (Avner *et al.*, 1973; Wolf *et al.*,
1973; Netter *et al.*, 1974). Polarity of recombination is restricted
to the ribosomal segment. This has led us to distinguish between
markers located in a polar region and markers located in nonpolar
regions. So far the only polar region described is the ribosomal
region linked to ω.

The model is based on the idea that, in the polar region of
heterosexual crosses, the acts of recombination are both nonreciprocal at the elementary level and dissymetrical at the population
level. Every time an ω^+ molecule pairs with an ω^- one, an obligatory event of recombination takes place, initiated always at the
ω locus and always taking the same direction. The formal mechanism
if presented in Fig. 1. Pairing between ω^+ and ω^- alleles specifically initiates a gene conversion process by an obligatory excision of the ω^- allele, followed by a sequential degradation of the
ω^- sequence and a resynthesis using the ω^+ sequence as template.
The final outcome of this process is a double-stranded molecule
presenting a segment of the ω^+ sequence and a segment of the ω^-
sequence. At every point the gene conversion process can be
arrested with a certain probability. Therefore, the probability
of gene conversion $\omega^- \rightarrow \omega^+$ is greater than that of $C^- \rightarrow C^+$, greater
than that of $S^- \rightarrow S^+$, and greater than that of $E^- \rightarrow E^+$. This scheme,
intentionally oversimplified, does not take into account the double-
stranded structure of DNA molecules. In particular, it does not
consider which strand is degraded and in which direction, whether
strands exchange or not during the process, what are the enzymes
involved, etc. It simply points out that (1) there is a finite
probability of converting one sequence into a copy of the other, so
that at the end of the process one allele has disappeared while the
other is represented twice; and (2) the products of the process are
always one parental molecule (ω^+) and one recombinant molecule (the
majority type).

If one makes the reasonable assumption that the number of

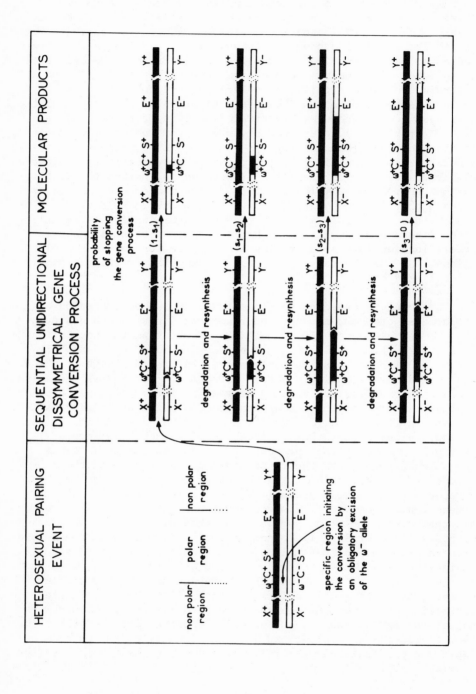

Figure 1. Schematic representation of the statistically dis-
symmetrical gene conversion occurring in the polar region adjacent
to the ω locus. The figure represents the elementary act of recombination in the ribosomal segment following the pairing of an
ω^+ and an ω^- molecule. The C, S, and E markers represent respectively the R_I, R_{II}, and R_{III} loci, which are genetically linked
and specify the mitochondrial ribosome. They are located in a
polar region under the control of ω. Other markers such as O and
P are located in nonpolar regions and are genetically unlinked to
the polar region although carried on the same molecule. They are
symbolized nonspecifically by X and Y. Absence of recombination
between either X or Y markers and the polar region in the molecular
products is arbitrary and made for convenience of drawing. Each
double-stranded DNA molecule of the pair is represented by a bar.
Solid bar, ω^+ parent; open bar, ω^- parent. Figure taken from
Dujon *et al.* (1973).

---

mating rounds is the same for polar and nonpolar regions, then the
logical conclusion is that in nonpolar regions the act of recombination has to be also nonreciprocal at the elementary level but statistically symmetrical at the population level. In other words
every elementary act produces a parental molecule concomitantly
with a recombined molecule. Otherwise the number of mating rounds
for polar regions would have to be much greater than for nonpolar
regions. The same kind of argument can be applied for nonpolar
crosses and leads also to the conclusion that every elementary act
has to be nonreciprocal.

     In conclusion, all regions of mtDNA undergo a nonreciprocal
recombination at the elementary level. In nonpolar crosses as well
as in nonpolar regions of polar crosses, these elementary acts occur
at the population level in two opposite directions with equal frequencies. In the polar region of polar crosses the nonreciprocal
elementary act is of the same nature as for other regions, except
that it occurs always in the same direction at the population level
and is always initiated at the ω locus.

EXPERIMENTAL TESTING OF THE MODEL

     A detailed comparison between quantitative predictions of
the model and experimental data have been presented by Dujon *et al.*
(1973). It suffices here to note that the estimation of parameters
such as s (probability of gene conversion for one allele) and m
(average number of mating rounds) can be derived from different sets
of experimental data, one from the output of alleles as a function
of input and the other from the frequency of recombinants as a
function of input. These two estimations are coherent. Furthermore,

these parameters are sufficient to account for other results, such
as three- or four-factor crosses.

DISCUSSION

The model has two main aspects. The first one, dealing with
the features of genetic exchanges and pairing process of mtDNA, is
not directly the topic of this article, and the reader should refer
to Dujon *et al*. (1973). The second aspect of the model dealing
with mechanism of recombination will be considered here in more
detail.

Existence of a polarity of recombination in the ribosomal
segment of heterosexual crosses is interpreted as the final result
of several rounds of matings, in each round recombination being
achieved by a nonreciprocal act which produces always one parental
sequence concomitantly with one recombined sequence. Assumption
that there is a similar average number of mating rounds for all
types of crosses and all segments of the mtDNA molecule leads to
the logical conclusion that each elementary act should give rise to
parental sequences together with recombined sequences. Therefore
the model postulates that every elementary act of recombination
between mtDNA molecules is nonreciprocal, one allele being converted
into a copy of the other. In nonpolar regions of mtDNA molecules,
the probability of gene conversion of both alleles is the same.
Consequently the two reciprocal recombinants are produced with equal
frequency at the population level. The same applies for polar
regions in nonpolar crosses (ω^+ X ω^+ or ω^- X ω^-). In polar regions
of polar crosses (ω^+ X ω^-), the pairing between the ω^+ and the ω^-
alleles specifically initiates gene conversion by an obligatory
excision of the ω^- allele. Then the degradation process is continued sequentially with a probability of stopping at every point.
Therefore the closer a marker is to ω the greater is its probability
of conversion.

A mechanism for the specific initiation at the ω locus could
be, for instance, a specific mismatching of base pair(s) which
triggers activity of an excision enzyme with high frequency. In
this sense the ω locus would act as a recombination promoter. The
possibility cannot be excluded definitely that nicking may not be
triggered by the mismatched region but can occur randomly to the
left of ω with high probability. However, this would not so easily
explain the fact that the great majority of recombinants, if not
all, have the ω^+ allele. Since density of genetic markers in nonpolar regions of the mtDNA molecule is too low, the existence of
other hypothetical recombination promoters and the question of
whether all elementary acts are initiated by a limited number of
such promoters or not cannot be discussed.

If one assumes a classical heteroduplex region, then the gradient of conversion frequency can be readily interpreted as arising either from heteroduplex regions of variable sizes with subsequent excision and repair of the complete heteroallelic area or from heteroduplex regions of constant size with subsequent excision and repair of a part of the heteroallelic area.

The mechanism is thus of the type *"breakage and copying."* The main consequence of such a mechanism is the necessity of synthesizing a segment of DNA to achieve the recombination process. However, this partial synthesis might become quantitatively important if recombination is very active. The fact that DNA synthesis is involved in recombination of mtDNA molecules may be hard to assess or disprove experimentally since this synthesis has to be distinguished from total replication. However, the synthesis of limited segments of DNA during recombination could be the reason, or one of the reasons, for the apparent dispersive replication reported for mtDNA of yeast (Sena *et al.*, 1973) and *Euglena* (Richards and Ryan, 1974).

This model, specifically aimed at explaining recombination in mitochondria, has some aspects in common to models proposed to explain prokaryotic recombination, eukaryotic gene conversion, and nonreciprocal genetic recombination among viruses (Holliday, 1964; Emerson, 1966; Stahl, 1969; Paszewski, 1970; Whitehouse, 1970; Boon and Zinder, 1971; Broker and Lehman, 1971; Gutz, 1971; Hurst *et al.*, 1972; Russo, 1973; Sobell, 1973). However, the major interests of mitochondria for studying mechanisms of recombination are the following. (1) It might be that there exists only one type of recombination in mitochondria, the nonreciprocal type, providing a simple tool for recombination studies at the level of enzymatic pathways (see Clark, 1971). (2) The comparison of size of converted segment to physical distances as determined by biochemical methods can be achieved. For instance, the distance between the C and E markers is about 1 to 3 µm (Faye *et al.*, 1973). This means that the gene conversion of the ribosomal segment might cover distances of some thousands of base pairs. (3) The nonreciprocal recombination proposed relates the recombination process between point mutations in a wild type (*i.e.* grande) to the phenomenon of petite induction, to suppressiveness, and to the known changes in the structure of mtDNA in petites. It is well established now that petites result from important deletion and numerous repetitions of genes within mtDNA molecules (Faye *et al.*, 1973). This finding together with the demonstration of genetic recombination between ρ^- mutants (Michaelis *et al.*, 1973) offers the possibility of studying formation of repetitive DNA and recombination of segments of repeated genes.

ACKNOWLEDGMENT

This model has been elaborated in collaboration with P. Slonimski and L. Weill.

The author takes pleasure in acknowledging P. Avner, M. Bolotin-Fukuhara, D. Coen, J. Deutsch, A. Kruszewska, W. Lancashire, G. Michaelis, P. Netter, E. Petrochilo, K. Wolf, and the students of the IIIème Cycle de Génétique Approfondie for kindly communicating their unpublished results and participating in many discussions.

The author is indebted to J. Gabarro for designing the computer programs.

This work has been supported by a grant ATP Différenciation Cellulaire n° 4304 from the C.N.R.S.

REFERENCES

Avner, P. R., D. Coen, B. Dujon and P. P. Slonimski. 1973. Mitochondrial genetics. IV. Allelism and mapping studies of oligomycin resistant mutants in *S. cerevisiae*. Mol. Gen. Genet. 125: 9.

Bolotin, M., D. Coen, J. Deutsch, B. Dujon, P. Netter, E. Petrochilo and P. P. Slonimski. 1971. La recombinaison des mitochondries chez *Saccharomyces cerevisiae*. Bull. Inst. Pasteur 69: 215.

Boon, T. and N. Zinder. 1971. Genotypes produced by individual recombination events involving bacteriophage f_1. J. Mol. Biol. 58: 133.

Broker, T. R. and I. R. Lehman. 1971. Branched DNA molecules: Intermediates in T4 recombination. J. Mol. Biol. 60: 131.

Clark, A. J. 1971. Toward a metabolic interpretation of genetic recombination of *E. coli* and its phages. Ann. Rev. Microbiol. 25: 437.

Coen, D., J. Deutsch, B. Dujon, P. Netter, E. Petrochilo, P. P. Slonimski and M. Bolotin-Fukuhara. 1974. Mitochondrial genetics VIII. in preparation.

Coen, D., J. Deutsch, P. Netter, E. Petrochilo and P. P. Slonimski. 1970. Mitochondrial genetics: I -- Methodology and phenomenology. Symp. Soc. Exp. Biol. 24: 449.

Deutsch, J., B. Dujon, P. Netter, E. Petrochilo, P. P. Slonimski, M. Bolotin-Fukuhara and D. Coen. 1974. Mitochondrial genetics VI. The petite mutation in *Saccharomyces cerevisiae*: Interrelations between the loss of the ρ^+ factor and the loss of the drug resistance mitochondrial genetic markers. Genetics in press.

Dujon, B., P. P. Slonimski and L. Weill. 1973. Mitochondrial genetics. IX. A model for recombination and segregation of mitochondrial genomes in *Saccharomyces cerevisiae*. Genetics Suppl. Berkeley Symposium, August 1973. Vol. 1.

Emerson, S. 1966. Quantitative implications of the DNA-repair model of gene conversion. Genetics 53: 475.

Faye, G., H. Fukuhara, C. Grandchamp, J. Lazowska, F. Michel, J. Casey, G. Getz, J. Locker, M. Rabinowitz, M. Bolotin-Fukuhara, D. Coen, J. Deutsch, B. Dujon, P. Netter and P. P. Slonimski. 1973. Mitochondrial nucleic acids in the *petite colonie* mutants: deletions and repetitions of genes. Biochimie 55: 779.

Gutz, H. 1971. Gene conversion: remarks on the quantitative implications of hybrid DNA models. Genet. Res. 17: 45.

Holliday, R. 1964. A mechanism for gene-conversion in fungi. Genet. Res. 5: 282.

Howell, N., M. K. Trembath, A. W. Linnane and H. B. Lukins. 1973. Biogenesis of mitochondria. XXX. An analysis of polarity of mitochondrial gene recombination and transmission. Mol. Gen. Genet. 122: 37.

Hurst, D. D., S. Fogel and R. K. Mortimer. 1972. Conversion-associated recombination in yeast. Proc. Nat. Acad. Sci. U.S.A. 69: 101.

Kleese, R. A., R. C. Grotbeck and J. R. Snyder. 1972. Recombination among three mitochondrial genes in yeast (*Saccharomyces cerevisiae*). J. Bacteriol. 112: 1023.

Michaelis, G., E. Petrochilo and P. P. Slonimski. 1973. Mitochondrial genetics. III. Recombined molecules of mitochondrial DNA obtained from crosses between cytoplasmic *petite* mutants of *Saccharomyces cerevisiae*: Physical and genetic characterization. Mol. Gen. Genet. 123: 51.

Nagley, P. and A. W. Linnane. 1972. Biogenesis of mitochondria. XXI. Studies on the nature of the mitochondrial genome in yeast. The degeneration effects of ethidium bromide on mitochondrial genetic information in a respiratory competent strain. J. Mol. Biol. 66: 181.

Netter, P., E. Petrochilo, P. P. Slonimski, M. Bolotin-Fukuhara, D. Coen, J. Deutsch and B. Dujon. 1964. Mitochondrial genetics VII. Allelism and mapping studies of ribosomal mutants resistant to chloramphenicol, erythromycin and spiramycin in *S. cerevisiae*. Genetics in press.

Paszewski, A. 1970. Gene conversion: observations on the DNA hybrid models. Genet. Res. 15: 55.

Rank, G. H. 1973. Recombination in three factor crosses of cytoplasmically inherited antibiotic-resistance mitochondrial markers in *S. cerevisiae*. Heredity 30: 265.

Richards, O. C. and R. S. Ryan. 1974. Synthesis and turnover of *Euglena gracilis* mitochondrial DNA. J. Mol. Biol. 82: 57.

Russo, V. E. A. 1973. On the physical structure of λ recombinant DNA. Mol. Gen. Genet. 122: 353.

Sena, E., J. Welch, D. Radin and S. Fogel. 1973. DNA replication during mating in yeast. Genetics 74 (suppl. 2): 248.

Sobell, H. M. 1973. Symmetry in protein nucleic acid interaction and its genetic implications. Advan. Genet. 17: 411.

Stahl, F. W. 1969. One way to think about gene conversion. Genetics 61 (suppl. 1): 1.

Suda, K. and A. Uchida. 1972. Segregation and recombination of cytoplasmic drug-resistance factors in *Saccharomyces cerevisiae*. Jap. J. Genet. 47: 441.

Visconti, N. and M. Delbrück. 1953. The mechanism of genetic recombination in phage. Genetics 38: 5.

Whitehouse, M. L. K. 1970. The mechanism of genetic recombination. Biol. Rev. 45: 265.

Wolf, K., B. Dujon, P. P. Slonimski. 1973. Mitochondrial genetics V. Multifactorial mitochondrial crosses involving a mutation conferring paromomycin-resistance in *Saccharomyces cerevisiae*. Mol. Gen. Genet. 125: 53.

THE ISOLATION OF MITOTIC *rec⁻* MUTANTS IN *SCHIZOSACCHAROMYCES POMBE*

Stephen L. Goldman* and Herbert Gutz[†]

* *The University of Toledo, Department of Biology, Toledo, Ohio 43606, and* [†] *The University of Texas at Dallas, Division of Biological Sciences, Dallas, Texas 75230*

The mechanisms governing the interaction of homologous DNA molecules that lead to the formation of genetic recombinants remain largely unknown in eukaryotes. Recent evidence (for review see Stern and Hotta, 1973) obtained from work with several species of *Lilium* indicates that the enzymatic control of recombination may be similar to that observed in bacteria and viruses. Given the fact that a portion of the genome directs the synthesis of enzymes that mediate recombination, additional information relating to its biochemistry could be obtained by selecting for mutants that alter genetic map distances. Presumably such an altered phenotype, *e.g.* absence of genetic recombination, would arise as a consequence of a modified or missing gene product that mediates exchange.

That this is a fruitful approach has already been demonstrated in *Neurospora*. Dominant genes that are locus specific and lower by as much as an order of magnitude intragenic meiotic map distances have been reported in this organism (Jessop and Catcheside, 1965; Catchside, 1966, 1968).

Although the selection of recombination-deficient mutants that exert their influence during meiosis is of great importance, the successful isolation of genes that modify exchange in a vegetative diploid cell is also of considerable interest. In this paper we describe an experimental procedure for the isolation of dominant *rec⁻* mutants of the fission yeast *Schizosaccharomyces pombe*. One

317

of the mutants obtained has been subjected to further genetic
analyses.

ISOLATION PROCEDURE FOR DOMINANT MITOTIC rec^- MUTANTS

Diploid strains homozygous for the mating type (h^-/h^-) containing the nonidentical $ade6$ alleles M216 and L623 were constructed according to the method described by Flores da Cunha (1970).
These mutants map on opposite ends of the $ade6$ gene and give weak
intrallelic complementation (Gutz, 1963, 1971). On minimal agar
(for media and other methods see Gutz, 1971) such diplonts still
form the red pigment characteristic for $ade6$ mutants. As a consequence of mitotic intragenic recombination, colonies of these
strains will form white papilla of $ade6^+$ segregants. It was therefore reasonable to assume that rec^- mutants will not form $ade6^+$
sectors on minimal agar and so will be detectable as papillaless
colonies.

The diploid strains were treated with ultraviolet (UV) light
prior to plating. Treatment with UV is known to increase the frequency of both classical mitotic crossover events and gene conversion and would therefore reduce the number of spontaneously occurring papillaless colonies (James, 1955; James and Lee-Whiting, 1955;
Nakai and Mortimer, 1969). These particular sectorless colonies
would correspond to the naturally occurring p_0 class of a Poisson
distribution. Almost all of the resulting colonies were red and
showed numerous white papilla, which upon subsequent testing proved
to be prototrophic for adenine.

We found one papillaless red colony on the minimal agar plates,
which was picked up for further experiments. The phenotype "papillaless colonies" proved to be stable when the strain was either
streaked or plated in dilutions to give no more than 150 colonies
per plate. Haploidization of this rec^- strain with p-fluorophenyl-
alanine showed that it was still disomic for the original $ade6$
heteroalleles, since the original parental alleles (M216 and L623)
are both present in the diploid. It therefore was supposed that
the strain carried a dominant mutation that suppresses recombination
between $ade6$ heteroalleles.

VERIFICATION OF THE GENOTYPE rec^-

To test the hypothesis further that this strain carries a gene
which blocks mitotic intragenic recombination, it was necessary to
obtain haploid isolates. The strain was crossed with an h^+/h^+
diploid under conditions that favor "twin meioses" (Gutz, 1967).
Twin meiosis means that after fusion of two diploid cells karyogamy

does not occur; each diploid nucleus undergoes a separate meiosis. Asci with eight haploid spores result.

From the h^+/h^+ X h^-/h^- cross, we dissected by micromanipulation several eight-spored asci. One ascus was obtained in which all eight spores were viable. From this ascus, the four h^- cultures (two being $ade6$-M216 and two being $ade6$-L623) were used to construct new diplonts with the original rec^+ strains. Half of the newly constructed diploids were expected to be recombinationless, $e.g.$ fail to form papillae, since the initial isolation procedure selected for dominant genes affecting mitotic intragenic recombination. Two of the four spore cultures used to construct new diploids produced papillaless colonies. In each case, the failure to produce sectors was associated with the two h^- $ade6$-M216 spore cultures.

Since the suppression of the formation of $ade6^+$ recombinants was associated with the two M216 cultures, it was necessary to determine whether the lack of mitotic intragenic recombination was due to mutational change in the $ade6$ locus or to a mutation in some other gene. To discriminate between the two possibilities one of the recombinationless h^- $ade6$-M216 cultures was crossed to the h^+ wild-type strain L975. Following the plating of free ascospores from this cross on complete media, 20 M216 cultures were isolated. Of the 20, 12 were h^+ for the mating type and eight were h^-. With these isolates, new diplonts were synthesized using the original L623 strains of compatable mating type. Of the 20 diplonts nine failed to form papillaless colonies, indicating the suppression of mitotic recombination within the $ade6$ locus. Thus the property "recombinationless" is carried by a rec gene that is not at or at least not closely linked to $ade6$. We call this locus $rec1$ in accordance with the nomenclature system used by Mortimer and Hawthorne (1966).

PARTIAL CHARACTERIZATION AND PROPERTIES OF $rec1$

It was also of interest to test whether or not $rec1$ affects meiotic intragenic recombination in the $ade6$ locus. It should be noted that in this experiment, as well as in the following, the same h^- $ade6$-M216 $rec1$ isolate was used as had been in the linkage determination. Table 1 shows the frequencies of prototrophic recombinants obtained when M216 rec^+ and the M216 rec^- strains were crossed to the same set of $ade6$ heteroalleles. In these experiments, free ascospores were plated on minimal media and on supplemented agar in such dilutions that the number of colonies per plate did not exceed 150 (for details see Gutz, 1971). The data shows that meiotic intragenic map distances are not affected by $rec1$.

Since in bacteria a number of recombinationless mutants are also UV sensitive (for review see Strauss, 1969) the response of a

Table 1. Frequencies of prototrophic spores in crosses of h^- ade6-M216 rec^+ and h^- ade6-M216 rec^- with nonidentical ade6 alleles (plating of free spores)

Crossed with ade6 mutants of mating type h^+*	M216 rec^+‡				M216 rec^-‡			
	Factor	MMA	MMA + adenine	Frequency of prototrophs X 10^6 (R)	Factor	MMA	MMA + adenine	Frequency of prototrophs X 10^6 (R)
L406	10^5	26	439	0.6	10^5	30	554	0.5
M216	10^5	0	150	0.0	10^5	0	122	0.0
M26*	10^4	162	135	120.0	10^4	172	142	121.0
M375	10^5	100	127	7.9	10^5	103	114	9.0
L539	10^4	172	110	156.0	10^4	168	109	154.0
L615	5×10^3	117	172	136.0	5×10^3	113	170	130.0
L432	5×10^3	300	150	400.0	5×10^3	113	54	420.0

* The mutants are listed in the order from "left" (L406) to the right hand end (L432) of the ade6 map (Gutz, 1963). The presence of M26 enhances the frequency of intragenic recombination within the ade6 locus.

‡ Factor (F) = (no. spores plated on MMA)/(no. spores plated on MMA + adenine).

R = (10^6 X no. colonies on MMA)/(F X no. colonies on MMA + adenine).

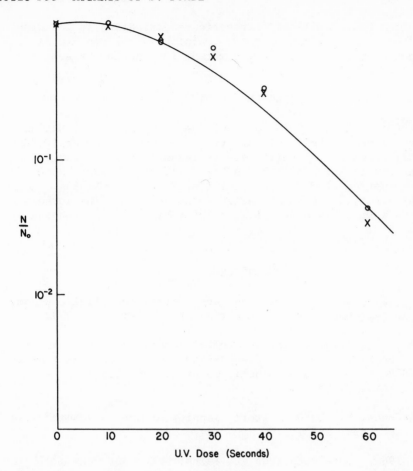

Figure 1.   Inactivation of h^- *ade*6-M216 rec^+ and h^- *ade*6-M216 *rec*1 by ultraviolet light. 0, h^- *ade*6-M216 rec^+; X, h^- *ade*6-M216 *rec*1.

*rec*1 strain to UV light was tested.   Fig. 1 shows that the mutant does not have an altered response to UV; its inactivation curve is nearly identical to that of the rec^+ strain from which it was derived.

It remains to be tested in future experiments whether *rec*1 has also an influence on intragenic recombination in other genes than *ade*6, as well as whether it affects intergenic mitotic crossing-over.

SUMMARY

A procedure which has led to the successful isolation of a dominant *rec*⁻ mutant in *Schizosaccharomyces pombe* is described.

This mutation blocks mitotic intragenic recombination in the *ade*6 locus and has been designated *rec*1. Meiotic intragenic map distances are not affected by *rec*1. The mutant is also not UV sensitive.

ACKNOWLEDGEMENTS

S. L. Goldman gratefully acknowledges support from a National Institutes of Health Postdoctoral Grant, Fellowship Number 7F02GM 41836-01A1, taken at the University of Texas at Dallas, and a Summer Faculty Fellowship from The University of Toledo. H. Gutz has been supported by NSF Grant GB-15148, NIH Grant GM13234, and by the University of Texas at Dallas Research Fund. The authors wish to thank Dr. William Lee Bischoff for his critical reading of the manuscript.

REFERENCES

Catcheside, D. G. 1966. A second gene controlling allelic recombination in *Neurospora crassa*. Aust. J. Biol. Sci. <u>19</u>: 1039.

Catcheside, D. G. 1968. The control of genetic recombination in *Neurospora crassa*. In (W. J. Peacock and R. D. Brock, eds.) Replication and Recombination of Genetic Material pp. 216-226. Australian Acad. Sci., Canberra.

Flores da Cunha, M. 1970. Mitotic mapping of *Schizosaccharomyces pombe*. Genet. Res. <u>16</u>: 127.

Gutz, H. 1963. Untersuchungen zur Feinstruktur der Gene *ade*7 and *ade*6 von *Schizosaccharomyces pombe* Lind. Habilitationsschrift, Technische Universität, Berlin.

Gutz, H. 1967. "Twin meiosis" and other ambivalences in the life cycle of *Schizosaccharomyces pombe*. Science 158: 796.

Gutz, H. 1971. Site specific induction of gene conversion in *Schizosaccharomyces pombe*. Genetics <u>69</u>: 317.

James, A. P. 1955. A genetic analysis of sectoring in ultraviolet-induced variant colonies of yeast. Genetics <u>40</u>: 204.

James, A. P. and B. Lee-Whiting. 1955. Radiation-induced genetic segregations in vegetative cells of diploid yeast. Genetics <u>40</u>: 826.

Jessop, A. P. and D. G. Catcheside. 1965. Interallelic recombination at the *his*1 locus in *Neurospora crassa* and its genetic control. Heredity <u>20</u>: 237.

Mortimer, R. K. and D. C. Hawthorne. 1966. Genetic mapping in *Saccharomyces*. Genetics 53: 165.

Nakai, S. and R. K. Mortimer. 1969. Studies of the genetic mechanism of radiation-induced mitotic segregation in yeast. Mol. Gen. Gen. 103: 329.

Stern, H. and Y. Hotta. 1973. Biochemical controls of meiosis. Ann. Rev. Genet. 7: 37.

Strauss, B. 1969. DNA repair mechanisms and their relation to mutation and recombination. In Curr. Top. Microbiol. Immunol. 44: 1.

RECOMBINATION IN HIGHER EUKARYOTES

INTERGENIC RECOMBINATION, DNA REPLICATION AND SYNAPTONEMAL

COMPLEX FORMATION IN THE DROSOPHILA OOCYTE

Rhoda F. Grell and J. W. Day

Biology Division, Oak Ridge National Laboratory, Oak

Ridge, Tennessee 37830

The transition from microbial systems to the higher eukaryotes
introduces a different order of time and physical dimensions. For
recombination studies the change confers both advantages and disadvantages. The increased complexity of the organism imposes difficulties in isolating meiocytes free of somatic cells and other germ
cells for the kinds of molecular approaches that have been used so
successfully in prokaryotes, but the increased complexity also en-
tails a temporal extension and compartmentalization of meiotic
events which, for some studies, simplifies their dissection and
examination.

An unanswered question, important to an understanding of the
mechanism of recombination, concerns its relation to normal DNA synthesis. The earlier simplified alternatives of copy-choice and
breakage-reunion models, the former coupled to DNA synthesis and
the latter independent of it, are no longer tenable. Both breakage
and synthesis apparently have a role in the recombination process.
Now one of the pertinent questions is whether synthesis is part of
normal replication or a discrete, independent event.

One approach to this problem has involved a comparison of the
S-phase in the meiocyte with the sensitive period for modification
of recombination frequencies. In all organisms so far examined,
the S-phase immediately prior to meiosis is exceptionally long
(Callan, 1973). This feature facilitates its localization and the
definition of its temporal relation to the sensitive period for
manipulating recombination frequencies. Among eukaryotes, the formal genetics of Drosophila is best known, making it the preferred
organism for recombinational analysis. Our initial studies with

327

Drosophila indicated that heat-induced changes in crossing-over were roughly coincident with DNA replication (Grell and Chandley, 1965). Subsequent reports with other organisms have both confirmed and denied this result, denials being most frequent when chiasma frequency rather than genetic exchange was the criterion for assay (*e.g.* Abel, 1965, 1968; Henderson, 1966; Lu, 1969; Maguire, 1968; Peacock, 1970).

Several years ago, we decided to examine the Drosophila oocyte in much greater detail in an attempt to obtain a more definitive answer. The work has involved a three-pronged attack combining genetic, autoradiographic, and electron-microscopic studies. The genetic approach undertook to measure the response to heat throughout the genome rather than in a single sensitive region. This procedure has permitted a delineation of the total responsive period and, at the same time, has revealed the variant responses that characterize different regions. These studies have generated a thermal recombination map reflecting the degree and duration of response of different segments of the genome. Parallel autoradiographic studies of the ovary at sequential times during oogenesis have defined fairly precisely the limits of the S-phase in the oocyte. Electron microscopy of the oocyte has placed the appearance and growth of the synaptonemal complex into its proper temporal niche.

The discussion of our results falls into three categories: first, the correspondence between the S-phase and the temperature-sensitive period for recombination; second, the effect of heat on positive interference; and third, the time of appearance of the synaptonemal complex and its relation to DNA replication and the heat-sensitive period.

A THERMAL RECOMBINATION MAP

A careful dissection of regional responses to temperature requires the recovery of a well-synchronized population of oocytes. To this end a method was devised called the "pupal system." A detailed description of the procedure has been published elsewhere (Grell, 1973). Briefly, it makes use of the synchrony in differentiation of the 30-40 egg strings constituting the two ovaries of the developing female. Within each of the 30-40 egg strings, the first oocyte reaches maturity at approximately the same time. Collection of the first 10-15 eggs per female, equivalent to 1/3 - 1/2 of her first set of 30-40 oocytes, from a group of females which developed and eclosed together, provides the synchronized sample.

Figure 1 gives the chronology of some events during female metamorphosis and oocyte development. At ∿120 hr the female begins puparium formation, which signals the transition from larval to pu-

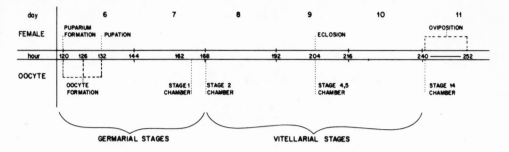

Figure 1. Chronology of events in developing females and their first oocytes.

pal stage. Pupation occurs at 132 hr. The pupal stage occupies about 3 days, at the end of which time the female eloses as an adult. Egg-laying begins about 36 hr later. Our cytological studies (Grell, 1967) have shown that oocytes also begin to appear at 120 hr and that they increase in number and reach a steady state of production at about 144 hr. Most of the sample that we recover is produced between 126 and 132 hr with a small contribution between 120 and 126 hr. Until 168 hr each egg string consists only of a small anterior portion called the germarium. At about 168 hr the most mature egg chamber, the stage-1 chamber, housing the most mature oocyte and its 15 nurse cells, is pinched off as a stage-2 chamber. This is the beginning of vitellarium formation. Growth of the oocyte occurs in the vitellarium, and by the time the mature stage-14 chamber is reached, the oocyte has increased in volume by a factor of 100,000 (King *et al.*, 1956). At eclosion the oldest chamber is at stage 4 or 5. The stage-14 chamber is formed about 36 hr after eclosion, when egg-laying begins. Thus, oogenesis for our sample occupies about 5 days.

To alter recombination in our sample, treatment must be given to the immature female. A rough determination of the heat-sensitive period for the first oocytes has localized sensitivity to the sixth and seventh days (120 - 168 hr), corresponding to about the first half of the pupal period (Grell, 1967). The responsive period was more precisely resolved by initiating treatment to different groups of females of identical genotype at sequential 6-hr time points, beginning no later than 120 hr and ending no earlier than 168 hr. Treatment was a temperature of 35°C given for 12 hr; a control temperature of 25°C was maintained at all other times. Initiation of 12-hr treatments at 6-hr intervals means that each treatment period except the first and last overlaps the preceding one by 6 hr and the following one by 6 hr, permitting more precise resolution of the initiation and termination of response.

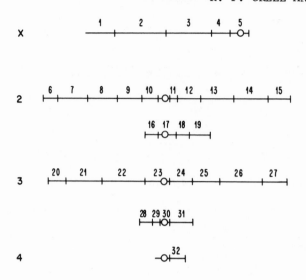

Figure 2. Thirty-two regions of the genome studied for crossover response to elevated temperature.

The total genome, comprising 32 segments, averaging 10 crossover units each, has been studied (Figure 2). The segments include five in the X chromosome, five in each arm of chromosome 2, four in each arm of 3, four each spanning the proximal region of chromosomes 2 and 3, and one in chromosome 4. Response in each of the 32 segments was measured during at least nine sequential time intervals.

Figure 3 presents the thermal recombination maps that have been generated for each of the five major arms. Each point on each curve represents the ratio of experimental to control value at the time interval indicated on the abscissa, so that increases fall above the control and decreases below. Each point is based on an average of 1500 flies in the experimental sample and 3000 in the control. The following are some of the salient features that appeared. Responses in the X (Fig. 3a) include marked decreases in four

Figure 3. Thermal recombination maps for the five chromosome arms. Treatments of 35°C for 12 hr were initiated at 6-hr intervals between 120 and 168 hr in all cases; earlier and later treatment periods were used in some cases. (a) X chromosome; (b) 2L; (c) 2R; (d) 3L; (e) 3R. (a-c) Regions 1 and 10, —△—; regions 2 and 9, —□—; regions 3 and 8, —▲—; regions 4 and 7, —o—; regions 5 and 6, —●—. (d,e) Regions 1 and 8, —□—; regions 2 and 7, —▲—; regions 3 and 6, —o—; regions 4 and 5, —●—.

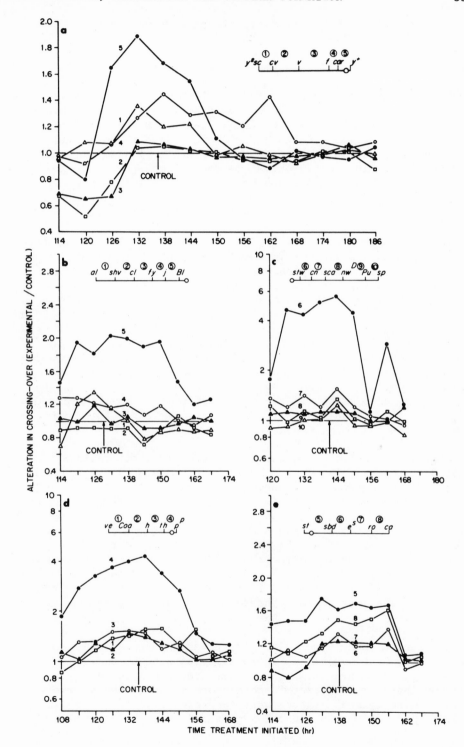

of the five regions with very early treatments initiated at 114 or
120 hr. Treatment after 120 hr produces a prominent increase in
centromeric region 5, lesser increases in distal region 1 and proximal region 4, and no increase in interstitial regions 2 and 3.
With the exception of region 4, increases span an 18-hr period between 132 and 150 hr. In chromosome 2 (Fig. 3b,c) maximal responses
occur in proximal regions 5 and 6, the predominant response in 2L
is early, and region 2 is unique in the genome in showing a consistent decrease. Region 6 shows a conspicuous dip at 156 hr and a
late response at 162 hr. Chromosome 3 (Fig. 3d,e) also shows maximal responses in the most proximal regions, 4 and 5. All regions
of 3L and 3R show a marked response, and responses terminate by
162 hr. With the exception of a proximal region in X and one in 2R,
all regions are at about control levels at 162 hr or earlier.

The composite pictures for each of the five arms (Fig. 4) reveal conspicuous differences in the degree, the time, the duration,
and the direction of their responses. The X chromosome is exceptional in exhibiting a significant decrease in total exchange, which
is maximal at 120 hr. The decrease in X was first detected by a
significant heat-induced increase in X nondisjunction (Grell, 1971a).
A search at that time for heat-induced autosomal nondisjunction gave
negative results, an outcome now understandable in light of the
failure of heat to decrease autosomal exchange or to increase autosomal univalents. Maximal responses for the five arms occur more
or less sequentially in the chronological order 2L, X, 3L, 3R, and
2R. The arms also differ in the degree of their responses according
to the seriation 3L>3R>2R>2L>X. Total response for all arms terminates at about 162 hr.

A comparison of the responses in the centromeric regions of X,
2, and 3 is shown in Figure 5. In each chromosome the centromeric
region shows the greatest enhancement in recombination, but the time
and degree of response differ in each case. Temporally, the X peaks
first with a treatment initiated at 132 hr, chromosome 3 somewhat
later with treatments at 138 and 144 hr, and chromosome 2 close to
the end of the period at 156 hr. The magnitude of the response
for the three regions varies markedly; the increases are 2-, 3.5-,
and 15-fold for the X, 2, and 3, respectively. The increase in 3
from a control level of 1.3 ± 0.24 to 19.6 ± 0.97 with a treatment
at 144 hr is the most dramatic heat-induced change so far encountered.

The fourth chromosomes virtually never undergo exchange in diploid females of Drosophila. The ability of heat to enhance crossing-over in the remainder of the genome prompted an attempt to induce crossing-over with heat in chromosome 4. Crossovers representing the two reciprocal classes were recovered at a frequency of
0.2-0.3%, but success in induction depended upon the treatment time.

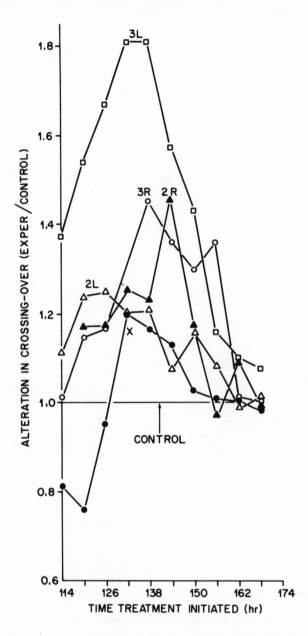

Figure 4. Total crossing-over in the five chromosome arms with 12-hr treatments at 35°C initiated at 6-hr intervals between 114 and 168 hr. X = ●, 2L = Δ, 2R = ▲, 3L = ☐, 3R = O.

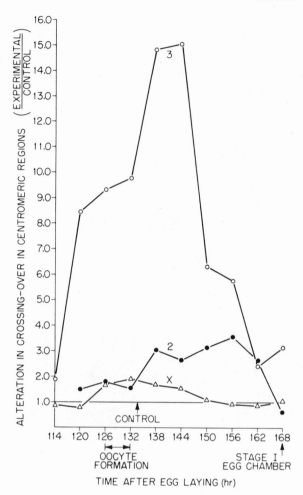

Figure 5. Crossing-over response of centromeric regions of X, 2, and 3 to 12-hr treatments at 35°C between 114 and 168 hr. Δ = X, ● = 2, O = 3 (after R. F. Grell, Chromosomes Today, vol. 4).

Figure 6. Autoradiographs of ovaries taken from pupae 144, 162, and 168 hr after egg-laying. TF = terminal filament. (a) 144-hr ovary showing seven ovarioles with posterior 16-cell cysts labeled. Arrow (→) indicates labeled cyst. (b) 162-hr ovary with label restricted to posterior sites within posterior 16-cell cysts. Arrow (→) indicates labeled posterior sites. (c) 168-hr ovary showing ovarioles with labeled stage-2 egg chambers representing second round of DNA replication in nurse cells. Arrows (→) indicate unlabeled oocyte at posterior end of chamber (after R. F. Grell, Chromosomes Today, vol. 4).

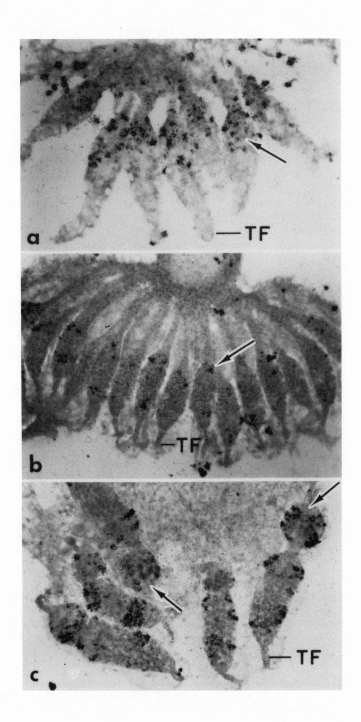

Maximal induction occurred when treatment was given between 132 and
156 hr, coinciding well with the time for maximal enhancement of
exchange in other regions of the genome (Grell, 1971b).

THE S-PHASE

A temporal comparison of the temperature-sensitive period with
the S-phase requires that the latter be well-defined. The duration
of DNA replication in the oocyte has been determined by two methods.
The first procedure involves a 45-min incubation in [^{3}H]thymidine
of ovaries taken from developing pupae at 6-hr intervals between
132 and 168 hr (Grell, 1973). Autoradiograms of Feulgen-stained
whole mounts were inspected for the presence of label in the oldest
16-cell cyst, which occupies the most posterior region in each
germarium. DNA synthesis in the 16-cell cyst, comprising the
oocyte(s) and nurse cells, has been found to be essentially synchro-
nous but possibly somewhat extended in the oocyte (Grell and Chandley, 1965). Labeling within the posterior cyst indicates then that
DNA replication is occurring in the oldest oocyte at the time of
exposure to [^{3}H]thymidine.

Autoradiograms of portions of ovaries taken from 144-, 162-,
and 168-hr pupae are shown in Figure 6. At 144 hr (Fig. 6a) the
posterior cyst in each of the seven ovarioles is heavily labeled;
by 162 hr (Fig. 6b) label is confined to restricted regions at the
posterior end of the posterior cyst, where the oocyte(s) lies, and
may represent continuing synthesis in the oocyte after its cessation
in the nurse cells; at 168 hr (Fig. 6c), stage-2 chambers representing the beginning of vitellarium formation are present. A second
replication is under way in the nurse cells, but the posterior
oocyte is devoid of label. From studies of this kind, the frequencies of posterior labeled cysts were found by two observers to be
significantly above 50% between 132 and 156 hr (Table 1).

A more sensitive method for determining the length of the S-
phase was devised by Day (1974). After incubation in [^{3}H]thymidine
for 1-2 hr, the pupal ovaries were transplanted into the abdomens
of adult females where they attached, usually to the gut, and frequently continued development. After 2-5 days the donor ovaries
were removed, and if vitellarial egg chambers were present autoradiograms were prepared. The diagnostic feature for this method
is the karyosome, formed by the condensation of all chromosomes
into a compact, densely staining body which is present between
stages 3 and 13 (King *et al.*, 1956). A labeled karyosome is an unambiguous indicator of DNA synthesis in the oocyte at the time of
exposure to [^{3}H]thymidine. Figure 7 shows an egg chamber derived
from a 144-hr ovary that was incubated in [^{3}H]thymidine and then
permitted to develop in an adult host for 4 days. The karyosome in

Table 1. Frequency of labeling in posterior cyst of ovarioles with increasing age*

Age (hr)	Set 1[†]					Set 2[†]				
	Slides inspected	L[†]	U[‡]	Total	L(%)	Slides inspected	L[‡]	U[‡]	Total	L(%)
132	14	214	108	322	66.5 ± 2.6	8	84	55	139	60.4 ± 4.1
138	11	154	82	236	65.3 ± 3.1	11	147	48	195	75.1 ± 3.1
144	26	436	166	602	72.4 ± 1.8	26	334	234	568	58.8 ± 2.1
150	12	154	50	204	75.5 ± 3.0	14	131	60	191	68.6 ± 3.4
156	4	85	49	134	63.4 ± 4.2	13	211	135	346	61.0 ± 2.6
162	5	30(63[§])	85	178	16.9(35.4[§])					
168	7	141[▽]	14	155	90.3[▽]					

* From R. F. Grell, Chromosomes Today, vol. 4.

[†] Independently scored by two individuals.

[‡] L, number of labeled cysts; U, number of unlabeled cysts.

[§] Indicates label restricted to several centers in posterior region of cyst.

[▽] Nurse cells only.

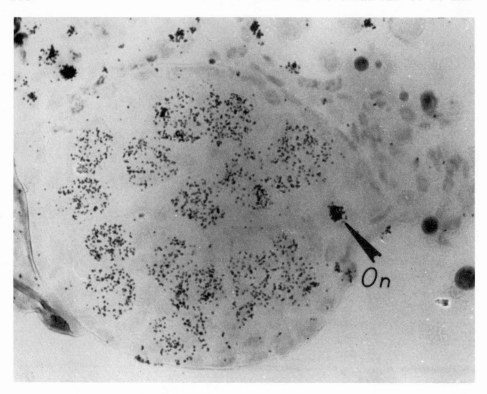

Figure 7. Autoradiograph of an ovary fragment from a 144-hr donor
pupa, incubated in [³H]thymidine, and transplanted to an adult host
for 4 days. *On* = labeled karyosome within oocyte nucleus.

the oocyte nucleus and the 15 nurse cell nuclei are all heavily
labeled. Studies carried out in this way fix the time of synthesis
between 132 and 162 hr, with maximal activity between 138 and 156
hr.

COINCIDENCE OF HEAT RESPONSE AND S-PHASE

     The coincidence between the temperature-sensitive period and
the S-phase is shown in Figure 8. The curve represents the response
of the total genome to heat treatment initiated at 6-hr intervals
between 114 and 168 hr. The increase begins between 126 and 132 hr
and terminates between 156 and 162 hr, encompassing about the first
30-36 hr in the life of the oocyte. The most sensitive period for
inducing crossing-over in chromosome 4 (132-150 hr) falls within
this period. The bar at the top indicates the duration of DNA synthesis as determined by the two methods described above. A comparison of the timetables for DNA replication and heat response shows

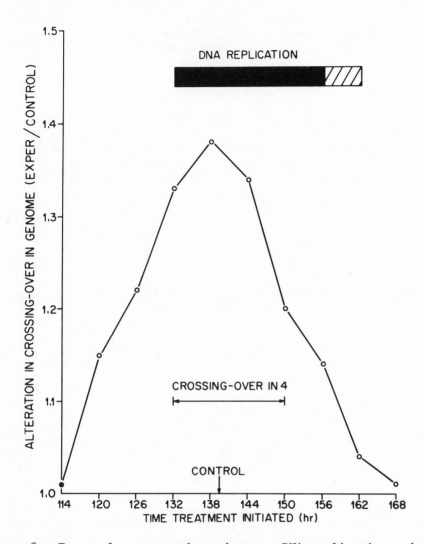

Figure 8.   Temporal correspondence between DNA replication and the
temperature-sensitive period for crossing-over.   Horizontal bar at
top represents duration of S-phase in the oocyte.   Black bar indicates duration as determined by method #1; black bar plus cross
hatch, duration as determined by the more sensitive method of Day
(1974).   Curve represents crossover response of total genome to
12-hr heat treatments at 35°C initiated at times shown on abscissa.
●, Measurement of response for 114-hr treatment does not include
2R.

that they are coincident over most and possibly all of their length. The curve peaks at 138 hr, indicating maximal response in the genome when heat is administered between 138 and 150 hr. This 12-hr period is coincident with the middle of the S-phase.

ALTERATIONS IN POSITIVE INTERFERENCE WITH HEAT

Positive interference is a well-recognized but poorly understood phenomenon which is generally considered to reflect a property of chromosome pairing. Any successful model of recombination in eukaryotes must provide some explanation for interference effects. Positive interference is most simply defined as the ability of one crossover to reduce or suppress other crossovers in its vicinity. To indicate the degree of interference between two regions, Muller (1916) coined the term "coincidence" and calculated the coefficient of coincidence as the ratio of observed doubles in the two regions to the number expected from chance distribution. If the quotient is 1 there is no interference; if it is significantly less than 1 there is positive interference; and if it is significantly more than 1 there is negative interference. Absolute interference has a quotient of 0. Positive interference becomes more pronounced as the distance between genes becomes shorter. In Drosophila, for segments 12 units or less, interference is generally complete; between 12 and 40 units there is partial interference; and for segments 40-50 units apart, interference disappears. These are generalizations, and the values vary in different parts of the genome.

If one calculates the coincidence value for any two regions subjected to heat treatment and divides this by the coincidence value for the same regions in the control, the effect of temperature on interference can be assessed. The expectation is for a decrease in interference between two regions as their length is increased by heat, and for an increase in interference in those cases where heat acts to decrease genetic length. An example of what we find is shown in Figure 9a. Changes in interference are plotted as a function of treatment time so that decreases fall above the control and increases below. The series of curves shows the effect of temperature on interference between region 5 in the X chromosome and each of the other four regions in X. Normally interference is complete between regions 4 and 5, since together they measure only 13 units. With heat treatment initiated at 120 hr, interference between 4 and 5 disappears and C_0 changes from 0 to >1.

Is the decrease in interference accompanied by the expected increase in the genetic length of the regions? The thermal recombination map (Fig. 9b) shows that it is not. Instead, crossing-over in both regions 4 and 5 is minimal and well below control level at 120 hr. The curve for regions 5 and 3 also shows reductions

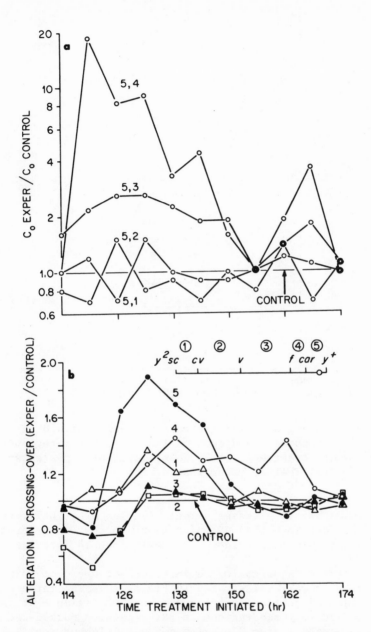

Figure 9. (a) Changes in interference between region 5 in the X chromosome and each of the other four regions in X with 12-hr temperature treatments of 35°C initiated at times shown on the abscissa. (b) Thermal recombination map of X.

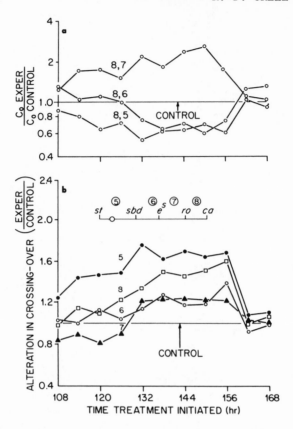

Figure 10. (a) Changes in interference between region 8 in the right arm of chromosome 3 and each of the other three regions with 12-hr temperature treatments of 35°C initiated at times shown on the abscissa. (b) Thermal recombination map of 3R.

in interference but to a lesser extent. On the other hand, regions 5 and 2, which are more than 40 units apart so that interference is normally absent, now show evidence of newly induced interference.

   The ability of heat to impose interference where it normally does not exist is well illustrated in Figure 10. The three curves show the effect of heat on interference between region 8 at the tip of 3R and the other three regions in 3R. Again, a marked decrease is observed between region 8 and its nearest neighbor region 7. Regions 8 and 6, however, show an increase in interference. A still greater increase is consistently observed between regions 8 and 5, where interference is normally absent. Furthermore, interference is greatest between regions 8 and 5 at 132 to 156 hr, when crossing-over in both regions is maximally increased, as shown in the thermal

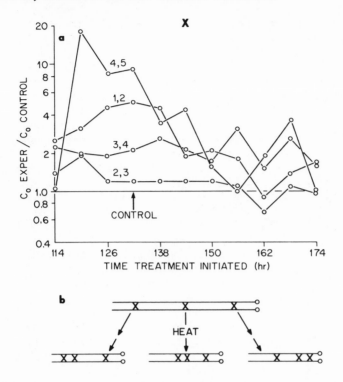

Figure 11. (a) Changes in interference between four sets of nearest neighbors in the X chromosome with 12-hr temperature treatments of 35°C initiated at times shown on the abscissa. (b) Model proposed to explain observed changes in interference, showing modification of normal distribution of nodes (effective pairing sites) with heat. Clustering in one region is postulated to occur at the expense of node establishment elsewhere in the chromosome, to occur preferentially in distal and proximal regions, and independently of amount of crossing-over.

recombination map (Fig. 10b). Conversely, interference is least between regions 8 and 7 during the same period, when crossing-over is also maximally increased. In other words, the effect of heat on interference does not seem to be correlated with its effect on crossing-over.

A somewhat different approach analyzes the response of all nearest neighbors in one arm. Figure 11a presents the results for the X chromosome. Each of the four sets of nearest neighbors shows a decrease in interference. The decreases are not uniform but are greater for distal and proximal nearest neighbors and less for medial ones, following the seriation 4,5>1,2>3,4>2,3. The decrease in

2,3 is maximal when crossing-over is minimal in both regions and is never accompanied by increases in exchange.

Similar analysis of the 18 nearest neighbors in the five chromosome arms shows that decreases in interference occur during all or most of the heat-sensitive period in 16 of them and increases in only two. Among five combinations representing distant regions where interference is normally absent, interference is newly imposed in four of them. A possible explanation for these results is shown in Figure 11b. The normal distribution of nodes or effective pairing sites or exchange points, shown at the top, is considered to be redistributed by heat to produce the arrangements shown below. Clustering of nodes in one segment of the chromosome occurs at the expense of their establishment in other segments. If clustering occurs preferentially in the distal and proximal region and is independent of the amount of crossing-over, a population of such chromosomes should give the results we observe. This model assumes that heat affects recombination in at least two ways: first by altering the position of crossovers, and second by altering the amount of crossing-over.

Although the responses of crossing-over and interference to heat appear unrelated in direction, they occupy approximately the same interval of time. Conventionally, it is assumed that pairing is completed before exchange occurs. If heat-induced changes in interference and in exchange reflect the times of pairing and crossing-over, respectively, then the two processes, instead of being separated in time, may be coordinated in time. If both processes are viewed as occurring over an extended time-span during premeiotic interphase and possibly beyond, establishment of pairing sites in one region could conceivably follow crossing-over in another.

TIME OF SYNAPTONEMAL COMPLEX FORMATION
IN THE DROSOPHILA OOCYTE

The assumption that pairing and exchange could occur or be initiated during premeiotic interphase is a departure from the classical picture of meiosis. Traditional thinking assumes that chromosomes are unpaired at interphase when replication occurs and that they begin to pair during the zygotene stage of prophase. To overcome this obstacle to the coupling of replication and recombination, Pritchard (1955) proposed that complete pairing is not a requirement for exchange; rather, exchange is accomplished in short, effectively paired regions during interphase when chromosomes are maximally extended. Tests with Drosophila have failed to confirm the Pritchard model, and have suggested that a rough alignment of homologs precedes the establishment of effective pairing sites (Grell, 1967).

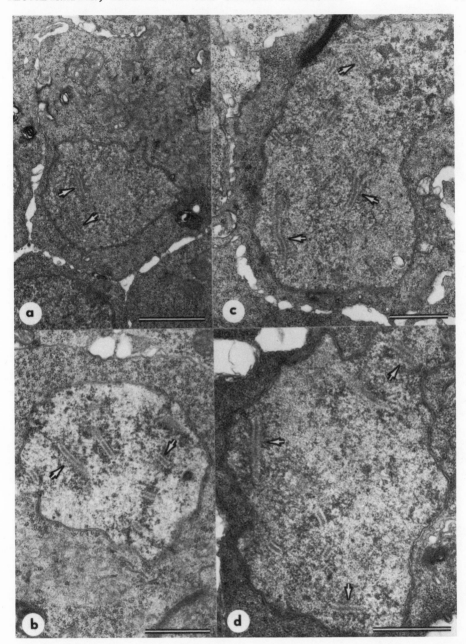

Figure 12. Electron micrographs of oocyte nuclei from pupae between 138 and 156 hr, showing synaptonemal complexes. (a) Oocyte from 138-hr pupa. (b) Oocyte from 144-hr pupa. (c) Oocyte from 150-hr pupa. (d) Oocyte from 156-hr pupa. Arrows (→) indicate synaptone-mal complexes. The bars (a-d) represent 1 μm.

346   R. F. GRELL AND J. W. DAY

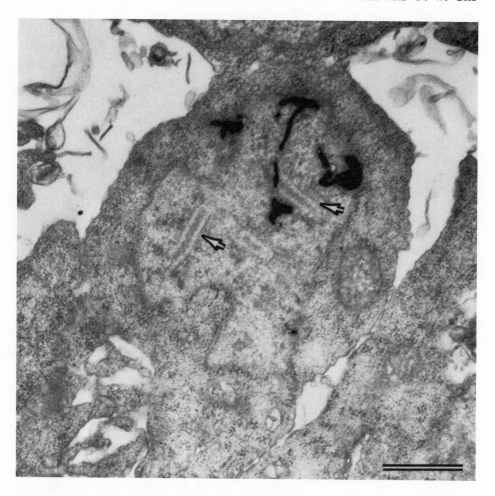

Figure 13. Electron micrograph-autoradiograph of oocyte nucleus
from a 144-hr ovary incubated in [³H]thymidine for 1 hr, showing
presence of both label and synaptonemal complexes in the same
nucleus. Arrows (→) indicate synaptonemal complexes. The bar
represents 1 μm.

        Considerable evidence exists, however, to suggest that homo-
logs may be roughly paired at premeiotic interphase or earlier
(for review see Grell, 1969). In this context, the synaptonemal
complex offers an extremely useful tool for analyzing pairing relationships. Whatever its functional role, the evidence from reconstruction studies is fairly convincing that the complex lies
between paired homologs along their longitudinal axis (Gillies,
1973; Wettstein and Sotelo, 1967; Moens and Perkins, 1969). To

conform with customary belief, the complex should not appear before zygotene, the presumed stage of pairing initiation. Our well-timed oocyte system provides a method for examining this assumption in Drosophila.

Figure 12 shows electron micrographs of oocyte nuclei taken from females between 138 and 156 hr, when DNA replication is in progress. At 138 hr the complex is well in evidence; at 144 hr considerable lengths of synaptonemal complex are visible; 150- and 156-hr oocytes contain still more complex.

The presence of the synaptonemal complex in oocytes between 138 and 156 hr implies, according to our timetable, that its formation and growth are coextensive with the S-phase. Unambiguous evidence for this conclusion is shown in Figure 13. An ovary from a 144-hr female was exposed to [^{3}H]thymidine for 1 hr. The autoradiograph shows the presence of label and the synaptonemal complex in the same nucleus.

If the presence of the synaptonemal complex during DNA replication implies that homologs are paired at the time of DNA replication, then there remains no apparent obstacle to the recoupling of replication and recombination.

ACKNOWLEDGMENTS

This research was conducted at the Biology Division, Oak Ridge National Laboratory and The University of Tennessee-Oak Ridge Graduate School of Biomedical Sciences, Oak Ridge, Tennessee 37830. The Oak Ridge National Laboratory is operated by the Union Carbide Corporation for the U.S. Atomic Energy Commission. J. W. Day is a postdoctoral investigator supported by subcontract No. 3322 from the Biology Division of Oak Ridge National Laboratory to The University of Tennessee.

REFERENCES

Abel, W. O. 1965. Uber den Beitpunkt des Crossing-Over und der Chromosomenverdopplung bei *Sphaerocarpus*. Z. Vererbungsl. 96: 228.

Abel, W. O. 1968. Time of crossing-over in *Sphaerocarpos*. Proc. 12th Int. Congr. Genet. 1: 70.

Callan, H. G. 1973. DNA replication in the chromosomes of eukaryotes. In (B. A. Hamkalo and J. Papaconstantinou, ed.) Molecular Cytogenetics, p. 31. Plenum Press, New York-London.

Day, J. W. 1974. Temporal relationship between premeiotic DNA synthesis and heat-induced recombination in oocytes of *Drosophila melanogaster*. In preparation.

Gillies, C. B. 1973. Ultrastructural analysis of maize pachytene karyotypes by three dimensional reconstruction of the synaptonemal complexes. Chromosoma 43: 145.

Grell, R. F. 1967. Pairing at the chromosomal level. J. Cell. Physiol. 70 (Suppl. 1): 119.

Grell, R. F. 1969. Meiotic and somatic pairing. In (E. W. Caspari and A. W. Ravin, eds.) Genetic Organization, vol. 1, p. 361. Academic Press, New York.

Grell, R. F. 1971a. Induction of sex chromosome non-disjunction by elevated temperature. Mutation Res. 11: 347.

Grell, R. F. 1971b. Heat-induced exchange in the fourth chromosome of diploid females of *Drosophila melanogaster*. Genetics 69: 523.

Grell, R. F. 1973. Recombination and DNA replication in the *Drosophila melanogaster* oocyte. Genetics 73: 87.

Grell, R. F. and A. C. Chandley. 1965. Evidence bearing on the coincidence of exchange and DNA replication in the oocyte of *Drosophila melanogaster*. Proc. Nat. Acad. Sci. U.S.A. 53: 1340.

Henderson, S. A. 1966. Time of chiasma formation in relation to the time of deoxyribonucleic acid synthesis. Nature 211: 1043.

King, R. C., A. C. Rubinson and R. F. Smith. 1956. Oogenesis in adult *Drosophila melanogaster*. Growth 20: 121.

Lu, B. C. 1969. Genetic recombination in Coprinus. I: Its precise timing as revealed by temperature treatment experiments. Can. J. Genet. Cytol. 11: 434.

Maguire, M. P. 1968. Evidence on the stage of heat induced crossover effect in maize. Genetics 60: 353.

Moens, P. B. and F. O. Perkins. 1969. Chromosome number of a small protist: Accurate determination. Science 166: 1289.

Muller, H. J. 1916. The mechanism of crossing-over. I-IV. Amer. Nat. 50: 284, 350, 421.

Peacock, W. J. 1970. Replication, recombination and chiasmata in *Goniaea australasiae* (Orthoptera:Acrididae). Genetics 65: 593.

Pritchard, R. H. 1955. The linear arrangement of a series of alleles in *Aspergillus nedulans*. Heredity 9: 343.

Wettstein, R. and J. R. Sotelo. 1967. Electron microscope serial reconstruction of the spermatocyte I nuclei at pachytene. J. Microscopie 6: 557.

STUDIES ON RECOMBINATION IN HIGHER ORGANISMS*

A. Chovnick, W. M. Gelbart, M. McCarron and J. Pandey

Genetics and Cell Biology Section, Biological Sciences Group, The University of Connecticut, Storrs, Connecticut 06268

Random-strand and half-tetrad recombination studies of rosy and maroon-like mutants have permitted us to investigate linked exchange in higher organisms. These studies involve the systematic recovery and analysis of the products of exchange events restricted to exceedingly short genetic intervals. Our observations lead us to conclude that all recombination involves a nonreciprocal transfer of information in the immediate region of the exchange event. These studies have been reported in great detail, and they have been the subject of recent review (Chovnick *et al.*, 1971; Finnerty, 1974).

Recent experiments bearing upon gene organization in higher organisms have generated an array of intriguing models (see reviews by Beerman, 1973; Davidson and Britten, 1973; Laird, 1973). Essentially, these investigations and the resultant models have served to focus attention upon major organizational features unique to the higher eukaryote gene. A more complete understanding of intragenic recombination in higher organisms requires a more rigorous definition of the specific genetic units used to study exchange. Some of our most recent work has been directed to this end.

The rosy locus (*ry*:3-52.0) of *Drosophila melanogaster* has been a key experimental system in our research effort. Rosy is a genetic

---

* This investigation was supported by a research grant, GM-09886, from the Public Health Service.

unit that controls the enzyme xanthine dehydrogenase (XDH), and
which has been restricted to salivary chromosome region 87D8-12
(Lefevre, 1971b).   Three observations place the structural information for XDH in or near rosy.   (1) The rosy eye color mutants
exhibit no detectable XDH activity (Glassman and Mitchell, 1959).
(2) Heterozygotes possessing one dose of ry^+ exhibit approximately
50% of normal enzyme activity, and flies carrying three doses of
ry^+ have 150% activity (Grell, 1962).   (3) Isoalleles differing
in their XDH electrophoretic mobility map to rosy or its immediate
vicinity (Yen and Glassman, 1965).

Large-scale recombination studies involving tests of rosy mutant heteroalleles are facilitated by the judicious application of
purine to the culture medium, permitting only rare ry^+ progeny to
survive.   From such experiments, a fine-structure map (Fig. 1) of
null enzyme rosy mutants was elaborated (Chovnick *et al.*, 1971)
that has served as the basis for experiments bearing upon the
mechanism of recombination in higher organisms.   Since none of these
rosy mutant alleles (Fig. 1) has a detectable altered XDH product,
they provide no information as to their structural (amino-acid
coding) or control (transcription- and translation-regulating)

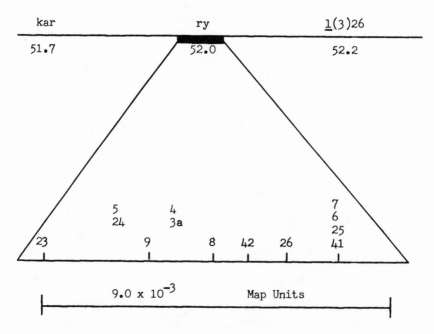

Figure 1.   A genetic map of the rosy region of chromosome 3.   The
map positions of various mutants used in this study are indicated,
and the genetic fine structure of the rosy locus is summarized.

roles. Moreover, important inferences have been drawn about the
mechanism of linked exchange based upon a simplistic view of the
relationship between distance as measured in recombination units
and nucleotide length. Thus, several questions about the organization of the rosy locus are pertinent to our analysis of recombination mechanisms: (1) What is the relationship of this map of
null-XDH rosy mutants to regulatory and structural components of
the locus? (2) What is the rate of recombination per nucleotide
length in the structural element, and how does this compare to
similar measurement in the control element? (3) How is the rosy
locus organized in terms of the number and kinds of DNA sequences
distributed within it?

We have recently begun to approach these questions. Initially,
we have concentrated on the identification of rosy variants for
which structural or control categorization is possible, and then
the subsequent localization of these variants on the existing map
(Fig. 1) of null-XDH rosy mutants. A number of classes of variants
are presently under investigation, but only one is considered in
the present report.

ELECTROPHORETIC VARIANTS AND WILD-TYPE ISOALLELES OF ROSY

As previously noted (Yen and Glassman, 1965; Charlesworth and
Charlesworth, 1973), electrophoretic variants of XDH, which map to
the rosy locus, are readily isolated from laboratory stocks and
natural populations of *Drosophila melanogaster*. We have established
a number of stable lines that exhibit single bands of XDH of uniform character upon electrophoresis (Fig. 2). Five discretely
different mobilities of XDH have been identified. They are designated by Roman numeral superscripts in order of increasing mobility,
XDH^I through XDH^V. Several mobility classes are each represented
by two different wild-type alleles. These alleles are derived from
different sources, and might well possess different coding sequences
leading to the same net charge on the XDH molecule.

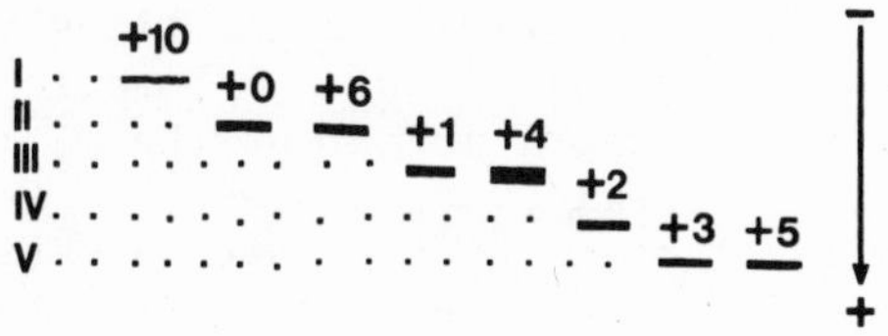

Figure 2. The ry^+ isoalleles used in this study, diagrammatically
arranged according to increasing electrophoretic mobility.

FINE-STRUCTURE MAPPING OF ELECTROPHORETIC SITES

In the absence of a selective procedure, it is impractical to directly map the genetic sites responsible for differences in electrophoretic mobility. Our experimental approach has been to induce null enzyme mutants upon each of the ry^+ isoalleles, and then to utilize the purine selective system to recover wild-type recombinants in mutant heteroallele mapping experiments. Wild-type recombinants recovered from experiments involving mutants of identical ry^+ ancestry invariably exhibit the parental electrophoretic class of XDH. Recombination experiments involving mutants induced on different ry^+ alleles permit us to follow the electrophoretic sites as unselected markers. Electrophoretic classification of the wild-type recombinant survivors permits localization of these electrophoretic sites as well as the null enzyme mutant sites (McCarron *et al.*, 1974).

In this experimental system, the ry^{+0} isoallele is our standard, and null enzyme mutants of ry^{+0} have been mapped relative to each other (Fig. 1). Our experimental logic is illustrated in Fig. 3. Utilizing a previously localized null enzyme rosy mutant of the ry^{+0} isoallele as a fixed reference point (ry^8), fine-structure recombination tests are carried out against a series of null enzyme mutants induced on a different isoallele (ry^{+1}). Some of these mutants are located to the left of our reference point (ry^{10X}), and others to the right (ry^{10Y}). In mutant heteroallele tests such as these (Fig. 3), each cross yields a single class of flanking marker crossover exceptions, and these provide for consistent mapping of the null enzyme sites. Moreover, analysis of the XDH electrophoretic characters of the recombinants yields a pattern of data that locates the relative position of the electrophoretic site(s) as well. Thus, for the crosses described in Fig. 3 involving ry^8, a mutant of the ry^{+0} isoallele (XDH^{II}), and a series of null enzyme mutants of the ry^{+1} (XDH^{III}) isoallele, the pattern of results indicates that the genetic basis for the electrophoretic difference maps to the right side of ry^8.

Figure 4 shows an important feature of allele recombination that was first observed in the effort to further localize the electrophoretic site indicated by the results illustrated in Fig. 3. In these experiments, four different ry^{100} series mutants were tested against ry^{41}, the rightmost mutant of the ry^{+0} isoallele (Fig. 1). All of the ry^{100} series mutants were located to the left of ry^{41}, and the results of these crosses are summarized in Fig. 4. There are three major features of these data: (1) The crossovers are all XDH^{III}, indicating that the electrophoretic site lies to the right of all crossover points. (2) The frequent occurrence (20/63) of coincident conversion (coconversion) of the electrophoretic site with conversion of ry^{41} is taken as a measure of proximity

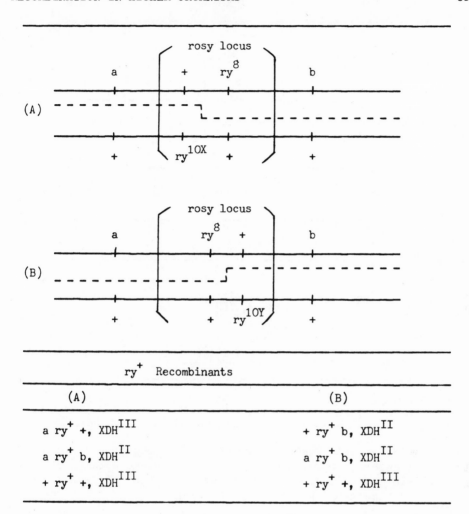

Figure 3.   Diagrammatic presentation of the results of a large-scale mutant heteroallele test involving null enzyme mutants of the ry^{+1} isoallele tested against ry^8, a mutant of the ry^{+0} isoallele that occupies a central location on the standard map of the rosy locus (Fig. 1).

of the electrophoretic site to ry^{41}.   (3) Conversion of ry^{41} does occur without conversion of the electrophoretic site, indicating that the two sites, in fact, are distinct.   Hence, we define the existence of a site, ry^{e111}, responsible for the electrophoretic difference between the ry^{+0} and ry^{+1} isoalleles.

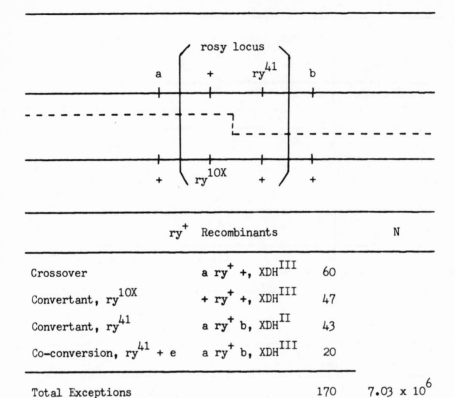

Figure 4. Diagrammatic presentation of the results of a large-scale mutant heteroallele test involving null enzyme mutants of the ry^{+1} isoallele tested against ry^{41}, a mutant of the ry^{+0} isoallele that occupies a marginal position on the standard map of the rosy locus (Fig. 1).

Following this experimental approach, we have carried out additional experiments designed to identify genetic sites responsible for the electrophoretic mobility differences between the ry^{+0} standard and the isoalleles ry^{+2}, ry^{+3}, ry^{+4}, and ry^{+5}. A detailed description of this work will be given in a separate report. Figure 5 summarizes the results of these experiments in the form of a genetic map of the rosy locus in which ry^5 and ry^{41} represent the left and right ends of the preexisting map of null enzyme mutants (Fig. 1). The relative positions of seven identified electrophoretic sites are indicated. It is of some interest that two site differences (rye^{507} and rye^{508}), distinguishing ry^{+0} and ry^{+5},

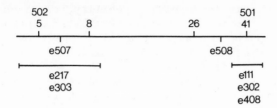

Figure 5.   The positions of the known electrophoretic sites relative to the standard null-XDH mutants ry^5, ry^8, and ry^{41} (see Fig.
1).

have been identified.   Similarly, two site differences were identified from the ry^{+0}-ry^{+3} tests (ry^{e303} and ry^{e302}).

ONE OR TWO STRUCTURAL ELEMENTS?

Consider next the distribution of the electrophoretic sites
elaborated in the present report (Fig. 5).   Clearly, structural
sites within the rosy locus are not confined to a small portion of
the map.   Indeed, at first glance one might conclude that most of
the standard rosy locus map (Fig. 1) represents a single structural
element coding for the XDH peptide.   However, a comparison of the
distribution of the seven identified electrophoretic sites (Fig.
5) with the distribution of known null activity mutant alleles
(Fig. 1) suggests that the genetic basis for electrophoretic variation in XDH may be restricted to two quite separable sectors of
the standard map.   The possibility exists that the structural
information for XDH resides in two elements, perhaps separated by
a control region of undefined length.   On this model, each structural element codes for a different peptide, which we designate as
the α and β subunits of XDH.   An active XDH molecule would be a
heterodimer consisting of one molecule of each subunit.   Let the
leftmost group of electrophoretic sites (Fig. 5) reside in the
coding element for the α subunit, and the rightmost group reside
within the β coding element.   Let α^S and α^F represent subunits of
slower and faster mobilities, respectively, and let β subunits be
similarly designated.   For consideration of this model, the XDH
moiety produced by ry^{+0} would then be $\alpha^S \beta^S$, while that produced
by ry^{+5} would be $\alpha^F \beta^F$.   The XDH electrophoretic pattern of ry^{+0}/ry^{+5}
heterozygotes consists of a heavy band of intermediate mobility
and light bands corresponding in mobility to ry^{+0} (XDH^{II}) and ry^{+5}
(XDH^V) homozygotes.   Observations such as these had led previously
to the suggestion that Drosophila XDH was a dimer consisting of two
units of a single peptide, the ry^+ product (Yen and Glassman, 1965).
We refer to this model as the single-subunit model.   On the one-

subunit model, in order of increasing mobility, these bands corre-
spond to XDH^{II}-XDH^{II} homodimers, XDH^{II}-XDH^{V} heterodimers, and XDH^{V}-
XDH^{V} homodimers. On the two-subunit model, the slowest-migrating
form is $\alpha^{S}\beta^{S}$, the intermediate is a combination of $\alpha^{S}\beta^{F}$ and $\alpha^{F}\beta^{S}$
molecules, and the fastest form is $\alpha^{F}\beta^{F}$. Thus, ry^{+0}/ry^{+5} heterozygotes exhibit identical electrophoretic patterns on either model.
However, a distinction between these two models is possible.

The two-subunit model predicts that $\alpha^{S}\beta^{S}/\alpha^{F}\beta^{F}$ and $\alpha^{S}\beta^{F}/\alpha^{F}\beta^{S}$
individuals will generate identical three-banded hybrid electrophor-
etic patterns. On the one-subunit model, these same heterozygotes
would be designated XDH^{II}/XDH^{V} and XDH^{int}/XDH^{int}, respectively;
the XDH^{II}/XDH^{V} heterozygote would be expected to produce the three-
banded hybrid electrophoretic pattern while the XDH^{int}/XDH^{int} individual would produce a single band of XDH^{int} mobility. Essentially,
the one-subunit model predicts a *cis-trans* difference, whereas the
two-subunit model predicts no such difference (see Fig. 6).

For the sake of this discussion, the ry^{+0}/ry^{+5} heterozygous
genotype may be rewritten as $rye^{507}S\ rye^{508}S/rye^{507}F\ rye^{508}F$. This
represents the *cis* configuration of electrophoretic sites. From
chromosomes recovered as coconversions in recombination tests, we
were able to generate ry^{+} allele combinations $rye^{507}S\ rye^{508}F$ and
$rye^{507}F\ rye^{508}S$ and thus to carry out the *cis-trans* test. Examination of XDH electrophoretic patterns revealed a clear-cut *cis-trans*
difference entirely consistent with the single-subunit model (Fig.
6). Hence, we conclude that most if not all of the standard genetic
map of the rosy locus (Fig. 1) represents a single, uninterrupted
DNA sequence, which is the XDH structural element. Moreover, we
submit that this structural element consists of a unique DNA sequence of some 3×10^{3} nucleotide pairs in length. That the struc-

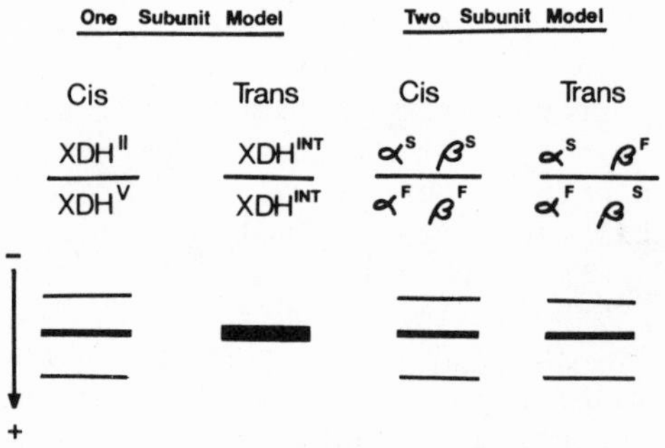

Figure 6. The predictions of the one- and two-subunit models.
Diagrams of the electrophoretic patterns expected on either model
are included. The *cis* configuration is $rye^{507}S\ rye^{508}S/rye^{507}F$
$rye^{508}F$; *trans* is $rye^{507}S\ rye^{508}F/rye^{507}F\ rye^{508}S$.

tural element is a unique DNA sequence is documented by our total
experience with fine-structure recombination experiments involving
some 2 X 10^3 ry^+ recombinants analyzed. We have seen no evidence
of the "unequal" crossing-over that would occur if repeat sequences
were present. The physical length of the structural element derives from the molecular weight of Drosophila XDH, which is estimated at 250,000 (Glassman et $al.$, 1966). Assuming the biologically
active XDH molecule to consist of two identical subunits (Yen and
Glassman, 1965), we are led to a subunit size of some 10^3 amino
acids, which requires a coding sequence of some 3 X 10^3 nucleotide
pairs. It is of interest to note that this estimate of the physical
length of the XDH structural element is strikingly similar to an
estimate based upon recombination data. Lefevre (1971b) correlates
0.01 map units with a length of 3.7-3.8 X 10^3 nucleotide pairs in
$D.$ $melanogaster$. The standard map of the rosy locus (Fig. 1) ex-
tends over 0.009 map units and thus 3.3-3.4 X 10^3 nucleotide pairs.

IMPACT OF COCONVERSION

The observation of coincident conversion described in the present analysis (Fig. 4) is an important and potentially most useful
feature of recombination involving exceedingly short genetic intervals. The significance of the phenomenon of coconversion was recognized quite early from fungal studies as demonstrating that the
conversion event involves a variable segment of DNA. Fogel et $al.$
(1971) have studied the frequency of coconversion as a function of
distance between the sites and have shown a linear relationship in-
versely proportional to distance. We have observed a similar relationship in the present investigation (manuscript in preparation).

The effect of coconversion on recombination in short intervals
in Drosophila can be seen in Table 1. Therein, a series of random-
strand mutant heteroallele recombination tests are summarized, in
which ry^{41} is tested against a series of mutants located at various
points along the map (Fig. 1). There are two major features of
this table: (1) Crossover frequencies are consistent with relative
map positions of the mutants. (2) Frequencies of conversion of the
ry^{41} allele appear constant in all heteroallele tests with the exception of tests against the closest allele, ry^2. The collapse
of the frequencies of all recombinant wild types in direct tests
of closely linked sites is a result of coconversion. Consider the
test ry^{41}/ry^2 in Table 1, Row 1. The results of this very large
experiment are unable to provide relative positioning of the mutants,
although the data indicate that they are not identical.

Table 1. Frequency (X 10^6) of ry^+ exceptional progeny resulting from the indicated heteroallele tests

Heteroallele pair	Analysis of ry^+ chromosomes		Total ry^+ progeny	$N/10^6$
	Crossovers	Conv-ry^{41}		
ry^{41}/ry^2	—	3.24	3.64	2.47
ry^{41}/ry^{26}	4.2	14.1	22.5	0.712
ry^{41}/ry^{42}	3.8	13.7	22.8	1.32
ry^{41}/ry^8	8.9	14.6	32.4	1.23
ry^{41}/ry^5	16.7	15.9	41.3	1.26

Table 2. Coconversions of ry^{41} and adjacent electrophoretic sites

Electrophoretic site	Conversions ry^{41}	Coconversions	Frequency of Coconversion
e111	63	20	0.32
e302	18	7	0.39
e408	8	2	0.25
Pooled	89	29	0.31
e508	9	0	

FINE-STRUCTURE MAPPING BY COCONVERSION WITH AN
UNSELECTED MARKER SITE

Following a logic that is formally analogous to recombination analysis in bacterial transformation and transduction, coconversion provides a sensitive tool for the ordering of closely linked sites in Drosophila that may not be resolvable by crossover analysis. Consider the results of the recombination test (Table 1) involving ry^{41}/ry^2 that yielded no crossovers but did produce both ry^{41} and ry^2 conversions. Had the experment included a closely linked unselected heterozygosity (*i.e.*, an electrophoretic site) in a known position, the relative positions of the mutant sites would have been apparent from the conversion classes. Consider the possibility that ry^{41} lies to the left of ry^2, and that the test involved heterozygosity for an electrophoretic site as well, indicated by the genotype $\dfrac{e^8 \quad ry^{41} \quad +}{e^J \quad + \quad ry^2}$. In such a genotype, conversion of ry^2 cannot involve a segment that picks up e^8. Thus, conversions of ry^2 will never involve coconversion for the electrophoretic site. On the other hand, because of the location of the electrophoretic site, there is no such restriction on coconversion for the electrophoretic site with conversion of ry^{41}.

A still more dramatic example of the resolving power of coconversion for site mapping in Drosophila is illustrated by the resolution of the location of the null-XDH mutant, ry^{501}, relative to ry^{41}. In Fig. 5, ry^{501} is placed above ry^{41} by virtue of the fact that in direct recombination tests no crossovers and no convertants of either ry^{41} or ry^{501} were recovered in 1.37 X 10^6 zygotes assayed. However, in direct tests of ry^{501} against ry^5, there was extensive recombination, as expected. Among the recombinants were four conversions of ry^{501}, and two of these involved coconversion of the electrophoretic site $e508$ as well. When ry^{41} was tested against ry^{502}, located at the far left end of the map, nine conversions of ry^{41} were recovered; none involved the $e508$ site. We infer from these observations that ry^{501} is located to the left of ry^{41}.

ESTIMATE OF SIZE OF CONVERSION SEGMENTS

Consider the array of electrophoretic sites at the right end of the rosy locus map of Fig. 5. The sites $e111$, $e301$, and $e408$ have been placed under the line directly under ry^{41} by virtue of experiments which (1) fail to exhibit crossovers between ry^{41} and the electrophoretic sites, and (2) the occurrence of coconversions with ry^{41}. Table 2 summarizes the results of experiments involving ry^{41} and each of the indicated electrophoretic sites. Thus, Table 2, Row 1 indicates that in all experiments involving ry^{41} and mutants of the ry^{100} series, a total of 63 convertants of ry^{41} were recovered, 20 of which were coconvertants involving the electro-

phoretic site, *e111*. Similar data were obtained for *e302* and *e408*.
It is indeed possible that these may be the same electrophoretic
site. In contrast, experiments involving ry^{41} and *e508* yielded
recombination data which placed *e508* to the left of ry^{41}, and there
were no coconversions of the *e508* site associated with nine recovered conversions of ry^{41}. Turning next to the ry^{26} site, we have
carried out experiments that provide opportunity to question the
frequency of coconversion of *e508* with conversion of ry^{26}. In
twelve such opportunities recorded thus far, there were no coconversions of the electrophoretic site associated with conversion of
ry^{26}. Based upon all of our past recombination experiments with
the rosy locus, we estimate the distance from ry^{26} to ry^{41} to
represent from 1/4 to 1/3 of the standard map of the rosy locus
(Fig. 1), or 750–1000 nucleotides. Placing *e508* approximately
halfway between ry^{26} and ry^{41} suggests that the interval from ry^{26}
or ry^{41} to *e508* measures some 375–500 nucleotides. That we have
seen no coconversions involving intervals as large as this in 21
opportunities suggests that the size range of conversion segments
among those conversions not associated with exchange for flanking
markers may not extend beyond several hundred nucleotides in this
experimental system.

CONCLUSION

In setting out to define more rigorously the rosy locus for
recombination studies, several questions were raised (see above),
for which some answers are available. We have provided evidence
that the rosy locus includes a single structural element coding
for the amino-acid sequence of the XDH polypeptide, and that most
if not all of the map of null enzyme mutants is included within that
element. The genetic data support the contention that the DNA in
this element is a single unique sequence, a viewpoint that is
consonant with current knowledge about the DNA complementary to
higher organism mRNA. A bonus from this effort was the demonstration of coconversion in Drosophila and the recognition of its potential value as a tool in fine-structure mapping. Moreover, with
the simple assumption that the existing map in fact represents the
XDH structural element, we are able to relate distance in recombination units to nucleotide length and to estimate the maximum size
of coconversion segments.

We anticipate that our current research soon will provide still
more accurate resolution of the limits of the XDH structural element, as well as a comparative analysis of recombination parameters
both in the structural element and in its immediate environment.

REFERENCES

Beermann, W.   1973.   Chromomeres and genes.   Cell Differentiation
4: 1.

Charlesworth, B. and D. Charlesworth.   1973.   A study of linkage
disequilibrium in populations of *Drosophila melanogaster*.   Genetics
73: 351.

Chovnick, A., G. H. Ballantyne and D. G. Holm.   1971.   Studies on
gene conversion and its relationship to linked exchange in *Drosophila melanogaster*.   Genetics 69: 179.

Davidson, E. H. and R. J. Britten.   1973.   Organization, transcription and regulation in the animal genome.   Quart. Rev. Biol. 48:
565.

Finnerty, V.   1974.   Gene conversion in Drosophila.   In (M. Ashburner and E. Novitski, eds.) Biology and Genetics of Drosophila, Vol.
1.   London, Academic Press, in press.

Fogel, S., D. D. Hurst and R. K. Mortimer.   1971.   Gene conversion
in unselected tetrads from multipoint crosses.   In (G. Kimber and
G. P. Rédei, eds.) Stadler Genetics Symposia, Vols. 1 and 2, pp.
89-110.   University of Missouri Agriculture Experiment Station,
Columbia, Mo.

Glassman, E. and H. K. Mitchell.   1959.   Mutants of *D. melanogaster*
deficient in xanthine dehydrogenase.   Genetics 44: 153.

Glassman, E., T. Shinoda, H. M. Moon and J. D. Karam.   1966.   *In
vitro* complementation between non-allelic Drosophila mutants deficient in xanthine dehydrogenase.   IV. Molecular weights.   J.
Mol. Biol. 20: 419.

Grell, E. H.   1962.   The dose effect of $ma-1^+$ and ry^+ on xanthine
dehydrogenase activity in *Drosophila melanogaster*.   Z. Vererbungsl.
93: 371.

Laird, C.   1973.   DNA of Drosophila chromosomes.   Ann. Rev. Genet.
7: 177.

Lefevre, G., Jr.   1971a.   Cytological information regarding mutants
listed in Lindsley and Grell 1968.   Drosophila Inf. Serv. 46: 40.

Lefevre, G., Jr.   1971b.   Salivary chromosome glands and the frequency of crossing over in *Drosophila melanogaster*.   Genetics 67: 497.

McCarron, M., W. Gelbart and A. Chovnick. 1974. Intracistronic
mapping of electrophoretic sites in *Drosophila melanogaster:*
Fidelity of information transfer by gene conversion. Genetics, in
press.

Yen, T. T. T. and E. Glassman. 1965. Electrophoretic vaiants of
xanthine dehydrogenase in *Drosophila melanogaster*. Genetics 52:
977.

GENIC CONTROL OF MEIOSIS AND SOME OBSERVATIONS ON THE

SYNAPTONEMAL COMPLEX IN *DROSOPHILA MELANOGASTER**

Adelaide T. C. Carpenter and Bruce S. Baker

Department of Zoology, Department of Genetics,

University of Wisconsin, Madison, Wisconsin 53706

Beginning with the work of Sandler *et al.* (1968) and Lindsley *et al.* (1968), a systematic attack on the genic control of meiosis in *Drosophila melanogaster* has been undertaken. Several successful screens for mutants that disrupt meiosis (meiotic mutants) have been reported (Sandler *et al.*, 1968; Sandler, 1971; Baker and Carpenter, 1972); to date, the term "meiotic mutant" has been operationally restricted to those mutants that disrupt genetically detectable parameters of chromosome behavior (*e.g.* disjunction and recombination). The effects of many of these, as well as previously known meiotic mutants, have been examined in detail (D. G. Davis, 1969; Robbins, 1971; B. K. Davis, 1971; Hall, 1972; Carpenter, 1973; Parry, 1973; Carpenter and Sandler, 1974; reviewed by Baker and Hall, 1974). There are at this time at least 40 loci whose wild-type alleles are necessary to ensure a normal meiosis in Drosophila males or females (Sandler and Lindsley, 1974).

Our aim in studying these mutants is to delimit the function of the wild-type allele of a locus in ensuring a normal meiosis by inference from the nature of the abnormalities in meiotic chromosome behavior caused by mutants at that locus. The meiotic events affected by mutants so far analyzed include the events of recombination, anaphase I separation (of homologous centromeres or of distributively paired chromosomes), anaphase II separation of sister centromeres, and the ability of chromosomes to move to the anaphase poles.

---

* Research supported by NIH Postdoctoral Fellowships to A.T.C.C. and B.B. Paper # 1740 of the Department of Genetics, University of Wisconsin.

Here the focus is on those mutants defective in recombination. To date, 14 mutants representing 11 loci have been analyzed. These mutations are all recessive, and all, when homozygous in females, result in decreased levels of recombination. (These mutants have no effect on male meiosis, presumably because recombination does not occur in wild-type *Drosophila melanogaster* males.) In addition, these mutations all increase the frequency of nondisjunction; however, a number of lines of evidence suggest that the increase in nondisjunction is a secondary effect of the decrease in exchange. Briefly, these are that (1) nondisjunction occurs at the first meiotic division; (2) nondisjunctional chromosomes are all nonrecombinant; and (3) when the various mutants are compared, it can be seen that the increase in nondisjunction is proportional to the decrease in recombination (Fig. 1). A more detailed account of this argument can be found in Baker and Hall (1974) and Sandler and Lindsley (1974).

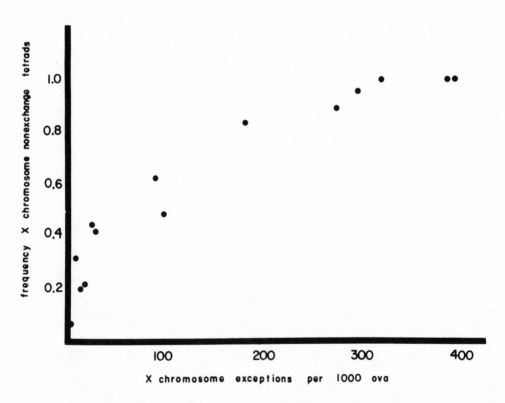

Figure 1. The relationship between the frequencies of exchange and nondisjunction of X chromosomes in mutants that reduce crossing-over. Redrawn from Baker and Hall (1974) with the addition of data for *abo* (Carpenter and Sandler, 1974) and *mei-W68* (B. S. Baker, unpublished observations).

The mutants that affect recombination can be divided into two classes — those affecting preconditions for exchange (functions ordinarily required for the physical recombination of DNA molecules, *e.g.* pairing) and those affecting exchange (functions directly involved in the formation of physically recombinant DNA molecules) — by two criteria. First, Sandler *et al.* (1968) and Lindsley *et al.* (1968), following Bridges (1915), suggested that the effect of the mutation on the coefficient of coincidence (C) could be used to separate the two classes; mutants defective in exchange should not have altered values for C, whereas mutants defective in preconditions for exchange might exhibit altered values for C. More recently, Carpenter and Sandler (1974) have suggested a second criterion — the effect of the mutant on crossing-over in different regions along a chromosome. That is, mutants defective in exchange should exhibit reduced crossing-over equally in all regions, yielding a map proportional to that in wild-type, whereas mutants defective in preconditions should exhibit reduced crossing-over more drastically in some regions than in others, yielding a distorted map.

By applying these tests to the 14 mutants which are defective in recombination, it is observed that in mutants at one locus (two alleles), crossing-over is reduced to the same extent in all intervals examined (Fig. 2a), and extant data are consistent with there being no alternation of C; therefore, the wild-type allele of this locus determines a function involved in exchange. Mutants at 9 loci (one with two alleles) exhibit distorted maps (Fig. 2a) and all but one have altered C; thus, the wild-type alleles of these loci determine functions involved in preconditions for exchange. Mutants at one locus (two alleles) exhibit no meiotic crossing-over, thus the above criteria are not applicable; however, from other considerations it has been suggested that this locus also specifies precondition for exchange (Hall, 1972).

Examination of the pattern of crossing-over in the mutants defective in preconditions for exchange allows us to delimit further the nature of the functions determined by the wild-type alleles of these loci. The patterns of crossing-over are quite similar in all of these mutants. In each mutant, crossing-over is reduced to the same extent in all distal euchromatic regions examined, whereas crossing-over is less severely depressed in the proximal euchromatic regions and in regions containing the centric heterochromatin (Fig. 2a). In wild-type, crossing-over is proportional to physical distance (DNA content; Lefevre, 1971) with the exception of the proximal regions, where crossing-over per unit physical distance is greatly reduced relative to more distal (euchromatic) regions (compare Fig. 2b and 2c). In fact, crossing-over in these mutants is more proportional to physical distance than it is in wild-type (Fig. 2d). This observation suggests that these mutations

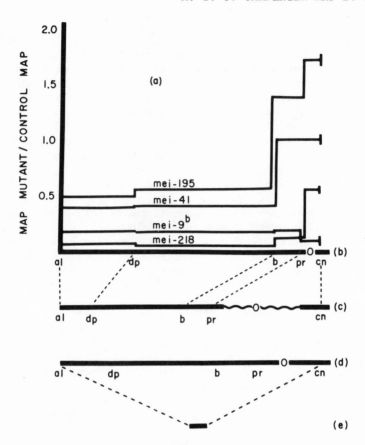

Figure 2. The pattern of crossing-over on chromosome *2L* observed
in the mutant defective in exchange (*mei-9ᵇ*) and representative
mutants defective in preconditions for exchange (*mei-218, mei-41,
mei-195*). (a) Ordinate: frequency of crossing-over in mutant
relative to wild-type for each interval. Abscissa: (b) wild-type
genetic map of *2L*; (c) map of relative physical distances between
markers used; (d) expanded genetic map of *al-cn* region of *2L* in the
presence of *mei-218* for comparison to physical map, c; (e) genetic
map of *al-cn* region of *2L* in the presence of *mei-218* on the same
scale as b. Circles indicate the centromere of chromosome *2*; wavy
lines indicate the centric heterochromatin. Genetic data from
Baker and Carpenter (1972).

are in loci whose wild-type alleles impose constraints on the location of exchanges; and the observation that the mutations cause an
overall decrease in recombination suggests that, in wild-type, these
constraints also serve to promote crossing-over (Baker and Carpenter,
1972).

It may be recalled that, in Drosophila, recombination occurs mitotically as well as meiotically, though at a much lower rate. Mitotic crossing-over is fairly proportional to physical distance (Garcia-Bellido, 1972). Thus, mitotic crossing-over is similar to meiotic crossing-over in mutants defective in processes involved in preconditions for meiotic exchange. Consequently, a major difference between meiotic and mitotic crossing-over may be that the wild-type alleles of these precondition loci function only meiotically. The observation that the mutant $c(3)G$, which completely eliminates meiotic crossing-over and is thought to be defective in a precondition for exchange (Hall, 1972), has no effect on mitotic crossing-over (LeClerc, 1946) is in accord with this notion.

Given our ability to dissect recombination processes genetically via mutants in the manner briefly described above, one would like to find the cytological and ultimately the molecular correlates of these genetically detectable functions. With this in mind, I (A.T.C.C.) have undertaken an electron microscopic study of meiosis in female Drosophila. In particular, I have been focussing attention on the synaptonemal complex (SC), a tripartite, ribbon-like structure present between synapsed homologs during prophase I (zygotene, pachytene) of meiosis; the presence of the SC correlates well with the occurrence of meiotic recombination in various organisms (Moses, 1968; but see Grell et al., 1972). The synaptonemal complex has been suggested to be a precondition for exchange (Moses, 1968; Westergaard and von Wettstein, 1972); thus, this structure is a likely candidate for the site of the defect in at least some of these mutants.

My studies involve three parameters of the SC in wild-type and mutant females: its times of appearance and disappearance, its length, and its fine structure. Drosophila females are particularly well-suited for this study, since developing oocytes are approximately linearly aranged with respect to developmental time in each ovariole, and oocyte nuclei are relatively small.

The technique I use is as follows. (1) Take serial sections (section thickness 60-80 nm) of the pertinent region of an ovariole --i.e., the entire germarium and the first 3-4 vitellarial cysts (see King, 1970, for terminology and diagrams of these structures) --from a 3- to 4-day-old inseminated adult female. (2) Examine the sections to locate the potential oocytes: photograph every sixth to tenth section of the germarium at low magnification and reconstruct each cyst by identifying its component 16 cells and their cytoplasmic connections (ring canals = rc) throughout the photographs. [In Drosophila females, both cells with 4 rc have SC in germarial cysts (King, 1970), as well as at least one of the 3-rc cells in some cysts (the latter has also been observed by Annalise Fiil and Søren Rasmussen, personal communications). Thus, both 4-rc cells per germarial cyst have been examined by reconstruction

(see below); in stage-1 and later cysts (see King, 1970, for staging
of vitellarial cysts), a single 4-rc cell is clearly the oocyte.]
(3) Photograph each section of oocyte nuclei and reconstruct the
SC (by tracing the nuclear outline and SC of each photograph onto
acetate sheets, stacking the sheets, and following each SC throughout its meanderings). (4) Finally, examine suitable sections for
fine-structure morphology. I have thus far analyzed 12 ovarioles
and reconstructed the SC in 30 oocytes, 8 of which are from the
same wild-type germarium (2 each from 4 cysts).

In wild-type germarial oocytes, there are five long (up to
20 μm) pieces of SC + associated chromatin, corresponding to the
X and the left and right arms of chromosomes *2* and *3*. The proximal
ends of these pieces converge on a single region of the nucleus
(the chromocenter); this region contains the proximal heterochromatin. SC is present in the chromocenter; in favorable reconstructions, the left and right arms of chromosomes *2* and *3* can be connected and the *X* heterochromatin proximal to the nucleolus identified. In some cells there is a short piece of chromocentral SC
clearly not associated with the *X*, *2*, or *3*; this is presumably the
tiny *4*th chromosome. Chromocentral (heterochromatic and *4*th chromosomal) complex differs in morphology from more distal (euchromatic)
SC; it is thinner (28–56 nm as opposed to 56–190 nm); its component
parts (lateral and central elements) are less distinct, and its
associated chromatin frequently appears to be more condensed (Figs.
3–6). However, heterochromatic and euchromatic SC are the same
width (120 nm). There does not appear to be an abrupt juncture be-

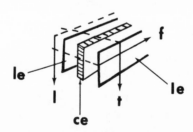

Figure 3. Sectioning planes of synaptonemal complex (diagramatic).
le, lateral element; *ce*, central element (transverse filaments
have been omitted for clarity); *l*, *t*, and *f*, lateral, transverse,
and frontal planes, respectively. "Width" is the distance between
the two lateral elements; it can be determined from *f* and *t* sections.
"Thickness" is the distance between the top and bottom of the complex in this diagram; it can be determined in *t* and *l* sections.
"Length" is the total length of the complex in a chromosome arm;
it can be determined from reconstruction of serial sections.

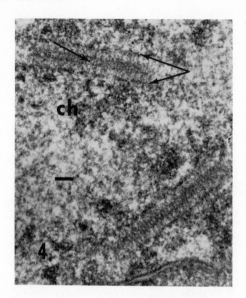

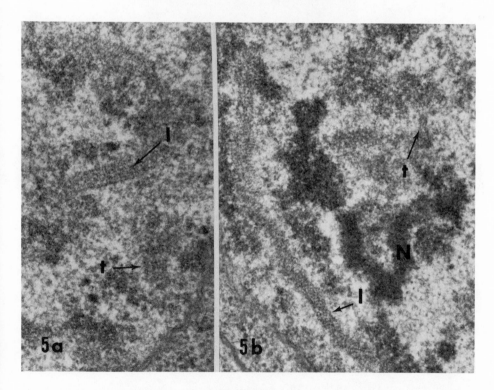

Figures 4-6. Fixation and post-staining procedures employed were essentially the same as those of Kubai (1973) except that the material
was dissected in Drosophila Ringer's solution instead of dilute fixa-
tive. All magnifications are 56,000X; the bar in Fig. 4 (cont. p. 373)

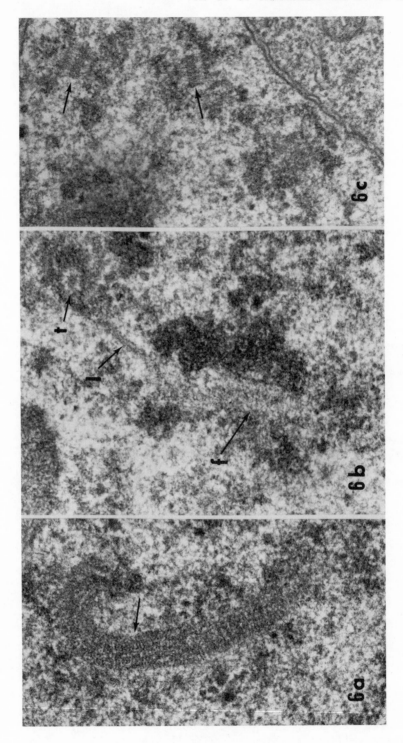

tween the euchromatic and the heterochromatic SC; rather, the SC
appears to become thicker and more distinct over some length as it
leaves the chromocentral region. The maximum thickness (*cf*. Figs.
5a and 6a) and total length of euchromatic SC vary between oocytes
from the same ovariole; both parameters appear to be correlated
with the position of the oocyte in the ovariole (*i.e.*, the developmental age) (Carpenter, in preparation).

There is a striking parallel between the observations on SC
morphology just described and the distribution of crossovers relative to physical distance discussed earlier. Near the centromeres,
the SC has the appearance here termed "heterochromatic"; it gradually becomes more "euchromatic" over some distance; the extensive
(20 µm or so) distal regions are entirely "euchromatic." There is
virtually no crossing-over in the proximal (centric) heterochromatin;
crossing-over per unit physical distance gradually increases in
euchromatic regions just distal to the proximal heterochromatin;
crossing-over per unit physical distance is high and constant in
the extensive distal euchromatin. The similarities between these
two types of observations suggest that they reflect different
aspects of the same basic phenomena — the imposition of constraints
on the location of recombinational events.

It is clearly of interest to determine whether any of the mutants which appear from genetic criteria to be defective in such
constraints fail to show the "euchromatic-heterochromatic" differentiation in SC morphology. Preliminary observations on the two
strongest precondition mutants (*mei-218* and *mei-41*; 8% and 48% of
wild-type crossing-over, respectively; Baker and Carpenter, 1972)
suggest that the SC of both appears normal in this respect. Moreover, the SC in *mei-218* appears to be of normal length. Further
examinations of these and other mutants affecting recombination are
in progress.

---

represents 0.1 µm. All planes of section have been determined by
the reconstruction of serial sections; all *l* sections presented
visualize the central element. Figure 4. Frontal sections through
two pieces of euchromatic SC. Arrows indicate central and lateral
elements; *ch*, chromatin. Figure 5. (a) Euchromatic *l* and *t* sections from an early germarial oocyte. (b) Heterochromatic *l* and *t*
sections from an early germarial oocyte; *N*, nucleolus. Figure 6.
(a) Euchromatic *l* section from a germarial oocyte posterior to
(older than) that in Fig. 5. (b) Heterochromatic *t*, *l*, and *f* sections from the oocyte in Fig. 6a. (c) Euchromatic *t* sections from
the oocyte in Fig. 6a.

ACKNOWLEDGMENTS

A.T.C.C. would like to express her gratitude for generous advice concerning the art of electron microscopy to Renate Bromberg, Joan B. Peterson, Dr. Donna Kubai, and most especially to Dr. Hans Ris, in whose laboratory the electron microscopic observations were performed.

REFERENCES

Baker, B. S. and A. T. C. Carpenter. 1972. Genetic analysis of sex chromosomal meiotic mutants in *Drosophila melanogaster*. Genetics 71: 255.

Baker, B. S. and J. C. Hall. 1974. Meiotic mutants: genic control of meiotic recombination and chromosome segregation. In (E. Novitski and M. Ashburner, eds.) Genetics and Biology of Drosophila I. Academic Press, New York. In press.

Bridges, C. B. 1915. A linkage variation in Drosophila. J. Exp. Zool. 19: 1.

Carpenter, A. T. C. 1973. A meiotic mutant defective in distributive disjunction in *Drosophila melanogaster*. Genetics 73: 393.

Carpenter, A. T. C. and L. Sandler. 1974. On recombination-defective meiotic mutants in *Drosophila melanogaster*. Genetics in press.

Davis, B. K. 1971. Genetic analysis of a meiotic mutant resulting in precocious sister-centromere separation in *Drosophila melanogaster*. Mol. Gen. Genet. 113: 251.

Davis, D. G. 1969. Chromosome behavior under the influence of claret-nondisjunctional in *Drosophila melanogaster*. Genetics 61: 577.

Garcia-Bellido, A. 1972. Some parameters of mitotic recombination in *Drosophila melanogaster*. Mol. Gen. Genet. 115: 54.

Grell, R. F., H. Bank and G. Gassner. 1972. Meiotic exchange without the synaptonemal complex. Nature New Biol. 240: 155.

Hall, J. C. 1972. Chromosome segregation influenced by two alleles of the meiotic mutant *c(3)G* in *Drosophila melanogaster*. Genetics 71: 367.

King, R. C. 1970. Ovarian Development in *Drosophila melanogaster*. Academic Press, New York.

Kubai, D. F.   1973.   Unorthodox mitosis in *Trichonympha agilis:* kinetochore differentiation and chromosome movement.   J. Cell Sci. 13: 511.

LeClerc, G.   1946.   Occurrence of mitotic crossing-over without meiotic crossing over.   Science 103: 553.

Lefevre, G., Jr.   1971.   Salivary chromosome bands and the frequency of crossing-over in *Drosophila melanogaster*.   Genetics 67: 497.

Lindsley, D. L., L. Sandler, B. Nicoletti and G. Trippa.   1968. Genetic control of recombination in Drosophila.   In (W. J. Peacock and R. D. Brock, eds.) Replication and Recombination of Genetic Material.   pp. 253-267.   Australian Acad. Sci., Canberra.

Moses, M. J.   1968.   Synaptinemal Complex.   Ann. Rev. Genet. 2: 363.

Parry, D. M.   1973.   A meiotic mutant affecting recombination in female *Drosophila melanogaster*.   Genetics 73: 465.

Robbins, L. G.   1971.   Nonexchange alignment: a meiotic process revealed by a synthetic meiotic mutant of *Drosophila melanogaster*. Mol. Gen. Genet. 110: 144.

Sandler, L.   1971.   Induction of autosomal meiotic mutants by EMS in *D. melanogaster*.   Drosophila Inf. Serv. 47: 68.

Sandler, L. and D. L. Lindsley.   1974.   Some observations on the study of the genetic control of meiosis in *Drosophila melanogaster*. *Proc. XIII Int. Congr. Genet.* in press.

Sandler, L., D. L. Lindsley, B. Nicoletti and G. Trippa.   1968. Mutants affecting meiosis in natural populations of *Drosophila melanogaster*.   Genetics 60: 525.

Westergaard, M. and D. von Wettstein.   1972.   The synaptinemal complex.   Ann. Rev. Genet. 6: 71.

COINCIDENCE OF MODIFIED CROSSOVER DISTRIBUTION WITH MODIFIED

SYNAPTONEMAL COMPLEXES

Peter B. Moens

York University, Downsview, Ontario, Canada

In eukaryotes the systematic nonoccurrence of reciprocal exchange in competent chromosomes is not predictable from molecular models of conversion or exchange. Modifications of crossover distribution include positive interference, species-specific limitations of crossovers per cell or per bivalent, the localization of crossovers in specific chromsosome segments, and the abolishment of crossovers in meiocytes of one or the other sex of members of one species. In each case the particular regulation of recombination represents an adaptation in the evolutionary strategy of the species. Unlike the process of recombination itself, these adaptations are often of recent origin, and differences occur between the species of a single genus or family.

The observations by Meyer (1964) that there is a direct correlation between the presence of crossing-over and the presence of synaptonemal complexes in the gametocytes of females and males of a number of Dipteran species, and that mutant *c3G Drosophila melanogaster* females lack both recombination and synaptonemal complexes, suggest that the complex may play a role in the regulation of crossover distribution. In spite of the large amount of information gathered on the synaptonemal complex since that time (Stern and Hotta, 1973; Moens, 1973; Moses, 1968; Westergaard and von Wettstein, 1972), it has not become clear whether such correlations are real or fortuitous. Some further observations that support the notion that there is a correlation, but are not decisive by any means, are described below.

Synaptonemal complexes are usually formed by the coalignment of the axial cores of pairs of homologous chromosomes at a distance

377

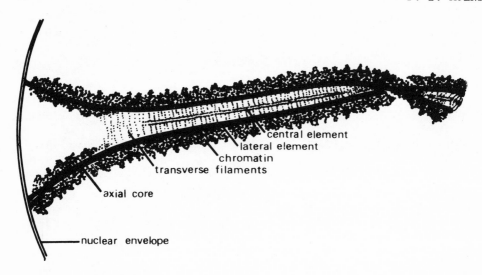

Figure 1. Diagram of a synaptonemal complex. It is formed by the pairing of two axial cores that are associated with the homologous chromosomes.

of 100 nm from each other (Fig. 1). In many organisms the cores are attached to the nuclear envelope, and synapsis essentially occurs between two loops closed by the nuclear envelope. Synaptonemal complexes have been traced through the entire length of bivalents by serial sectioning and water-spreading of meiotic nuclei of protists, fungi, plants, insects, and mammals (Westergaard and von Wettstein, 1972; Counce and Meyer, 1973). In each case one or more crossovers should have been encountered in each bivalent but none were recognized, possibly because of the lack of preconceived notions of the fine structure of an exchange.

Prior to chromosome synapsis, each axial core is associated with two sister chromatids. When the cores of a set of homologous chromosomes become aligned to form the lateral elements of a synaptonemal complex (Fig. 2A), reciprocal exchanges must cause some of the newly constituted chromatids to be associated alternately with one and then with the other lateral element (Fig. 2B, C). For no compelling reasons, it has in general been assumed that at the site of a reciprocal exchange the nonexchange chromatids remain associated with the uninterrupted lateral elements. There is no real objection to the equally likely assumption that the lateral elements remain associated with the crossover chromatids. A reciprocal exchange would produce a half-twist in the synaptonemal complex due to breakage and rejoining of lateral elements. The joining of lateral elements that are associated with nonsister chromatids is a common occurrence in the triploid lily (Moens, 1969).

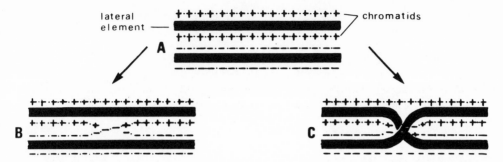

Figure 2. (A) Prior to crossing-over each lateral element is associated with two continuous sister chromatids. (B) At the site of a reciprocal exchange the lateral element may follow the continuity of the noncrossover chromatids or (C) the crossover chromatids. In the latter case, a half-twist could be formed in the synaptonemal complex. In some cases the structure of the complex may be related to the position and frequency of reciprocal exchanges.

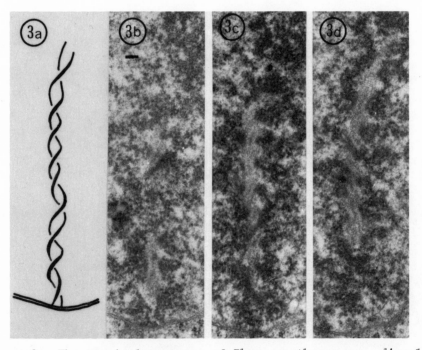

Figure 3. The terminal segments of *Rhoeo spathacea* var. *discolor* bivalents all have a series of tight coils. Because this plant is a permanent translocation heterozygote, crossing-over takes place only in the translocated terminal segments. Bar on 3b is 100 nm.

(The spacing of twirls or coils may be a function of the composition of the synaptonemal complex at any given site.)

The fine structure of a synaptonemal complex at the site of a
crossover can be studied to advantage if the crossovers are localized in a specific region of the chromosome and if that region can be
identified by electron microscopy. For example, the onion *Allium
fistulosum* has chiasmata on both sides of each centromere but not
elsewhere in the bivalent. In the permanent translocation heterozygote *Rhoeo spathacea* var. *discolor* (Swartz) Stearn, crossing-over
is limited to the distal translocated segments, and some grass-
hoppers of the genera *Chloealtis* and *Stetophyma* have terminal chiasmata. Electron microscopy of the terminal chromosome segments
of *R. spathacea* var. *discolor* shows tight coils of the synaptonemal
complex (Fig. 3) (Moens, 1972). Assuming that the chromosomes were
not relationally coiled prior to pairing, the coils could have been
generated in one of two ways: either the attachment sites of each
complex at the nuclear envelope underwent rotation, or the lateral
elements broke and rejoined at several closely spaced sites. Bent
lateral elements at the site of a potential coil (Fig. 4) suggest
that the latter possibility is a real one. *Rhoeo spathacea* var.

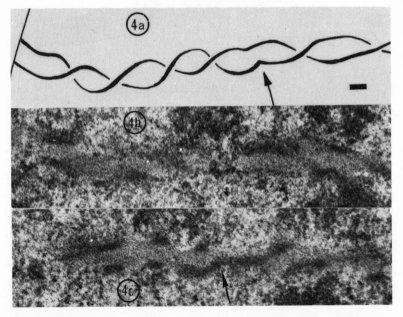

Figure 4. A series of tight coils in a *Chloealtis conspersa* bivalent. The arrows mark the position of a potential coil. Such configurations suggest that coils may result from breakage and rejoining rather than rotation of the attachment point at the nuclear
envelope. The bar on 4a is 100 nm.

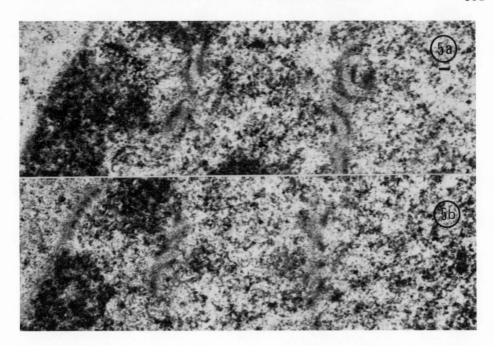

Figure 5. An example of several tight coils in the *C. conspersa*
bivalent. No coils were found in the earlier stages of meiotic
prophase, nor were they found in the grasshopper *Chorthippus longicornis*, which has no localized chiasmata.

concolor is closely related to *discolor* but has no translocations
and forms six bivalents at meiosis. Of the fertile offspring from
crosses between the two varieties, half form rings and half form
bivalents (Wimber, 1968). In *concolor* the chiasmata are presumably
not localized in the terminal segments, and it would be interesting
to find out if this correlates with a lack of coils in the terminal
segments. The plants, however, are difficult to obtain (Dr. D. E.
Wimber, personal communications).

    The grasshopper *Chloealtis conspersa* has three large meta-
centric chromosome pairs with terminal chiasmata that nearly always
form closed circles at meiotic prophase. Electron microscopy of
spermatocyte nuclei at pachytene shows that tight coils can be
found in the terminal portions of some of the bivalents (Figs. 4
and 5). Such coils have not been found in nuclei at the earlier
zygotene stage. The grasshopper *Chorthippus longicornis* has a
similar karyotype but does not have terminal chiasmata. No coils
have been found in the terminal segments of the bivalents.

Coincident, but possibly unrelated modifications occur in a number of other organisms. Jones (1973) reports that in the grasshopper *Stethophyma grossum*, which has chiasmata in the proximal end of the bivalent but not in the distal end, one end of the synaptonemal complex is strikingly asymmetrical and rigid due to the pronounced enlargement of one of the two lateral elements. In the ascomycetous fungus *Podospora anserina*, which has no detectable synaptonemal complexes (Zickler, 1973), there is nearly total interference (one crossover per chromosome arm) (Rizet and Englemann, 1949), while *Ascobolus immersus* has pronounced synaptonemal complexes (Zickler, 1973) but genetic interference that is weak if present at all (Stadler *et al.*, 1970).

Clearly, no single structural modification of the synaptonemal complex can account for the observed variation in the distribution of exchange events along the paired chromosomes. Yet the many observed structural modifications suggest modifications of the functions of the complex, perhaps those of chromosome synapsis and recombination.

ACKNOWLEDGMENTS

Financial support is from the National Research Council of Canada. I thank Dr. K. Rothfels of the Department of Botany, University of Toronto, for some of the live material and some of the illustrations and for discussion of the observations.

REFERENCES

Counce, S. J. and G. F. Meyer. 1973. Differentiation of the synaptonemal complex and the kinetochore in *Locusta* spermatocytes studied by whole mount electron microscopy. Chromosoma 44: 231.

Jones, G. H. 1973. Light and electron microscope studies of chromosome pairing in relation to chiasma localization in *Stethophyma grossum* (Orthoptera: Acrididae). Chromosoma 42: 145.

Meyer, G. F. 1964. A possible correlation between the submicroscopic structure of meiotic chromosomes and crossing over. In (M. Titlbach, ed.) Electron Microscopy 1964, Vol. B. pp. 461.

Moens, P. B. 1969. The fine structure of meiotic chromosome pairing in the triploid *Lilium tigrinum*. J. Cell Biol. 40: 273.

Moens, P. B. 1972. Fine structure of chromosome coiling at meiotic prophase in *Rhoeo discolor*. Can. J. Genet. Cytol. 14: 801.

Moens, P. B. 1973. Mechanisms of chromosome synapsis at meiotic prophase. Int. Rev. Cytol. 35: 117.

Moses, M. J. 1968. Synaptinemal complex. Ann. Rev. Genet. 2: 363.

Rizet, G. and C. Englemann. 1949. Contribution à l'étude génétique d'un Ascomycète tetrasporé: *Podospora anserina*. Rev. Cytol. Biol. Vég. 2: 202.

Stadler, D. R., A. M. Towe and J. L. Rossignol. 1970. Intragenetic recombination of ascospore color mutants in *Ascobolus* and its relationship to the segregation of outside markers. Genetics 66: 429.

Stern, H. and Y. Hotta. 1973. Biochemical controls of meiosis. Ann. Rev. Genet. 7: 37.

Westergaard, M. and D. von Wettstein. 1972. The synaptinemal complex. Ann. Rev. Genet. 6: 71.

Wimber, D. E. 1968. The nuclear cytology of bivalents and ring-forming *Rhoeos* and their hybrids. Amer. J. Bot. 55: 572.

Zickler, D. 1973. Fine structure of chromosome pairing in ten Ascomycetes: meiotic and premeiotic synaptonemal complexes. Chromosoma 40: 401.

SYNAPTONEMAL COMPLEX KARYOTYPING IN SPREADS OF MAMMALIAN SPERMATOCYTES

Montrose J. Moses and Sheila J. Counce

Departments of Anatomy and Zoology, Duke University

Medical Center, Durham, North Carolina 27710

The synaptonemal complex is a concomitant of meiotic chromosome synapsis and crossing-over in eukaryotes (Moses, 1969), and as such could serve as the basis for bivalent karyotype analysis at a higher level of resolution than hitherto possible. For example, Gillies (1972), on *Neurospora*, Moens (1974), on *Locusta* spermatocytes, and Carpenter (this volume), on *Drosophila* oocytes, are already realizing this potential from three-dimensional reconstructions of electron micrographs and serial sections. Moens and Perkins (1969) have used the method to establish the chromosome number of a protist. We have recently begun to apply karyotype analysis of these complexes to mammalian meiosis, using a new and somewhat less tedious technique.

The basis of our method is a recent study by Counce and Meyer (1973). They demonstrated that spermatocytes of *Locusta* spread on a weak saline hypophase, picked up on electron microscope grids, fixed with formalin, rinsed with detergent, and stained with phosphotungstic acid in ethanol show the complexes selectively contrasted so that they stand out clearly from the surrounding chromatin that would otherwise obscure them. In such preparations Counce and Meyer observed that kinetochores also were contrasted, and further, that they constituted differentiations of the lateral elements of the synaptonemal complex.

In the present study our first objective was to show that these relationships also hold for mammalian cells. Complexes from human, hamster, and lemur spermatocytes have the same features observed in the Locust. Figure 1 is an electron micrograph of complexes from a hamster spermatocyte, showing attachment points to the nuclear envelope, along with (a) terminal, (b) submedial, and (c) medial kinetochores. As has been established in serial section studies,

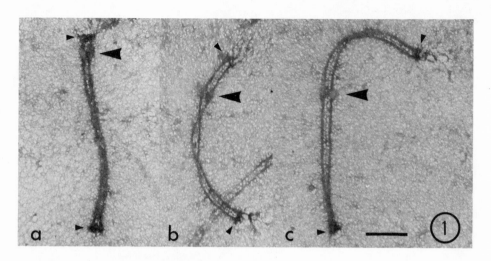

Figure 1.   Three autosomal synaptonemal complexes from a spread
hamster pachytene spermatocyte stained by Counce and Meyer's method.
Each complex is seen for its entire length, which also represents
the length of the bivalent of which it is a part.   The filamentous
complex consists of two parallel lateral elements, each flanking and
equidistant from a finer central element, connected by transverse
filaments.   The dense terminal plaques (small arrowheads) are the
attachment points to the nuclear envelope, which evidently serve to
keep the complexes in place during flattening and spreading of the
nucleus.   The kinetochores (large arrowheads), one per chromosome,
are seen as pronounced thickenings of the lateral elements.   The
characteristic positions of the kinetochores identify the chromosomes
as (a) telocentric, (b) submetacentric, and (c) nearly metacentric.
Marker represents 1 μm.

Figure 2.   Entire pachytene nucleus from a whole-mount spread of
hamster spermatocytes.   Each bivalent can be characterized by the
length of its synaptonemal complex, and the position of the kinetochore.   Postive identification must be made at a higher magnification
than shown here.   Marker represents 5 μm.

Figure 3.   Tracing of complexes from the same nucleus as in Fig. 2
(but made at a higher magnificantion and reduced to the same magnification as above).   The complexes have been lettered arbitrarily
for identification.   There are 21 autosomal complexes (bivalents)
and an XY pair; the short Y and the long X are indicated.   The X and
Y are synapsed for part of their length, the lateral elements of the
complex in this region becoming single axial cores where the sex
chromosomes are unpaired.

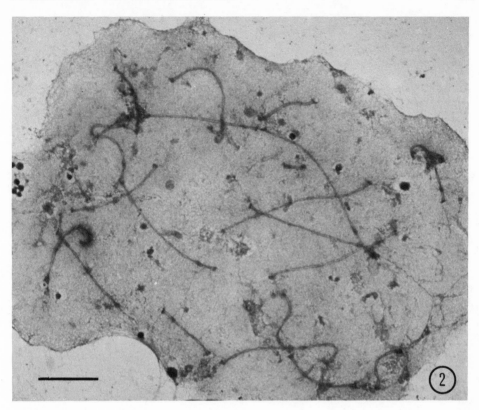

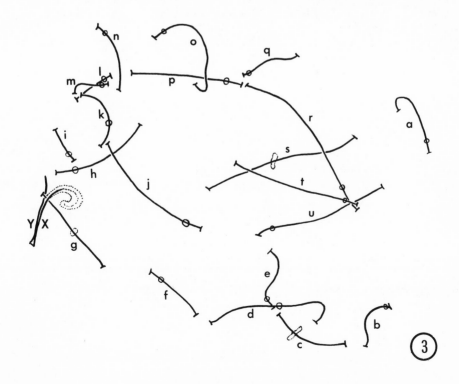

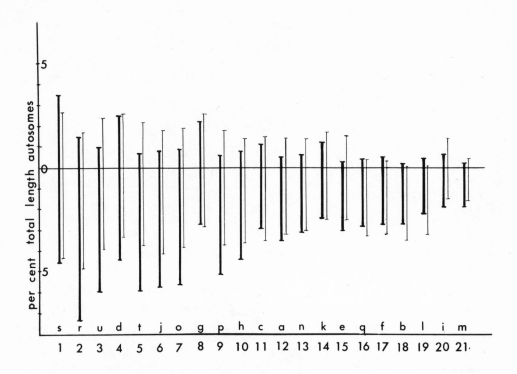

Figure 4. An ideogram of the pachytene synaptonemal complex (bivalent) autosomes in Figs. 2 and 3, constructed by ranking the complexes by length and aligning the kinetochores. For comparison,
lengths and centromere positions were measured from published karyotypes of somatic cells. The data for each chromosome are presented
as percent of the summed lengths of the autosomes; for comparison
they are shown as light lines adjacent to the comparable complexes
(heavy lines). The distribution of complexes resembles that of the
somatic karyotype. Letters refer to complexes in Figs. 2 and 3.

the lateral and central elements are continuous along the length of
the bivalent. Kinetochores have not yet been described in sectioned
mammalian pachytene chromosomes; in fact, in one report it was stated
that centromeres could not be observed in sections of hamster spermatocytes (Woollam *et al*., 1966). Thus the spreading method may have
distinct advantages where location of the kinetochore is important.

Also, in our preparations we often observe pachytene nuclei
which are visible in their entirety, slightly spread and flattened.
In many cases, all of the synaptonemal complexes of the complement
of bivalent chromosomes are present and clearly distinguishable.

An entire hamster spermatocyte nucleus at pachytene is shown in Fig. 2. All the complexes of the complement of bivalent chromosomes are present and clearly distinguishable, including the XY pair. Each bivalent can be identified by its length and the position of its kinetochore. A tracing of this micrograph (Fig. 3) shows the complement of complexes more clearly. The diploid chromosome number for the golden hamster (*Mesocricetus auratus*) is 44: 21 autosomal pairs, and X, and a Y. There are exactly 21 synaptonemal complexes and an XY pair, the latter synapsed at one end.

An ideogram can be made of such a complement by first arranging the complexes according to length and then identifying the metacentric and submetacentric complexes (Fig. 4). When these are matched with a mitotic chromosomal ideogram, the agreement is good. In the golden hamster (Fredga and Santesson, 1964), chromosomes 4, 8, 14, and 20 are metacentric, or nearly so. The longest autosome is submetacentric. Chromosomes 16-19 are telocentric. The corresponding complexes have comparable characteristics. In some nuclei, depending upon stage, the nucleoli are attached to the complexes and serve as further identification criteria.

The methods of serial section reconstruction and of spreading actually complement each other. Each has its own advantages and disadvantages and can give information that the other cannot. Three of the chief advantages of the new spreading procedure are its relative simplicity and rapidity and the ease of identifying kinetochores. For these reasons, the method promises broad applicability to a range of hitherto unapproachable questions of chromosome structure and behavior in meiosis, such as the manner and extent of XY pairing, chiasma formation, and the identification and fate of chromosomal rearrangements. Studies are presently underway in our laboratory on these problems in several mammals, including man and mouse.

ACKNOWLEDGEMENTS

The authors gratefully acknowledge the assistance of Ms. Katherine Moses in this study. Research supported in part by grants from the National Science Foundation (#GB-40562) and United States Public Health Service (NIH: # CA-1-4236).

REFERENCES

Counce, S. J. and G. F. Meyer. 1973. Differentiation of the synaptonemal complex and the kinetochore in *Locusta* spermatocytes studied with whole mount electron microscopy. Chromosoma <u>44</u>: 231.

390

M. J. MOSES AND S. J. COUNCE

Fredga, K. and B. Santesson. 1964. Male meiosis in the Syrian, Chinese, and European hamsters. Hereditas 52: 36.

Gillies, C. B. 1972. Reconstruction of the *Neurospora crassa* pachytene karyotype from serial sections of synaptonemal complexes. Chromosoma 36: 119.

Moens, P. B. 1974. Quantitative electron microscopy of chromosome organization at meiotic prophase. Cold Spring Harbor Symp. Quant. Biol. in press.

Moens, P. B. and F. O. Perkins. 1969. Chromosome number of a small protist: accurate determination. Science 166: 1289.

Moses, M. J. 1969. Structure and function of the synaptonemal complex. Genetics 61 (Suppl.): 41.

Woollam, D. H. M., E. H. R. Ford and J. W. Millen. 1966. The attachment of pachytene chromosomes to the nuclear membrane in mammalian spermatocytes. Exp. Cell Res. 42: 657.

AN EXTRACHROMOSOMAL SUPPRESSOR OF MALE CROSSING-OVER IN

DROSOPHILA ANANASSAE

Claude W. Hinton

Department of Biology, The College of Wooster,

Wooster, Ohio 44691

In *Drosophila ananassae*, crossing-over in males produces populations of strands having properties comparable to those recovered from females: complementary classes are recovered equally, recombination frequencies are additive, and chromosome interference is positive or absent. On the other hand, the frequency of exchanges in males is generally much lower than in females, and the distribution of exchanges also differs between the sexes (Table 1). The occurrence of crossing-over in males is dependent upon a dominant allele located 8 map units to the right of *ru*, a recessive allele mapped 5 units to the left of *ru*, and another recessive located in the left arm of chromosome 2. Miscellaneous observations indicate the existence of still undefined loci that regulate the frequency and regional distribution of exchanges in males (Hinton, 1970 and unpublished).

In screening for genes that control crossing-over in males, reciprocal crosses between tester and tested stocks are routinely compared to detect sex linkage. There are usually no differences between F_1 males from reciprocal crosses, but a recently encountered exception provides the basis for the analysis described in this report. The *bri pe stw ru* tester stock, previously diagnosed to be homozygous for the three alleles prerequisite to male crossing-over, was reciprocally crossed to an undefined stock bearing the *pc* marker (the mutants used as markers in these crosses are described by Hinton, 1974). On test crossing to *bri pe stw pc ru* females, the F_1 males from cross A (Table 2) consistently produced recombinant progeny. In contrast, the recovery of very few, if any, recombinant progeny from individual F_1B males suggested the possibility of an X-linked suppressor of crossing-over in the *pc* stock. The consistent difference between F_1A and F_1B males could

391

Table 1. Recombination frequency and distribution in the third
chromosome of *Drosophila ananassae*

Test-crossed sex	Progeny scored	Recombination frequency					
		bri	*pe*	*stw*	*pc*	*ru*	Sum
Females	2030	0.076	0.389	0.231	0.216		0.912
Males	3514	0.001	0.022	0.007	0.013		0.042

not be explained simply by a Y-linked suppressor from the tester
stock, because F_1 males from crosses of tester males to numerous
other stocks do produce recombinants.

According to the X-linked suppressor hypothesis, both F_1A and
F_1B females should be heterozygous and should transmit the suppressor to half of their sons. To test this expectation, F_1 females
were backcrossed to *bri pe stw ru* tester males, and their wild-type
(*pc/bri pe stw ru*) X_1 sons were selected and test-crossed. The results, shown in Table 2, are incompatible with segregation of an
X-linked suppressor; the 30 X_1A males displayed continuously distributed recombination frequencies with a mean and range comparable
to F_1A males, whereas 60 X_1B males repeated the performance of F_1B
males. Since both X_1A and X_1B males shared Y chromosomes from the
tester stock, the possibility of a Y-linked suppressor is again
excluded. Moriwaki *et al.* (1970) attributed an observed second-
chromosome recombination frequency difference between F_1 males from
reciprocal crosses to the Y chromosome, but their analysis proceeded
no further.

Having eliminated either an autosomal or sex-linked allele as
the basis for the observed suppression of male crossing-over, the
difference between reciprocal crosses can be assigned to an extrachromosomal suppressor present in the *pc* stock and transmitted only
by females. Thus, crossing-over occurred in both F_1A males and X_1A
sons of F_1 females whose cytoplasm originated from the tester stock,
but where the cytoplasm was derived from the *pc* stock, as in F_1B
males and X_1B sons of F_1 females, crossing-over was negligible. A
test of this interpretation is provided by backcrossing F_1 males to
females from the tester stock; it is expected that the wild-type
(*bri pe stw ru/pc*) X_1A and X_1B sons, sharing suppressor-free cytoplasm, will both produce recombinant progeny. This expectation is
clearly confirmed by the test-cross data (Table 2) showing that X_1B
sons of F_1 males produce at least as much recombination as their
X_1A controls. The existence of a maternally transmitted extrachromosomal suppressor is further indicated by the following observations.

Table 2. Recombination frequencies in *Drosophila ananassae* males derived from reciprocal crosses and recurrent backcrosses

Source of test-crossed males	Reciprocal cross A (bri pe stw ru ♀♀ X pc ♂♂)				Reciprocal cross B (pc ♀♀ X bri pe stw ru ♂♂)			
	Number of		Recombination frequency (bri-ru)		Number of		Recombination frequency (bri-ru)	
	Males tested	Progeny scored	Mean	Range	Males tested	Progeny scored	Mean	Range
F_1	9	1153	0.075	0.04-0.11	9	1157	0.003	0-0.01
	12	3970	0.042	0.02-0.07	12	4411	0.0005	0-0.003
	30	4914	0.067	0.01-0.11	10	1762	0.003	0-0.02
	20	5485	0.054	0.02-0.12	7	2144	0.003	0-0.01
X_1 sons of F_1 females	30	9425	0.057	0.02-0.09	40	10641	0.002	0-0.01
					20	7137	0.0001	0-0.002
X_1 sons of F_1 males	24	5903	0.045	0.02-0.12	16	4136	0.044	0.02-0.08
					10	1477	0.072	0.02-0.14
X_2 sons of X_1 females	9	3514	0.042	0.02-0.09	10	3851	0.002	0-0.01
X_6 sons of X_5 females	9	3178	0.092	0.04-0.16	9	3594	0.002	0-0.01

Wild-type (*pc/bri pe stw ru*) daughters of F_1A and F_1B females were
selected and recurrently backcrossed to males from the tester stock,
and this procedure was repeated in successive generations. Wild-
type X_2 and X_6 males, when test-crossed, maintained the recombination frequency difference observed between F_1A and F_1B males. It
appears that the suppressor can be transmitted through females with
undiminished effectiveness for at least six generations.

For the purpose of establishing a tester stock bearing the
suppressor, crosses were made between X_3 *bri pe stw ru* males and
females to produce replicate stocks, two from X_2B females presumed
to carry the suppressor and two controls from X_1A females. Then,
to confirm the presence of the suppressor in the derived B lines,
F_1 *bri pe stw ru/pc* males, obtained by crossing females from the
derived stocks to *pc* males, were test-crossed (lower 2 entries in
Table 3). The control male recombination frequencies of 0.060 and
0.080 are inflated due to the unexpected occurrence of 0.021 and
0.027, respectively, recombinants in the *stw-pc* interval as compared
to about 0.007 typically observed for this region in these crosses
(Table 1). Be that as it may, the recombination frequency mean
(0.042) and range (0.02-0.08) for F_1 males from one derived B line
are indistinguishable from those for F_1A males (Table 2), and those
for F_1 males from the other B line, while reduced, are clearly not
as low as those for F_1B males. This unanticipated failure to establish the suppressor in homozygous *bri pe stw ru* stocks could be
rationalized with the assumption that the *pc* stock third chromosome,
which was selected in each backcross generation, is necessary for
the persistence of the suppressor. That assumption has been examined
by crossing X_5A and X_5B *bri pe stw ru* females directly to males from
the *pc* stock and by test-crossing their F_1 sons. Their distinctly
intermediate mean recombination frequency of 0.018 suggests that the
persistence of the suppressor is a function of the number of generations intervening between homozygosis and testing.

It is of interest to know what effect the suppressor of male
crossing-over has on crossing-over in females. An initial observation of suspiciously high third-chromosome recombination frequencies
in F_1B females (Table 4) indicated that crossing-over might be increased in the presence of the suppressor, but no control F_1A females
were tested. Comparison of X_2A with X_2B females reveals slightly
higher recombination frequencies in the presence of the suppressor
of male crossing-over, and this result is paralleled by X-chromosome
recombination frequencies in F_1A and F_1B females. Obviously, female
recombination frequencies are not decreased by the suppressor of
male crossing-over. In this regard, the suppressor appears to be
analogous to the three genes that control crossing-over in males:
although critical experiments to detect small effects have not been
made, a variety of incidental observations have shown that crossing-
over in females is not grossly altered by allelic substitutions at
any of the three loci.

Table 3. Diminution of the extrachromosomal suppressor of male crossing-over in the absence of the third chromosome from the *pc* stock

Generations after *bri pe stw ru* homozygosis	Source of *bri pe stw ru* females crossed to *pc* males							
	Control lines (A)				Suppressed lines (B)			
	Number of		Recombination frequency (*bri-ru*)		Number of		Recombination frequency (*bri-ru*)	
	Males tested	Progeny scored	Mean	Range	Males tested	Progeny scored	Mean	Range
1	10	4268	0.052	0.02–0.09	29	10910	0.018	0.005–0.04
2	9	2888	0.060	0.02–0.12	9	2835	0.026	0.01–0.04
	9	2821	0.080	0.03–0.12	9	3076	0.042	0.02–0.08

Table 4. Comparison of recombination frequencies in females with
(B) or without (A) the extrachromosomal suppressor of male
crossing-over

Test-crossed females		Progeny	Recombination frequencies					
Source	Number	scored	*bri*	*pe*	*stw*	*pc*	*ru*	Sum
F_1B	7	1054	0.103	0.385	0.292	0.333		1.113
X_2A	7	2030	0.076	0.389	0.231	0.216		0.912
X_2B	10	3116	0.087	0.388	0.264	0.221		0.961
			cop	f^{49}	Bx^2	w^g		Sum
F_1A	10	1388	0.128	0.153	0.063			0.343
F_1B	10	1348	0.151	0.160	0.092			0.403

The demonstration of an extrachromosomal suppressor of male
crossing-over through formal genetic analysis yields no information
with respect to either the specific biological identity of the suppressor or the mechanism of its action. There are precedents for
maternally transmitted extrachromosomal factors in other *Drosophila*
species, and the phenotype in the present case is no more exotic
than CO_2 sensitivity conferred by the sigma virus (L'Heritier, 1970),
lethality of male embryos induced by the sex ratio spirochaete
(Oishi and Poulson, 1970), or sterility of hybrid males associated
with Mycoplasma (Kernaghan and Ehrman, 1970). But to the extent
that recombinational and mutational phenomena may share mechanisms
(*e.g.* see Green, 1970), the most intriguing precedents are the
extrachromosomal mutator elements invoked by Levitan (1963) and by
Minamori and Sugimoto (1973). Whatever its biological nature, it
is expected that the extrachromosomal suppressor will provide an
interesting and useful probe into the mechanism of crossing-over.

SUMMARY

        Reciprocal crosses between two stocks of *Drosophila ananassae*
produce F_1 males having typical recombination frequencies of either
0.05 or 0.003, measured in the third chromosome. Genetic analysis
of this difference reveals an extrachromosomal suppressor that is
maternally transmitted and dependent upon a specific third chromosome for its maintenance. Recombination frequencies in females are
not reduced in the presence of the suppressor of male crossing-over.

ACKNOWLEDGEMENTS

I am grateful for the support of this work by National Insti-
tutes of Health Grant GM16536 and for the technical assistance of
Nancy Gfeller. On the occasion of his appointment to Professor
Emeritus, I wish to acknowledge my indebtedness to Maurice
Whittinghill who introduced me to *Drosophila* and the mysteries of
crossing-over.

REFERENCES

Green, M. M.   1970.   The genetics of a mutator gene in *Drosophila
melanogaster*.   Mutation Res. <u>10</u>: 353.

Hinton, C. W.   1970.   The identification of two loci controlling
crossing over in males of *Drosophila ananassae*.   Genetics <u>66</u>: 663.

Hinton, C. W.   1974.   The cytogenetics of *Drosophila ananassae*.
In (M. Ashburner and E. Novitski, eds.) Biology and Genetics of
Drosophila.   Vol. 1.   In press.

Kernaghan, R. P. and L. Ehrman.   1970.   An electron microscopic
study of the etiology of hybrid sterility in *Drosophila paulistorum*
I. Mycoplasma-like inclusions in the testis of sterile males.
Chromosoma <u>29</u>: 291.

Levitan, M.   1963.   A maternal factor which breaks paternal chromosomes.   Nature <u>200</u>: 437.

L'Heritier, P.   1970.   Drosophila viruses and their role as evolutionary factors.   In (T. Dobzhansky, ed.) Evolutionary Biology.
Vol. 4.   pp. 185-209.   Appleton, New York.

Minamori, S. and K. Sugimoto.   1973.   Extrachromosomal element delta
in *Drosophila melanogaster*.   IX. Induction of delta-retaining
chromosome lines, by mutation and gene mapping.   Genetics <u>74</u>: 477.

Moriwaki, D., Y. N. Tobari and Y. Oguma.   1970.   Spontaneous crossing over in the male of *Drosophila ananassae*.   Jap. J. Genet. <u>45</u>:
411.

Oishi, K. and D. F. Poulson.   1970.   A virus associated with SR-
spirochaetes of *Drosophila nebulosa*.   Proc. Nat. Acad. Sci. U.S.A.
<u>67</u>: 1565.

X-RAY AND ULTRAVIOLET LIGHT SENSITIVITIES OF A METHYL

METHANESULFONATE-SENSITIVE STRAIN OF *DROSOPHILA MELANOGASTER**

P. Dennis Smith and Carol G. Shear

Department of Biology, Emory University, Atlanta,

Georgia 30322

Genetic recombination is a multifaceted biological phenomenon with a variety of expressions on a wide range of biological systems. These expressions have in common the interaction of genetic elements to produce reorganized molecules, and this reordering process serves as a fundamental mechanism for introducing biological diversity to these systems. Radding (1973) has classified the types of recombinational interactions observed into three general categories: general recombination, site-specific recombination, and nonhomologous recombination. Two approaches have been employed for the analysis of these genetic exchange interactions. The more classic methodology utilizes systems which focus on the analysis of recombinational events by an examination of the exchange products of genetic interactions. More recently systematic investigations of recombinational interactions have aimed at illuminating the underlying genetic and biochemical control mechanisms (*e.g.* see Clark, 1973). This latter approach drew attention to the demonstrable relationship between recombination deficiency and mutagen sensitivity and suggested that mutagen sensitivity could be an effective indicator not only of deficiencies of DNA repair ability but also of abnormalities of recombination proficiency.

ISOLATION OF A DROSOPHILA MUTAGEN-SENSITIVE STRAIN

Our laboratory is currently engaged in studies aimed at analyzing the genetic control of recombination and DNA repair in

---

*No. II in a series. Paper no. I is in Mutation Research <u>20</u>: 215.

the complex eukaryote, *Drosophila melanogaster*, utilizing specific
screening procedures for the isolation of mutagen-sensitive strains.
The present report describes recent studies of an X-linked strain,
designated mut[S], originally isolated on the basis of sensitivity
to the monofunctional alkylating agent methyl methanesulfonate
(Smith, 1973). The mutant strain exhibits no morphological abnormalities, resembling the Oregon-R wild-type strain from which it
was derived. Early in our studies, it was observed that homozygous
mut[S] females were highly infertile; Table 1 indicates the degree
of this infertility. Although homozygous mut[S] females were allowed
to oviposit for a period of 5 days and laid very large numbers of
eggs, these females produced, on the average, just over two viable
progeny per female. Cytological examination of the internal anatomy
of a number of mut[S] females indicated no apparent structural abnormalities of the reproductive organs. Similar fertility studies
of both young and old males (Table 2) indicated no significant
reduction in fertility. The very low numbers of viable progeny
coupled with the lack of apparent abnormalities in the female
reproductive system and the female-specific nature of the infertility suggests that the mutagen-sensitivity locus may also be
involved with normal meiotic events, possibly disjunction.

CROSS-SENSITIVITY TO RADIATIONS AND ALKYLATING AGENTS

Sensitivities to mutagens in both prokaryotic and eukaryotic
organisms have been associated with defects in specific DNA repair
mechanisms, either photoreactivation, excision repair, or recombinational repair (Beers *et al.*, 1972). Two of these systems, photoreactivation and excision repair, have been demonstrated to function
in Drosophila (J. B. Boyd and J. M. Presley, personal communication;
Trosko and Wilder, 1973). We have examined the cross-sensitivity
of our methyl methanesulfonate-sensitive strain to other mutagenic
agents (Fig. 1). Oregon-R wild-type males and mut[S] males were mated
to attached-X females to establish two stocks, and the percent
survival of males was determined with respect to the survival of
attached-X female siblings. These data indicate that the mut[S]
strain is very sensitive to the alkylating agents and to X-irradiation and apparently moderately sensitive to ultraviolet light.
Direct photoreactivation of Drosophila embryonic cells has recently
been demonstrated (Levin and Jordan, 1973), and we have used a
similar system to assay third-instar larvae for *in vivo* photoreactivation ability. After exposure to ultraviolet light (1000 ergs/
mm^2; 254 µm), replicate larval cultures were either maintained in
total darkness or exposed to photoreactivating light (1 hr, 2 GE
F1578 BLB bulbs, 10 inches from larvae) then maintained in the dark
until eclosion. Nonphotoreactivated mut[S] males exhibited 14.5%
survival, while photoreactivated mut[S] males showed 31% survival.
These *in vivo* measurements of photoreactivation ability argue against
a major defect in this pathway.

Table 1. Fertility of mut^S females

Genotype	Total	No. fertile	% fertile
+/+	110	106	96
+/mut^S	67	67	100
mut^S/mut^S	337	198 [a]	59

[a] Average number of progeny per female = 2.15.

Table 2. Fertility of mut^S males

Genotype	Age (days)	Total	No. fertile	% fertile
+	1	118	118	100
	15	94	89	95
mut^S	1	103	94	91
	15	99	99	100

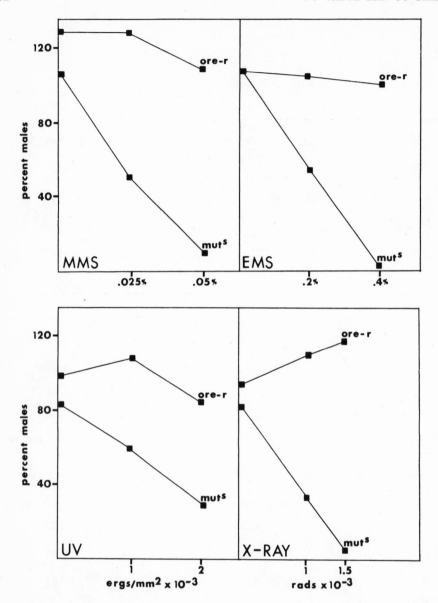

Figure 1. Comparative cross-sensitivities of Oregon-R wild-type
and mut[s] males to various mutagenic agents. Percent males were
measured as the number of surviving males to number of surviving
C(1)DX, yf females X 100. Alkylating agents were added as 1-ml
doses to 2-day-old developing cultures. Radiation was applied to
third-instar larvae. MMS = methyl methanesulfonate, EMS = ethyl
methanesulfonate.

SUMMARY

Our laboratory is concerned with studies of the genetic controls of recombination and DNA repair in the higher eukaryote, *Drosophila melanogaster*. These investigations have focused on mutagen sensitivity as a feasible approach to these problems, and the present report describes the cross-sensitivity of a mutagen-sensitive strain to the alkylating agents MMS and EMS and to X-irradiation and ultraviolet light. *In vivo* survival experiments suggest a defect in a DNA repair system, probably not photoreactivation. Studies of female infertility suggest that the mutagen-sensitive strain may also exhibit associated meiotic difficulties.

ACKNOWLEDGMENTS

These studies were supported by Public Health Service Research grant GM-18485 from the National Institutes of Health.

REFERENCES

Beers, R. F. Jr., R. M. Herriott and R. C. Tilghman (eds.). 1972. Molecular and Cellular Repair Processes. Johns Hopkins University Press, Baltimore.

Clark, A. J. 1973. Recombination deficient mutants of *E. coli* and other bacteria. Ann. Rev. Genet. 7: 67.

Levin, V. L. and M. S. Jordan. 1973. Photoreactivation of *Drosophila melanogaster* embryonic cells. Photochem. Photobiol. 17: 461

Radding, C. M. 1973. Molecular mechanisms in genetic recombination. Ann. Rev. Genet. 7: 87.

Smith, P. D. 1973. Mutagen sensitivity of *Drosophila melanogaster*. I. Isolation and preliminary characterization of a methyl methane-sulphonate-sensitive strain. Mutat. Res. 20: 215.

Trosko, J. E. and K. Wilder. 1973. Repair of UV-induced pyrimidine dimers in *Drosophila melanogaster* cells *in vitro*. Genetics 73: 297.

MODELS OF RECOMBINATION

Red-MEDIATED RECOMBINATION IN BACTERIOPHAGE LAMBDA

Franklin W. Stahl and Mary M. Stahl

Institute of Molecular Biology, University of Oregon,

Eugene, Oregon 97403

INTRODUCTION

Among unreplicated encapsidated lambda chromosomes "crossovers" are nonuniformly distributed along the chromosome (Jordan and Mesleson, 1965). They are concentrated at the ends, especially the right end (Fig. 1). Among replicated chromosomes, however, crossovers are uniformly distributed as judged from the congruity of the linkage map and the microscopically examined chromosome (Fig. 2). The explanation for this difference between replicated and unreplicated chromosomes is that recombination throughout lambda, except at the ends, is dependent on extensive DNA synthesis (Stahl *et al.*, 1972a). The dependence of recombination on synthesis and the resulting nonuniform crossover distribution along unreplicated chromosomes is conspicuous only in the presence of the Red system, the general recombination system of the phage (Stahl *et al.*, 1974).

We presented a model (Stahl *et al.*, 1973) to rationalize these facts. In addition, the model took account of the partial dependence of replication on the Red system (Enquist and Skalka, 1973), the fact that many heterozygotes at gene O extend to gene R near the end of the chromosome (Russo, 1973; White and Fox, 1974), and the conclusion (Stahl *et al.*, 1972b) that unreplicated phage chromosomes are absolutely dependent upon recombination in order to be matured.

Our model combined ideas of Cassuto *et al.* (1971), of Sigal and Alberts (1972) and Meselson (1972), and of Boon and Zinder (1969) in such a way that the Red system acted on a pair of lambda circles to yield a structure of rolling circle topology. One reacting circle comprised the tail and the other the circle of the

F. STAHL AND M. STAHL

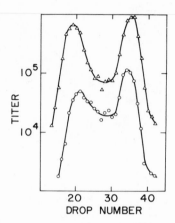

Figure 1. The density distributions of unreplicated phages from
a cross in which one parent was heavy and the other light. The
following cross was performed at 42°C in a host (FA22) in which λ
DNA replication is blocked by the high temperature:

$$susA11 \underline{\hspace{7cm}} + \begin{bmatrix} ^{13}C, & ^{15}N \end{bmatrix}$$

$$by$$

$$+ \underline{\hspace{7cm}} susR5 \begin{bmatrix} ^{12}C, & ^{14}N \end{bmatrix}.$$

Both parents were temperature sensitive for replication ($ts0$) as
well to insure the tightness of the replication block (a "double-
block" experiment). The total progeny phage ($\triangle$) banded in two
peaks, whose modes defined the densities of particles that inherited
unreplicated heavy (^{13}C, ^{15}N) and light (^{12}C, ^{14}N) chromosomes,
respectively. The bimodality of the density distribution of the
sus^+ recombinants ($\circ$) arising between these terminally located
genes indicates that most of the "crossing-over" was concentrated
at the ends of the chromosomes (Stahl $et\ al.$, 1974). The data in
this figure are from an unpublished study by J. M. Crasemann.

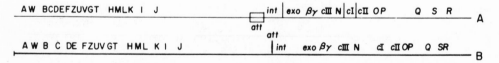

Figure 2. Comparison of λ maps. (A) Map based on recombination
frequencies from standard crosses with all recombination systems
present. (B) Map based on electron micrography of deletions and
substitutions (from Davidson and Szybalski, 1971).

rolling circle; the two parts were united by a potentially heteroduplex overlap. We supposed that the Red system catalyzed the
following sequence of events:

   (a) By an unspecified mechanism, a single strand was transferred from one duplex into a gap in the other (diagram 1),
yielding

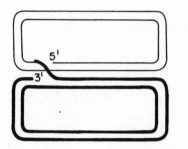

diagram 1

   (b) By coordinate action of polymerase and the 5'-specific
lambda exonuclease component of the Red system, the strand transfer
was extended (diagram 2) giving

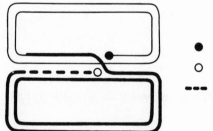

● λ EXONUCLEASE
○ POLYMERASE
--- NEW DNA

diagram 2

   (c) We supposed that the nuclease action and hence the strand
transfer would stop upon approach of the exonuclease to a nick on
the opposite strand. This supposition was promoted by the feeling
that the duplex would melt out as the exonuclease approached such
a nick, and that the relatively low activity of the enzyme for the
resulting single-strand DNA (Little, 1967) would effectively halt
its procession. The resulting structure (diagram 3) would look
like this:

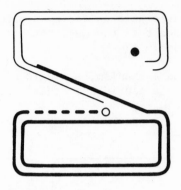

diagram 3

(d)   The completion of a maturable recombinant chromosome
would now require that the dimer in diagram 3 acquire the enzymatic
wherewithal to roll.   In particular, fork propagation must progress
until the tail contains a pair of duplex *cos*'s (sites of action of
the Ter system, which generates the sticky ends of the mature λ
chromosome); a chromosome embraced by a pair of duplex *cos*'s is
"finished" and maturable (see especially Feiss and Margulies,
1973).   Our notion was that crossovers near the middle of the
mature phage gene sequence would have to replicate further to reach
a *cos* than would those near the end.   This would result in a lesser
dependence of recombination on replication for crossovers whose
overlaps extended almost to the end of the chromosome.   Thus, the
model supposed that a bit of replication *was* available to "unreplicated" phage, even in "double block" conditions (McMilin and Russo,
1972) (see Figs. 1 and 3).   That rather awkward feature of the model
was paired off with the attraction of being able to account for all
Red-mediated exchange, replicating-dependent or "not", by a single
pathway.

C. M. Radding (personal communication) then pointed out to us
that our model predicts a particular structure for the hets found
at the terminal crossovers in replication-blocked crosses.   The
sequence of events depicted above leads exclusively to mature phage
(diagram 4) of the type

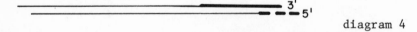

diagram 4

where the light and heavy-lined segments are from different parents
(and the dashed line is a bit of newly synthesized DNA).   Then
Radding reminded us that these structures are exactly those that
White and Fox (1974) did *not* find in the majority among the progeny
of *red⁺rec⁺* replication-blocked crosses.   They found instead primarily the reciprocal structure (diagram 5).

diagram 5

Thus, our model could not be correct for the primary mode of operation of Red in rec^+ replication-blocked crosses. However, it remained possible that Red operating in rec^- cells might produce structures of the type predicted by our model. The next section of this paper describes an experiment showing that even in $recA^-$ cells, the replication-blocked Red system produces mature chromosomes whose structures are exclusively those of the predominant type found by White and Fox (1974) for red^+rec^+ crosses.

EXPERIMENTAL

An experiment to distinguish between the two types of overlaps diagrammed in the previous section was designed for us by Ray White. It is a streamlined version of the analysis first conducted by White and Fox (1974).

Under replication-blocked $recA^-$ conditions ($dnaB^-$ $susP^-$) we conducted the following cross:

$$\underline{\hspace{6cm}}\; c26\; +\; P3\; +\; \text{[heavy label]}$$

by

$$\underline{\hspace{6cm}}\; +\; O29\; +\; P80\; \text{[light label]},$$

where the markers in the O and P genes are sus mutants and the c marker can be scored by inspection of the plaque. The progeny was centrifuged to equilibrium in cesium formate, the bottom of the tube was punctured, and the emerging fractions were collected and then assayed for total phage (c and c^+ on C600) and for sus^+ recombinants (on the su^- strain 594) (Fig. 3). The peak fractions 42 and 52 were then analyzed as follows: they were adsorbed to bacterial strain 594 at multiplicities (less than 10^{-3}) sufficiently low to make double infections negligible. The unadsorbed phage titer was reduced with anti-lambda antiserum, and the complexes were plated on the su^+ indicator C600 so as to give about 10 plaques per plate. The plates were incubated at 37°C, and as soon as the plaques were clearly visible 50 well isolated plaques were picked (primary pickates) each into 1 ml broth. The plates were again incubated and inspected the next day to permit rejection of any primary pickate that might have been picked close to a tardy neighbor. Each of the primary pickates was then spotted on 594 to permit rejection of any that were not sus^+ recombinants. The remaining primary pickates were diluted and plated on C600. The resulting plates were examined for c and c^+ plaques. Primary pickates that manifested less than 1% of a minority type out of more than 300 plaques examined were (arbitrarily) considered to be nonheterozygous at the c locus. Primary pickates giving 1% or greater of phage of

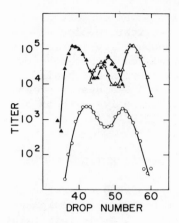

Figure 3.   The density distributions of unreplicated phages from a
recA⁻ cross in which one parent was heavy and the other light.
The following cross was performed at 39°C in a *recA⁻* host (FZ14)
in which λ DNA replication is blocked by the high temperature:

$$\frac{c \; + P3 \; + \; \left[^{13}C, \; ^{15}N\right]}{}$$

by

$$\frac{}{+ \; 029 \; + \; P80 \; \left[^{12}C, \; ^{14}N\right]}.$$

Since both parents were *susP⁻* and the host was *su⁻*, this cross was
"double-blocked" for replication.   The total *c* (▲) and *c⁺* (△)
phage each emerged in two peaks.   The modes of the outermost peaks
define the densities of particles that inherited unreplicated heavy
and light chromosomes, respectively.   The innermost peaks are the
products of Int-mediated crossing-over at *att* (see Stahl *et al.*,
1972b, 1974).   The *sus⁺* recombinant distribution (O) is bimodal
because these recombinants arise by two routes; terminal, Red-
mediated recombination generates heteroduplexes in which the majority material contribution comes from either the heavy (*c,P3*) or
the light (029,P80) parent.   Mismatch repair of these heteroduplexes
can result in *sus⁺* particles, able to grow on 594 (see White and
Fox, 1974; Stahl *et al.*, 1974).   The *sus⁺* recombinants in drops 42
and 52 were analyzed for heterozygosity (Table 1).

----

a minority type were defined as heterozygous at the *c* locus and
were further characterized as follows: Five clear (*c*) plaques and
five turbid (*c⁺*) plaques were picked (secondary pickates) from
replating of each of the primary pickates het at the *c* locus.   Each
of these 10 secondary pickates was then tested for the 029, the
P3, and the P80 markers.   Frequently, all five clears were of identical genotype, and all five turbids were identical.   In every case,

it was possible to assign a unique genotype to the chromosome which
had replicated to give the primary pickate. The results of these
analyses are summarized in Table 1.

The most useful feature of the data in Table 1 is that 029
hets are found only in the light peak (drop 52), while (less significantly) P3 hets are found only in the heavy peak (drop 42).
In order for any c-locus het to have passed through the su^- strain

Table 1. Summary of genotypes of plaques picked from light and
heavy recombinant peaks of Figure 3

	Drop #42	Drop #52
Number of plaques picked	50	50
Plaques rejected by detection of tardy neighbors	2	2
Plaques rejected as unable to spot on a su^- bacterium	7	3
Plaques plated out to detect c-locus heterozygosity	41	45
Pure c plaques	27	13
Pure c^+ plaques	0	4
c-locus hets	14	28
Genotypes of c-locus hets		
$\dfrac{c \; + \; + \; +}{+ \; + \; + \; +}$	11	3
$\dfrac{c \; + \; P3 \; +}{+ \; + \; + \; +}$	3	0
$\dfrac{c \; + \; + \; +}{+ \; 029 \; + \; +}$	0	25

594 to make a plaque on C600, it must have been wild type in both
gene O and P on the transcribed DNA chain. Since O and P are
transcribed rightward, this is the 5'-ended strand. Thus, in
those hets where any parental markers remain opposite the wild-type
strand, we can ask whether they are markers from the parent that
contributed the majority of the material. If so, then the recombinant must have looked like diagram 5. If not, then the recombinant must have looked like the one predicted by the model, diagram
4.

Hets from the light peak (52) contain material contributed
primarily from the $O29$ and $P80$ parent. Those that still have any
parental markers have $O29$. Hence, the 5'-ended strand of the recombinant must have been contributed by the other parent. The complementary argument holds for the hets that are predominantly heavy
(peak 42). Thus, one may conclude that Red by itself gives rise
to the same recombinant structure that is generated by Red and Rec
together (diagram 5).

In the following section we present a variant of our original
model that conforms to the finding presented. In addition we discuss an observation that (at least in retrospect) can be interpreted in support of the new model.

THE MODEL

We suppose that the following structures (diagram 6) arise:

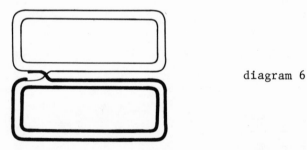

diagram 6

These structures ("figure 8's") differ from those in the old model
(diagram 1) by being at least grossly reciprocal. In addition we
suppose that chains of either polarity may be involved in the exchange. [It is interesting to note that the original exchange may
indeed have involved chains of a particular polarity. However,
ligation at the exchanged points followed by migration back across
the points results in a structure in which the "exchanged" segments
are now of "opposite polarity" to those originally exchanged. Thus,
our model is compatible with the "Aviemore Model" (Radding and
Meselson, personal communication), which supposes isomerization

(Sigal and Alberts, 1972) of structures like those in diagram 2.
This line of thought implicitly recognizes that some Red recombinants may arise via the route specified by our old model. However,
such recombinants are not the ones found among unreplicated progeny.] The junction in diagram 6 is free to migrate and, in our
model, will do so until a nick is encountered. We presume this
nick to be "accidental" in that it is not caused by an identified
recombination gene. We shall not systematically consider all
possible combinations of nicks, polarities, and migration distances
and directions with respect to the initial exchange position. The
one most easily diagrammed (diagram 7), which illustrates the
basic features of the interesting (recombinant-yielding) outcomes,
is the following:

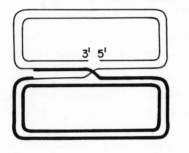

diagram 7

A nick at the exchange point has stopped the reciprocal branch
migration. (It is at this point that we suppose the Red and Rec
systems to respond contrastingly. *Escherichia coli*'s Rec system,
because it is endonucleolytic, can convert the structure in diagram
7 into a reciprocal break-reunion double-size circle. The Red
system, endowed only exonucleolytically, cannot.)

    For the sake of clarity we now diagram a sequence of events
with the understanding that "in reality" the events are apt to
overlap in time. First (diagram 8), the lambda exonuclease
digests the 5' end until it approaches a nick, opening the circle
and stopping the procession as in the old model.

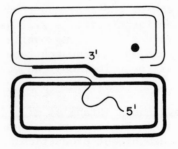

diagram 8

Strand migration and simple elongation by a polymerase at the
3'-ended chain (diagram 9) gives

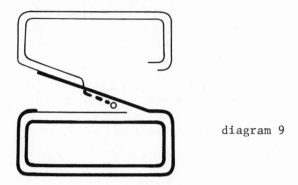

diagram 9

Now, moving a *cos* out onto the tail of the dimer will require
acquisition of a full replication complex, if the *cos* on the closed
circle is far from the fork. If, however, the events described to
this point have brought the fork close to a *cos*, simple chain
elongation may succeed in penetrating the circular duplex sufficiently to generate a complete recombinant molecule on the tail of
the dimer (diagram 10).

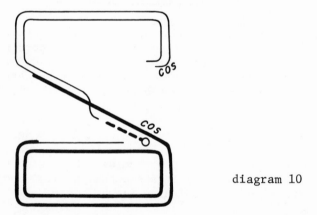

diagram 10

A recombinant (near the end of the map) can then be encapsidated.
The resulting mature recombinant particle will have the requisite
features -- little DNA synthesis and long overlaps of the proper
(White-Fox) polarity [within which mismatch repair (White and Fox,
1974; Wildenberg, personal communication) can occur].

    An additional bit of information can be interpreted in support
of our new model. We have shown (Stahl *et al.*, 1974) that mutation
in the *gam* gene of lambda results in a reduction of the terminal,
replication-independent recombinant production. Loss of *gam* function in a *recB⁻* host, however, is without effect (Stahl and Stahl,

1974) as may reasonably have been expected (see Sakaki *et al.*, 1973). Thus, the formation of terminal recombinants among unreplicated phage is *recBC* nuclease sensitive. This sensitivity suggests an intermediate involving single-chained DNA, a conspicuous feature of our present model. In diagram 8, cutting either the (thin-lined) strand hanging down or the (heavy-lined) strand it displaces would result in a loss of terminal recombinant production.

DISCUSSION

The dependence of most Red recombination on extensive DNA synthesis can be accounted for by the proposition that circular monomers interact in a Red-mediated event to produce structures of rolling circle topology. Two kinds of circles are distinguishable, depending on the chain polarities at the replicating fork. We may call the two kinds "Rolling Circles" and "Unrolling Circles", depending on whether the continuously synthesized chain is on the circle or the tail, respectively. Our old model (Stahl *et al.*, 1973) supposed that Red, at least when acting alone, produced exclusively Rolling Circles. Our experiments have now shown that a prediction of that model is wrong, and we have retrenched to a model in which unreplicated recombinants are matured exclusively from Unrolling Circles, while acknowledging that Red may in fact be capable of generating both kinds of structures.

Unfortunately, the most basic assumption of our model remains questionable. We have supposed that the replication enzymes operate on Red-produced structures, but we have not ruled out the obvious alternative that Red acts on replication-produced structures. One argument against the latter point of view has been presented (Stahl *et al.*, 1973), but more decisive experiments are needed (*e.g.* see Wilkins and Mistry, 1974).

ACKNOWLEDGMENTS

The experimental work reported herein was supported by Research Grant GB 8109 from the National Science Foundation and by Program Project Grant GM 15423 (Aaron Novick, Project Director) from the National Institutes of Health. Charles Radding and Ray White have continued to provide tough criticism and helpful guidance. Ken McMilin held our hands through the execution of the strand polarity experiment. We are indebted to Jean Crasemann for providing previously unpublished data for Figure 1. Bob Malone and Daryl Faulds helped us with the manuscript.

REFERENCES

Boon, T. and N. D. Zinder. 1969. A mechanism for genetic recombination generating one parent and one recombinant. Proc. Nat. Acad. Sci. U.S.A. 64: 573.

Cassuto, E., T. Lash, K. S. Sriprakash and C. M. Radding. 1971. Role of exonuclease and β protein of phage λ in genetic recombination, V. Recombination of λ DNA in vitro. Proc. Nat. Acad. Sci. U.S.A. 68: 1639.

Davidson, N. and W. Szybalski. 1971. Physical and chemical characteristics of lambda DNA. In (A. D. Hershey, ed.) The Bacteriophage Lambda. p. 45. Cold Spring Harbor Laboratory, Cold Spring Harbor, New York.

Enquist, L. W. and A. Skalka. 1973. Replication of bacteriophage λ DNA dependent on the function of host and viral genes. I. Interaction of *red*, *gam* and *rec*. J. Mol. Biol. 75: 185.

Feiss, M. and T. Margulies. 1973. On maturation of the bacteriophage lambda chromosome. Mol. Gen. Genet. 127: 285.

Hershey, A. D. (Editor). 1971. *The Bacteriophage Lambda*. Cold Spring Harbor Laboratory, Cold Spring Harbor, New York.

Jordan, E. and M. Meselson. 1965. A discrepancy between the physical and the genetic maps of bacteriophage lambda. Genetics 51: 77.

Little, J. W. 1967. An exonuclease induced by bacteriophage λ. II. Nature of the enzymatic reaction. J. Biol. Chem. 242: 679.

McMilin, K. D. and V. E. A. Russo. 1972. Maturation and recombination of bacteriophage lambda DNA molecules in the absence of DNA duplication. J. Mol. Biol. 68: 49.

Meselson, M. 1972. Formation of hybrid DNA by rotary diffusion during genetic recombination. J. Mol. Biol. 71: 795.

Russo, V. E. A. 1973. On the physical structure of lambda recombinant DNA. Mol. Gen. Genet. 122: 353.

Sakaki, Y., A. E. Karu, S. Linn and H. Echols. 1973. Purification and properties of the γ-protein specified by bacteriophage λ: an inhibitor of the host recBC recombination enzyme. Proc. Nat. Acad. Sci. U.S.A. 70: 2215.

Sigal, N. and B. Alberts. 1972. Genetic recombination: the nature

of a crossed strand-exchange between two homologous DNA molecules.
J. Mol. Biol. 71: 789.

Stahl, F. W., S. Chung, J. Crasemann, D. Faulds, J. Haemer, S.
Lam, R. E. Malone, K. D. McMilin, Y. Nozu, J. Siegel, J. Strathern
and M. Stahl. 1973. Recombination, replication, and maturation
in phage lambda. In (C. F. Fox and W. S. Robinson, eds.) Virus
Research. p. 487. Academic Press, New York.

Stahl, F. W., K. D. McMilin, M. M. Stahl, J. M. Crasemann and S.
Lam. 1974. The distribution of crossovers along unreplicated
lambda bacteriophage chromosomes. Genetics submitted.

Stahl, F. W., K. D. McMilin, M. M. Stahl, R. E. Malone, Y. Nozu
and V. E. A. Russo. 1972b. A role for recombination in the production of "free-loader" lambda bacteriophage particles. J. Mol.
Biol. 68: 57.

Stahl, F. W., K. D. McMilin, M. M. Stahl and Y. Nozu. 1972a. An
enhancing role for DNA synthesis in formation of bacteriophage
lambda recombinants. Proc. Nat. Acad. Sci. U.S.A. 69: 3598.

Stahl, F. W. and M. M. Stahl. 1974. A role for *rec*BC nuclease
in the distribution of crossovers along unreplicated chromosomes
of phage λ. Molec. Gen. Genet. in press.

White, R. L. and M. S. Fox. 1974. On the molecular basis of
high negative interference. Proc. Nat. Acad. Sci. U.S.A. in press.

Wilkins, A. S. and J. Mistry. 1974. Phage lambda's generalized
recombination system -- study of the intracellular DNA pool during
lytic infection. Molec. Gen. Genet. in press.

A REPLICATOR'S VIEW OF RECOMBINATION (AND REPAIR)

Ann Skalka

Roche Institute of Molecular Biology, Nutley, New

Jersey 07110

During the course of studies on the growth of *gamma* λ mutants in *rec*[+] and *rec*[-] cells, L. W. Enquist and I (Enquist and Skalka, 1973) observed a growth defect in λ *red* mutants that was independent of the *rec* condition of the host. *Red* mutants synthesize their DNA at only 1/3 to 1/2 the wild-type rate, and concatemers formed at late times are on the average shorter than normal. *Red*[-] DNA also seems to be packaged with somewhat less than the wild-type efficiency, and phage bursts are only about 30 to 40% that of wild type (Table 1). The importance of *red* genes to λ growth is further emphasized by the occurrence of a number of bacterial mutants on which λ *red* mutants do not plate at all. This class, called *feb*[-], includes *pol*A[-] and *lig*[-] strains (Zissler *et al.*, 1971). The following section summarizes results from studies of DNA synthesis and phage production in *red*[-] and *gam*[-] infection of these *feb*[-] hosts.

As the data in Fig. 1 show, infection of a *pol*A[-] host by either the single or double (*red*[-]*gam*[-]) mutant phage produced about 40-55 phage equivalents of DNA, but only about five plaque-forming phage per cell. Results from sedimentation and electron microscopic analysis of this DNA are described in Table 2. The data (details of which will be reported elsewhere) indicated that greater than 60% of each of the three mutant phage DNAs was in the form of monomeric circles — most of these contained an interruption in one or the other of their strands. In the *red*[-]*gam*[+] infection, monomeric linears were also formed. Concatemers, presumed to issue from a rolling-circle replicating structure characteristic of late DNA synthesis, are not formed. Thus it appears that in the *pol*A[-] host, *red* as well as *gam* mutants are somehow locked in the "early" mode of replication (Carter *et al.*, 1969; Enquist and Skalka, 1973).

421

Table 1. Growth of mutants after infection of various host
bacterial strains[a]

	Hosts				
	rec^+ (W3110)	rec^- (204)	$recA^-B^-$ (KL254)	$polA^-$ (W3110)	lig^- (N2668)
Phage Genotype	Yield relative to wild type phage				
red^+ gam^+ (wild type)	$1.0(167)^b$	1.0(60)	1.0(90)	1.0(140)	1.0(60)
red^- gam^+	0.34	0.40	0.38	.04	.05
red^+ gam^-	0.37	0.36	1.07	.03	n.d.[c]
red^- gam^-	0.16	0.09	0.30	.02	n.d.[c]

[a] Growth was in supplemented liquid minimal medium. The multiplicity of infection was 1-2 phages per bacteria, and burst sizes
were determined by standard one-step growth techniques. Except for
lig^- infection, red mutations were either the missense bet 113 or
amber bet 270 and the gam mutations, the missense ($gam5$) or $amber$
gam 210. In the lig^- infection, λ $int6red3$ $i21$ clear was used.

[b] Numbers in parenthesis indicate actual burst size.

[c] Not done.

Similar results (Table 2) were obtained with a red mutant grown in
a lig^- host (N2668 of Gottesman et $al.$, 1973). Thus it appears
that it is not just polymerase I but the function of the polymerase
+ ligase repair pathway that may be essential for concatemer production by red^- phage.

     The results with gam^- phage in the $polA^-$ or lig^- host (Table
2) are mostly interpretable within the framework of a model based
on the known interaction between gam protein and the hosts' rec BC
nuclease (Enquist and Skalka, 1973). The model states that a
critical step in the production of rolling circles, or their concatemer products, is uniquely sensitive to this nuclease. Thus,
in the absence of inhibition by $gamma$ protein, concatemers are not
formed. The observation that gam mutants plate on $recB^-$ lig^- but
not on lig^- bacteria (Gottesman et $al.$, 1973) is consistent with
this interpretation. However, although this model predicts a defect in late replication for gam^- phage, Enquist and Skalka (1973)
concluded, in part from results shown from wild-type host, that
some concatemers can arise from the red or rec-mediated recombination. The absence of such molecules in the $polA^-$ host suggests

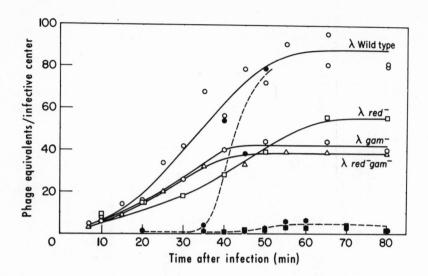

Figure 1. Phage equivalents of λ DNA were measured by hybridiza-
tion of ³H-labeled DNA with λ DNA on membrane filters. The host
was *thy⁻*, and ³H-labeled *thy* (4 μg/ml) was present from the time
of infection. Details of the techniques and calculations have
been published (Enquist and Skalka, 1973). Dashed line shows formation of free plaque-forming particles in each infection.

that DNA polymerase I might be required in either recombination
pathway (or both). Several schemes for a molecular mechanism of
general recombination do include a role for DNA polymerase I
(Radding, 1973). An alternative (or additional) possibility is
that some *red* and/or *rec* recombination intermediates do not survive
in *gam⁻* infected *polA⁻* cells.

The host cells in the *red⁻gam⁺* infection (Table 2) are pheno-
typically *rec⁻* because the *gam* protein can be expected to inhibit
the *rec*BC nuclease. Although general recombination is defective,
the model mentioned above predicts that in this infection the switch
to late replication should occur as in the wild-type infection.
Because in the *red⁻* infection we observe only monomeric circles and
linears, but no concatemers at late times, we must conclude that
some activity of either *pol* or *red* is required for the switch to
late replication. Since *red⁺gam⁺* phage grow better in *polA⁻* hosts
than *red⁻gam⁺* in *pol⁺* hosts (see Table 1), it appears that *red* is
better than *pol* at supplying this hypothetical activity.

Results with the double mutant (*red⁻gam⁻*) in the *polA⁻* host
(Table 2) are the same as with the *gam* single mutant alone. Thus
the *gam⁻* phenotype is epistatic over the *red⁻* phenotype.

Table 2. Phage DNA synthesized in $polA^-$ or lig^- hosts

Phage genotype	Wild-type host		$polA^-$ host		lig^- host	
	Rel. amt. (%)[a]	Structure	Rel. amt. (%)[a]	Structure[b]	Rel. amt. (%)[a]	Structure
$red^+ gam^+$	100	concatemers	100	concatemers	100	concatemers
$red^- gam^+$	60	concatemers (short)	50	circular and linear monomers	50	circular and linear monomers
$red^+ gam^-$	45	circular monomers (and some concatemers)	40	circular monomers	n.d.[c]	n.d.[c]
$red^- gam^-$	30	circular monomers (and some concatemers)	40	circular monomers	n.d.[c]	n.d.[c]

[a] Percentages relative to $red^+ gam^+$ calculated from maximal amounts (60–100 phage equivalents) accumulated in experiments similar to that described in Fig. 1.

[b] Details of structural analysis of density purified phage DNA have been published (Skalka, Poonian and Bartl, 1972).

[c] Not done.

THE MODEL

COMPLEMENTARY ACTIVITY OF THE *red* RECOMBINATION AND THE POLYMERASE-LIGASE REPAIR PATHWAYS IN THE PRODUCTION OF ROLLING-CIRCLE REPLICATION INTERMEDIATES

During its first few rounds, the λ chromosome is replicated as a circle from a fixed origin and often in both directions (Schnös and Inman, 1970). High-resolution electron microscopy has revealed structural details consistent with the notion that, at the replication fork, one parental strand of DNA is copied continuously and the other discontinuously. Discontinuous copying occurs on opposite parental strands of forks going in opposite directions (Inman and Schnös, 1971). Thus, in molecules with two replication forks new strands are built up continuously on one (the 3') end and discontinuously on the other (the 5') end. Said another way, a parental strand that is copied continuously at a fork going in one direction is copied discontinuously at the fork going in the opposite direction. The model shown in Fig. 2 is based on the assumption that one of two different sequences of events is initiated when a growing fork encounters a nick on one of the parental strands. The sequence of events and the type of product formed depend on whether the nick is on the strand being copied continuously or on the strand being copied discontinuously in the region of that fork. Since λ can have two growing forks going in either (or both) directions, the events can be described by placing a nick in a particular location — here, on the ℓ strand somewhere between genes A and R.

Let us first consider the results when the nick is approached by the leftward fork — *i.e.*, when the nick is on the strand being copied continuously. When the replication apparatus reaches this nick, the arm that contains the nicked parental strand will be broken. The leftward fork will stop because the replication apparatus falls off the broken end. On the other (discontinuously copied) parental strand of this fork, a gap will remain as large, perhaps, as the average length of an Okazaki fragment. This gap can be repaired by the sequential action of DNA polymerase I and ligase. If such repair occurs, the structure can become a rolling circle with a growing point at the unimpeded rightward fork. If this repair does not occur (*i.e.*, in *pol*A⁻ or *lig*⁻ hosts), the rightward fork can continue around the circle — displacing a linear monomer when it reaches the gap (or nick). In *gam*⁻ infected cells the broken arm (a double-stranded, free-ended structure) is digested by the *rec*BC nuclease, thereby destroying the nascent rolling circle. The end product of such digestion is presumably a nicked or gapped circle, which might subsequently be repaired.

Now for the rightward fork. Here the break is on the strand being copied discontinuously, and the replication apparatus passes

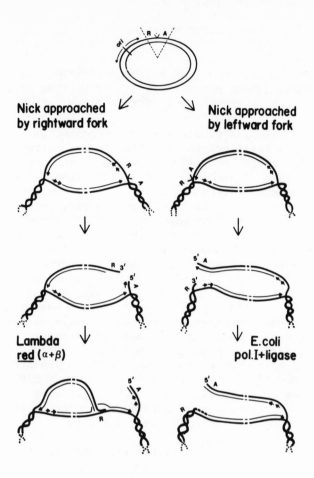

Nick approached
by rightward fork

Nick approached
by leftward fork

Lambda
red (α+β)

E.coli
pol.I+ligase

Figure 2. A model: Molecular mechanisms for the complementary
activity of the *red* recombination system and polymerase I-ligase
repair system in the production of rolling-circle replicating
structures.

right by it, displacing a replicated arm containing a parental
strand with a 3' end. Unless the nick has occurred at the start
of an Okazaki initiation site, the 3' end of the broken arm will
contain a single-stranded region — presumably of length the average
size of an Okazaki fragment. The replication fork continues along,
generating a second double-stranded arm that contains a parental
strand with a 5' end, identical to the arm generated by the leftward fork. If BC nuclease is active (in *gam⁻* infection), both arms
will be digested. In *gam⁺* infection, if nothing further happens
(*i.e.* in *red⁻polA⁻* infection), the two forks will continue around
the circle, generating one circle and one linear monomer at their
termination.

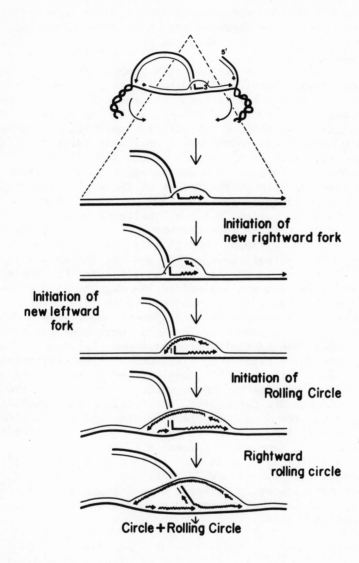

Figure 3.   Rolling circle from a *red*-promoted "D loop."

        Various models of *red*-mediated recombination involve a single-
stranded presynaptic intermediate (Radding, 1973). Such a structure
is contained at the terminus of the arm with the parental 3' end.
I propose that the *red* recombination system acts on this region and
its complementary sequence (here on the other parental strand, but
not necessarily) to form a *red*-mediated synaptic complex. Several
molecular mechanisms (see Radding, 1973; also Radding, this symposium) can be envisioned to resolve this complex into a "postsynap-
tic" structure containing old DNA linked to new and a new replication fork. (It is presumably through the generation of new replication forks that *red* affects the *rate* of λ DNA synthesis.)   Since
my results suggest that the *red*-mediated events, which affect phage
growth, do not involve DNA polymerase I or ligase [wild-type (*red*$^+$)
λ makes almost wild-type (*rec*$^+$) levels of DNA in *polA*$^-$ or *lig*$^-$
cells), I should like to propose a mechanism (Fig. 3) by which this
structure is resolved through the action of the replication apparatus itself. The proposed synaptic complex, as shown, has many of
the features of the so-called "D loops," believed to be the sites
of initiation of DNA replication (Kasamatsu *et al.*, 1971; Inman and
Schnös, 1973). These "D loops" contain only DNA. Some models of
λ replication invoke oligoribonucleotide primers (Hayes and Szybalski, 1973a,b). If such is the case, we must assume that the replication apparatus can also use a 3'-ended DNA segment as a primer.
The apparatus would then initiate synthesis from this point to form
a new rightward fork. The initially discontinuous leftward copy
from this fork continues around to form the continuous copy at a
new leftward fork. The initially discontinuous copy from the new
leftward fork continues rightward, displaces the parental strand
that initially formed the synaptic complex, and forms a third new
fork. Thus from an initial two forks we have five. After the first
four (opposite forks) are terminated, the double strand containing
what was originally the 3'-ended primer is attached to the 5'-ended
free tail. The last fork becomes the growing point of a rolling
circle. It cannot be terminated unless it encounters a nick. Thus
the replication apparatus at this fork is in a sense "trapped"; it
is unavailable to initiate at new "D loops" or *ori* sites. If the
number of such apparatuses is limited, such "trapping" is sufficient
to explain why λ circle (early) replication stops when rolling-circle
(late) replication begins.

        The termination of the first four of these forks and formation
of the rolling circle from the fifth can be visualized more easily
by drawing the *red*-promoted "D loop" at a complementary sequence
on a different circle rather than on the parental circle as was
shown in Fig. 3. This final diagram (Fig. 4) also illustrates how
some genetic recombinants might arise. The 3'-ended single-stranded
region from the arm of the first circle is in the area of gene R.
Therefore the join between the two genotypes represented in the
figure (RA and R'A') is between genes R and A'. If the original

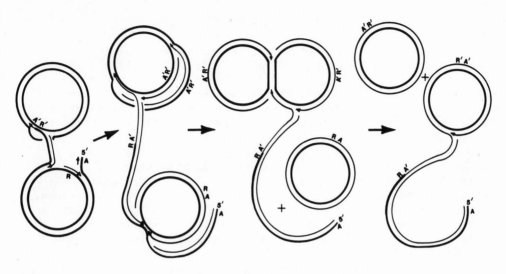

Figure 4. Rolling circle from a *red*-promoted "D loop" on a second circle. Arrows show the direction of *continuous* copying.

nick was not exactly at a cohesive end (*cos*) site or if it was any place else on the chromosome, maturation of DNA by cutting at the *cos* sites in the concatemer tail of the rolling circle will generate a (nonreciprocal?) recombinant phage.

The schemes shown in Figs. 2 to 4 provide no obvious role for the 5'→3' exonuclease activity of λ *exo* — an activity presumed to be involved in *red*-mediated recombination. It could be that this activity is necessary to achieve a proper "fit" in the synaptic complex. Alternatively, the exonuclease might be necessary (as mentioned above) in other pathways which can resolve synaptic complexes. In that case its role in this scheme would perhaps be passive — as part of a complex of enzymes which function together to accomplish several activities. The schemes do, however, predict the existence of another type of activity for the *red* system or for host proteins associated with the *red* system. This hypothetical activity is necessary to catalyze or stabilize an opening of the DNA duplex so that the single-stranded 3' end of the parental DNA can form a synaptic complex. Such activity could be assigned to a phage protein analogous, perhaps, to the gene 32 protein of T4 or the DNA binding protein of T7. The *beta* protein or an *exo-beta* complex, alone or in concert with the *Escherichia coli* binding protein, might possess such activity. Such possibilities might be testable. All of the *red* mutants that I have employed are, in fact, missing either just *beta* or *beta* and *exo*. Analysis of DNA synthesized by *red* mutants missing only λ exonuclease might provide some clues to the role of each of their proteins.

POST SCRIPTS

(1) For purposes of discussion, the nick essential to the scheme in Fig. 2 has been placed in a particular location. This is not critical to the model, and random (infrequent) breaks could generate rolling circles in a similar way--but these would have random starting points and roll in either direction. It seems unlikely that λ would leave such an important function completely to chance (although chance might suffice if the responsible endonuclease were missing). The ℓ strand between genes R and A seems a likely location for such a nick for the following reasons: (a) The resulting rolling circles roll in the direction in which they are probably packaged (N. Sternberg and R. A. Weisberg; M. Syvanen, personal communications) and in the direction in which at least one report suggests they are replicated (LePecq and Baldwin, 1968). (b) The *ter* endonuclease presumed to be encoded in the head gene A (Wang and Kaiser, 1973) might have the capacity under certain conditions to make a nick at this location. Coupling the nicking and formation of concatemers to packaging seems an economical twist. (c) Since the *ori* is closer to the right end, most of the time the nick will be approached first by the rightward fork, generating a substrate for the *red* pathway. This is the most efficient way for λ to make rolling circles, since it allows the initiation of new replication forks and thereby increases the rate of DNA synthesis.

(2) red^-pol^- ≈ $1/rec^-pol^-$ (?). Lambda, due to the peculiarities of its maturation and packaging system, needs concatemers to survive (Enquist and Skalka, 1973; Dawson, Skalka and Simon, in preparation). It does not seem unreasonable, then, that the phage has learned to produce a protein (*gamma*) that inhibits the potential threat to its concatemers embodied in the host's BC nuclease. *E. coli* has a circular chromosome, which probably must remain circular if the cell is to remain viable. For *E. coli*, then, the converse may be true. It might, in fact, need the BC nuclease to prevent the potential disaster created by the formation of linear (broken) chromosomes or rolling circles. An inability to prevent or control this kind of disaster (a *rec* mutation) coupled to the inability to repair interruptions which lead to it (a $polA^-$ mutation) may be a condition that leads to a slow but inevitable death (Monk and Kinross, 1972; Monk *et al.*, 1973). When viewed from this angle, both *red* and *rec* functions take on a new and interesting character. It seems possible that this view might have some relevance to analyses which consider the molecular mechanism involved in pathways that lead to genetic exchange.

REFERENCES

Carter, B. J., B. D. Shaw and M. G. Smith. 1969. Two stages in the replication of bacteriophage λ DNA. Biochim. Biophys. Acta 195: 494.

Enquist, L. W. and A. Skalka. 1973. Replication of bacteriophage λ DNA dependent on the function of host and viral genes. I. Interaction of *red*, *gam*, and *rec*. J. Mol. Biol. 75: 185.

Gottesman, M. M., M. L. Hicks and M. Gellert. 1973. Genetics and function of DNA ligase in *Escherichia coli*. J. Mol. Biol. 77: 531.

Hayes, S. and W. Szybalski. 1973a. Control of short leftward transcripts from the immunity and *ori* regions in induced coliphage lambda. Molec. Gen. Genet. 126: 275.

Hayes, S. and W. Szybalski. 1973b. Synthesis of RNA primer for lambda DNA replication is controlled by phage and host. In (B. A. Hamkalo and J. Papaconstantinou, eds.) Molecular Cytogenetics. p. 277. Plenum Press, New York.

Inman, R. B. and M. Schnös. 1971. Structure of branch points in replicating DNA; presence of single-stranded connections in λ DNA branch points. J. Mol. Biol. 56: 319.

Inman, R. B. and M. Schnös. 1973. D-Loops in intracellular λ DNA. In (R. D. Wells and R. B. Inman, eds.) DNA Synthesis In Vitro. p. 437. University Park Press, Baltimore.

Kasamatsu, H., D. L. Robberson and J. Vinograd. 1971. A novel close-circular mitochondrial DNA with properties of a replicating intermediate. Proc. Nat. Acad. Sci. U.S.A. 68: 2252.

LePecq, J. B. and R. L. Baldwin. 1968. The starting point and direction of λ DNA replication. Cold Spring Harbor Symp. Quant. Biol. 33: 609.

Monk, M. and J. Kinross. 1972. Conditional lethality of *rec* A and *rec* B derivatives of a strain of *Escherichia coli* K-12 with a temperature-sensitive deoxyribonucleic acid polymerase I. J. Bacteriol. 109: 971.

Monk, M., J. Kinross and C. D. Town. 1973. Deoxyribonucleic acid synthesis in *rec* A and *rec* B derivatives of an *Escherichia coli* K-12 strain with a temperature-sensitive deoxyribonucleic acid polymerase I. J. Bacteriol. 114: 1014.

Radding, C. M. 1973. Molecular mechanisms in genetic recombination. Ann. Rev. Genet. 7: 87.

Schnös, M. and R. B. Inman. 1970. Position of branch points in replicating λ DNA. J. Mol. Biol. 51: 61.

Skalka, A., M. Poonian and P. Bartl. 1972. Concatemers in DNA replication: Electron microscopic studies of partially denatured intracellular lambda DNA. J. Mol. Biol. 64: 541.

Wang, J. C. and A. D. Kaiser. 1973. Evidence that the cohesive ends of mature λ DNA are generated by the gene A product. Nature New Biol. 241: 16.

Zissler, J., E. Signer and F. Schaefer. 1971. The role of recombination in growth of bacteriophage lambda. I. The *gamma* gene. In (A. D. Hershey, ed.) The Bacteriophage Lambda. p. 455. Cold Spring Harbor Laboratory, Cold Spring Harbor, N.Y.

CONCERNING THE STEREOCHEMISTRY OF STRAND EQUIVALENCE IN GENETIC RECOMBINATION

Henry M. Sobell

Department of Chemistry, The University of Rochester, River Campus Station, Rochester, New York 14627 and Department of Radiation Biology and Biophysics, The University of Rochester, School of Medicine and Dentistry, Rochester, New York 14620

In their article describing the nature of crossed-strand exchange between homologous DNA molecules (a likely intermediate in genetic recombination), Sigal and Alberts (1972) have demonstrated the stereochemical feasibility of a connection in which all bases remain paired without undue bond strain or unfavorable contacts. They have provided the important additional observation that such a junction can migrate by a rotary diffusion mechanism; this would involve the exchange of two identical bases above or below the cross-connection, with an accompanying rotation of both helices in the same sense about their helical axes. Such a process could be rapid enough to account for the formation of extensive regions of hybrid DNA during genetic recombination (Meselson, 1972).

Of particular interest is an added suggestion by Sigal and Alberts concerning the nature of strand equivalence in genetic recombination: "If each of the rods supporting the two space-filling helices were cut at the level of the cross connection, the top sections of both double helices could be swiveled around each other without bond breakage. This would yield an identical cross strand exchange in which the top section, formerly on the left, is now on the right and vice versa. Moreover in this new strand exchange, the pair of 'outside strands' in the original strand exchange will become 'bridging strands,' while the original bridging strands will become outside strands. *The two forms of this strand exchange must*

433

be in rapid equilibrium at physiological temperatures. Therefore, any mechanism for terminating pairing by cutting bridging strands at the cross connection should generate DNA molecules with flanking genetic markers in parental configuration (XY and xy) at the same frequency as DNA molecules with flanking markers recombined (Xy and xY)" (Sigal and Alberts, 1972, p. 792, italics added). This interesting suggestion, however, was not further substantiated with the use of molecular models. This is unfortunate, since the kinetic properties of this interconversion would be expected to reflect its detailed stereochemistry.

     The purpose of this paper is to document the detailed stereo-chemical nature of strand equivalence in crossed-strand exchange between homologous DNA molecules. This study has suggested that the

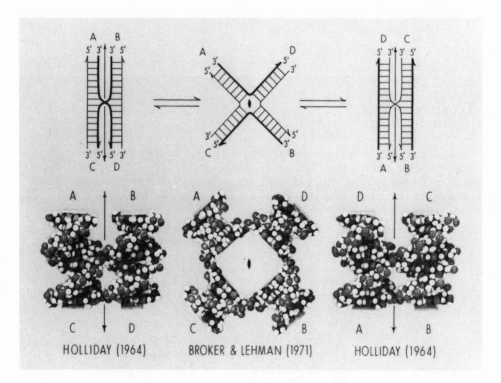

Figure 1. Schematic illustrations of the interconversion between the two forms of crossed-strand exchange leading to strand equiva-lence in genetic recombination, and their space-filling model (CPK) representations. In order to exchange bridging strands in the Holliday (1964) crossed-strand exchange shown on the left to the one shown on the right, one must pass through the fourfold junction described by Broker and Lehman (1971).

kinetics of interconversion between the two forms of crossed-strand
exchange may be significantly slower than that envisioned by Sigal
and Alberts. This finding may have important implications with
regard to current models for genetic recombination.

THE STEREOCHEMICAL NATURE OF STRAND EQUIVALENCE IN
CROSSED STRAND EXCHANGE

Figures 1 and 2 summarize the basic features of the stereochemical interconversion of bridging strands in a Holliday structure leading to strand equivalence. In order to interconvert
bridging strands in a crossed-strand exchange, one must rotate
helical DNA sections above and below the crossed-strand exchange
in a counterclockwise manner, simultaneously bending them apart to
obtain the fourfold structural intermediate described by Broker and
Lehman (1971). This fourfold junction can then be converted to an
identical Holliday structure with new bridging strands by continuing the combined operations of rotation and bending of helical DNA
sections in the same sense (see Fig. 2). Before interconversion,

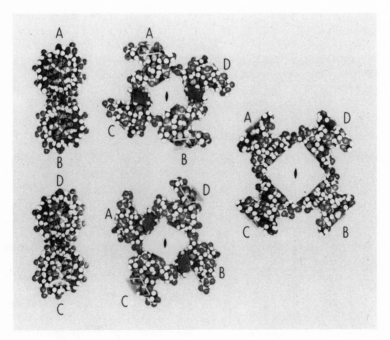

Figure 2. Sequence of conformational changes leading to the interconversion of bridging strands in a Holliday (1964) crossed-strand
exchange, using the space-filling (CPK) molecular representations.

section A lay "above" C, B "above" D. After interconversion, section D lay "above" A, C "above" B. It should be noted that DNA
sections formerly "on top" of the crossed-strand exchange (*i.e.*,
A and B) now lie "below" the new (and completely identical) crossed-
strand exchange. Furthermore, the interconversion process conserves
twofold symmetry at each step and, in this regard, obeys a simple
but elegant symmetry conservation rule.

What can be said about the probable kinetics of such an interconversion process? DNA molecules spanning thousands of Angstroms
almost certainly would require many seconds (even minutes) to undergo a conformational change such as this. One cannot envision a
rapid interconversion on the millisecond time scale at physiological
temperatures unless the conformational change was energetically
driven by some structural protein or endonucleolytic enzyme. Models
for genetic recombination which require the rapid interconversion
of bridging strands at migrating hybrid DNA junctions may require
modification along these lines. My own model for genetic recombination requires no such modification.

STRAND EQUIVALENCE AND THE HOLLIDAY SYNAPTIC STRUCTURE

My recombination model begins with the postulate that there
exist branch migratable regions at the ends of genes or operons
(promoters), which act (after "nicking") as pairing regions for
synapsis (for previous details, see Sobell, 1972, 1973). Synapsis
between homologous DNA molecules then occurs through a series of
branch migration steps to give the central structural intermediate
shown in Fig. 3. This intermediate structure has two fourfold
Broker-Lehman junctions; each independently can give rise to a
crossed-strand exchange before final closure by ligase to give a
total of *four* different Holliday synaptic structures. These structures can then migrate into the structural genome and be resolved
by nucleolytic action to effect genetic recombination. Two Holliday synaptic structures would be expected to contain pairs of
bridging strands of the same polarity (*i.e.*, 5'-3', 5'-3' in one
crossed-strand exchange and 5'-3', 5'-3' in the other crossed-strand
exchange; or 3'-5', 3'-5' in one crossed-strand exchange and 3'-5',
3'-5' in the other crossed-strand exchange). Synaptic structures
of these types (types I) can give rise to single-strand exchange
events; this results in a parental configuration of flanking markers
in recombinant molecules. Two Holliday synaptic structures are
expected to contain pairs of bridging strands with a mixed polarity
(*i.e.*, 5'-3', 5'-3' in one crossed-strand exchange and 3'-5', 3'-5'
in the other crossed-strand exchange; or 3'-5', 3'-5' in one crossed-strand exchange and 5'-3', 5'-3' in the other crossed-strand
exchange). Synaptic structures of these types (types II) can give
rise to double-strand exchange events, resulting in a recombinant

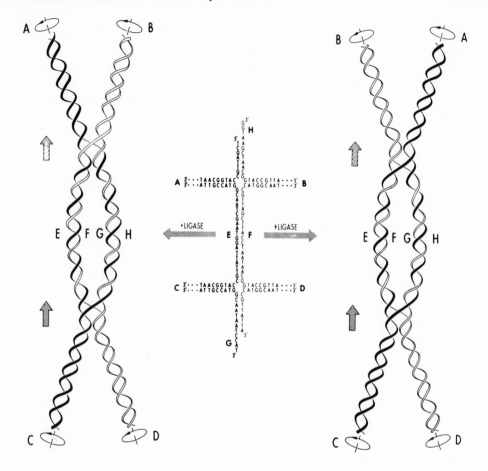

Figure 3. Utilization of the stereochemical information shown in
Figs. 1 and 2 to form the two types of Holliday synaptic structures

configuration of flanking markers in recombinant molecules. It
should be noted that type I synaptic structures must have an integral multiple of *ten* base pairs in each hybrid DNA section, while
type II synaptic structures must have an integral multiple of *five*
base pairs in each hybrid DNA section. Since all four types of
synaptic structures can form with equal probability, one would expect to find equal frequencies of parental and recombinant flanking
marker configurations in genetic recombination, in accord with the
data for gene conversion in yeast (see, *e.g.*, Hurst *et al.*, 1972).

ACKNOWLEDGMENTS

This work has been supported in part by grants from the National Institutes of Health, the American Cancer Society, and the Atomic Energy Commission. This paper has been assigned report no. UR-3490-501 at the Atomic Energy Project, the University of Rochester.

REFERENCES

Broker, T. R. and I. R. Lehman. 1971. Branched DNA molecules: intermediates in T4 recombination. J. Mol. Biol. 60: 131.

Holliday, R. 1964. A mechanism for gene conversion in fungi. Genet. Res. 5: 282.

Hurst, D. D., S. Fogel and R. K. Mortimer. 1972. Conversion-associated recombination in yeast. Proc. Nat. Acad. Sci. U.S.A. 69: 101.

Meselson, M. 1972. Formation of hybrid DNA by rotary diffusion during genetic recombination. J. Mol. Biol. 71: 795.

Sigal, N. and B. Alberts. 1972. Genetic recombination: The nature of a crossed strand exchange between two homologous DNA molecules. J. Mol. Biol. 71: 789.

Sobell, H. M. 1972. Molecular mechanism for genetic recombination. Proc. Nat. Acad. Sci. U.S.A. 69: 2483.

Sobell, H. M. 1973. Symmetry in protein-nucleic acid interaction and its genetic implications. Advan. Genet. 17: 411.

THE EVOLUTION OF RECOMBINATION MODELS

Rollin D. Hotchkiss

The Rockefeller University, New York, New York 10021

The search for a general model or description of genetic recombination has stirred many investigators over the years, and has been recently intensified as we seem to be coming within reach of some manipulable components of the system. It seems to me that this search, though conceptual, has had its own evolution like any material system.

What do we mean, first of all, by a general model of genetic recombination? I venture to say that it would be a model whose general features encompass specific observations from a broad variety of different recombination systems, and it would present a mechanism whose successive steps follow one another in some obligatory and predictable fashion. Whether a mechanism should also be taken to be concerted or directed toward recombination is at the very least debatable. It seems wiser to consider them as pathways that may lead to recombination, as one result of the alternative modes of resolving tangled DNA complexes entraining biparental components. Of course, general remarks can be contrived about any set of observations, but most such remarks will not deserve consideration as models or theories. Perhaps a theory can be said to be general when the empirical corrections, variations, or exceptions to it are "mere details" — i.e. occur at a lower level in the hierarchy of "causes" and effects than those specified in the model. And it is useful if it consolidates observations under an easily learned scheme, and productive if it leads to experiments that test its own scheme, or at least experiments that narrow down one's predictions.

Successive ideas in genetics have all come as a kind of "exception" to earlier generalizations. Linkage was an exception to

free assortment; recombination was an exception superimposed upon
total linkage. Now we have exceptions to random recombination, and
these have for a time tended to obstruct the unification of ideas
of mechanism derived in different systems. I have argued elsewhere
(Hotchkiss, 1971) that, in essence, all of these aberrations of recombination consist of the observation of a number of recombinants
within some subpopulation that is larger or smaller than that expected on some basis that is "satisfactory" in other applications.
Of course, this assumed basis may or may not already include different amounts of the distortion — therefore, expectations can in
various systems be higher or lower than the final observations. One
notes that recombination models through the last decade have increasingly tried to take account of these apparent exceptions at the
new level: gene conversion in particular, interference, nonadditivity, map distortion, polarity, and the like.

The original notion of breakage-and-rejoining implicit in the
ideas of Sturtevant and Morgan seemed to imply almost miraculous
exactness when the maps they made possible began to acquire enormous
detail. Perhaps for this reason, around the 1950s "copy-switch"
models were resurrected for recombination — but these in turn seemed
excluded when it became clear that in a number of systems, including
eukaryotic ones, actual preexisting segments of DNA or chromosome
strands exchanged places. But most recent models include some
features of both breakage-rejoining and copying of the wrong template. The harmony came about with the recognition of the complementary double-stranded nature of DNA.

The models of Whitehouse and of Holliday (Holliday, 1964;
Whitehouse and Hastings, 1965) have been valuable in the teaching
of genetics, since they restate in concise form the nature of findings in recombination, although without much predictivity. Furthermore, they were early in taking explicit and general advantage of
the duplex DNA structure to reduce the problems of register and
precision in a recombination by having single strands find their
place in a foreign duplex for the site of exact complementary fit.
The Whitehouse models could more easily permit single-strand copy
choice to create new heterozygosity; but both invoked — at an early
time — excision and repair to explain, especially, the possibility
of conversion or of making an extra copy of a parental allele. But
it was Holliday's model that outlined most simply and clearly how
the switching of single homologous strand ends could produce a complex potentially capable of yielding in fewer steps the observed
products. I think it is fair to say that the Holliday structure
with joined homologous single strands is at least one step, and that
it is the principal basis for biparental joining ultimately called
for in all modern recombination models. It is, in a sense, the only
sophisticated way in which two homologous DNAs can become covalently
joined.

Conversion was once considered to be a special, exceptional event, as rare as the systems in which it can be unequivocally detected. But now it can be considered as the "local noise" produced at the borderline of a classical recombination. In most systems there is no marker available at the site, and no possibility of making a balance sheet to demonstrate such a conversion. Thus these conversions could account for mapping disturbances, etc., at this junction for most recombinations; but provision is required for at least some few recombinations in which they are minimal or absent. A further implication of this ubiquitousness of conversions would be that "silent" conversions at least — I have called them "molecular" conversions (Hotchkiss, 1973) — are even more common than recombinations. For, among detected conversions, it is now established that just about one-half (Whitehouse, 1969; Fogel *et al.*, 1971) are not accompanied by recombination.

These last findings have led to the postulation, in several recent models, of a symmetrical resolution step equally likely to resolve the biparental complex with or without outside marker recombination (Holliday, 1974; Sigal and Alberts, 1972). It should be pointed out that, in comparisons of symmetries and configurations, the similarities or differences have to be separately evaluated at three different levels: the physical strands as such, strands with respect to origin, and strands with respect to information carried on them. These resolution steps have received new elegance since they have been explained upon the basis of the explicit helix isomerism described by Sigal and Alberts (1972) for a whole series of intermediates of different origin. The intermediate favored in most of the recently proposed models is similar to the Holliday intermediate.

Although the symmetry of the resolution step can explain the genesis of recombinant and nonrecombinant products, there are other signs that recombinations are not totally reciprocal — such observations as polarity, unequal frequency of reciprocal products, marker effects, and other local effects. For this reason, some of us have been emphasizing a nonreciprocality in the way in which the two parental DNA components enter into the *formation* of an intermediate complex (Paszewski, 1970; Boon and Zinder, 1969; Hotchkiss, 1971, 1973). By considering the two parentals as taking different roles, something like the donor and recipient in the first exchange of parts, one can understand the unequal contributions of the parents and still retain the symmetrical resolution.

This evolution has taken us all the way from symmetrical complexes, which were first proposed to undergo unexplained unsymmetrical repair or resolution steps, around to unsymmetrical complexes, which are now pictured as generally undergoing random escape steps in resolution.

The dynamics by which the symmetrical resolutions become available are the structural dynamics of helix isomerization — the lateral migration of cross-links and strand rotation about the cross-links. As such, these processes probably partake of the very considerable similarity in DNA from one organism to another. The dynamics of the asymmetric steps (especially in the earlier stages) probably derive from the components that are more likely to be different in different species and mutants of the same species. These are the various "nicking" endonucleases, the exonucleases, polymerases, and even perhaps the ligases, now widely held to accomplish the relevant molecular changes in the DNA substance. A few of us have been suggesting lately that the relative rates of polymerase and excision steps could determine the extent and outcome of various steps in recombination (Hotchkiss, 1973; Holliday, 1974). I think this kind of relative differential might underlie the differences Clark finds in his pathways of recombination (see Gillen and Clark, this volume).

As unsolved questions in this area, I should like to suggest that we know too little as yet about the potential "bridge-clipping" mechanisms and homology requirements in various strand migrations. While the resolution of a double-bridge complex is intuitively simple to portray, we still do not know whether it may be a simultaneous event with steric restrictions, a concerted pair of endonucleolytic breakages, or a pair of successive reactions (Hotchkiss, 1971) with their own interpolated probability of completion. Any postulated recognition system must somehow avoid clipping the kind of single bridges that presumably occur at a replication fork.

Secondly, the very essence of heterologous recombination — the possibilities for hybrid formation, bridge migration, and strand repair — all depend upon how the strands and DNA enzymes perceive base mismatches and physical mispairing (gaps or loops). If the strand segments newly pairing as the result of displacement, exonucleolytic erosion of an existing strand, or migration can be stampeded into accepting approximations that a polymerase might never permit — or conversely if they reject them — there may be limitations upon the strand migrations we draw in our molecular schemes. If we can learn more about these matters, we can know and not merely assume what the probabilities are for forming, extending, incorporating, or terminating hybrid regions with various configurations. That is, we may then better understand what we now call marker effects.

In summary, the quantitative variations of recombination, once considered aberrations, are increasingly viewed as resulting from the not always random differences in activity levels of the several enzymes of DNA repair, while the more commonly random steps are increasingly believed to derive from the essentially random diffusion of cross-links and base pairs within the DNA molecules. The former, more specific steps are probably involved in originating and fixing an intermediate and the latter, more random ones in achieving its resolution into recombinant products.

REFERENCES

Boon, T. and N. D. Zinder. 1969. Proc. Nat. Acad. Sci. U.S.A. 64: 573.

Fogel, S., D. D. Hurst and R. K. Mortimer. 1971. In (G. Kimber and G. P. Rédei, eds.) Stadler Genetics Symposia, Vols. 1 and 2, pp. 89-110. University of Missouri Agricultural Experiment Station, Columbia, Mo.

Holliday, R. 1964. Genet. Res. 5: 282.

Holliday, R. 1974. Genetics, in press.

Hotchkiss, R. D. 1971. Advan. Genet. 16: 325.

Hotchkiss, R. D. 1973. In (G. Kimber and G. P. Rédei, eds.) Stadler Genetics Symposia, Vol. 5, pp. 145-160. University of Missouri Agricultural Experiment Station, Columbia, Mo.

Paszewski, A. 1970. Genet. Res. 15: 55.

Sigal, N. and B. Alberts. 1972. J. Mol. Biol. 71: 789.

Whitehouse, H. L. K. and P. J. Hastings. 1965. Genet. Res. 6: 27.

Whitehouse, H. L. K. 1969. Towards an Understanding of the Mechanism of Heredity, 2nd ed., p. 317. St. Martins Press, New York.

CONTRIBUTORS

BAKER, B. S., Department of Genetics, University of Wisconsin, Madison, Wisconsin 53706

BANKS, G. R., National Institute for Medical Research, Mill Hill, London NW7 1AA, England

BASEE, S. K., The Public Health Research Institute of the City of New York, Inc., New York, New York 10016

BENBOW, R. M., MRC Laboratory of Molecular Biology, Hills Road, Cambridge, England CB2-2QH

BLATTNER, F. R., McArdle Laboratory for Cancer Research, University of Wisconsin, Madison, Wisconsin 53706

BOREL, J. D., McArdle Laboratory for Cancer Research, University of Wisconsin, Madison, Wisconsin 53706

CARPENTER, A. T. C., Department of Zoology, University of Wisconsin, Madison, Wisconsin 53706

CHOVNICK, A., Genetics and Cell Biology Section, Biological Sciences Group, The University of Connecticut, Storrs, Connecticut 06268

CHUNG, S., Department of Molecular Biology, University of California, Berkeley, California 94720

CIRIGLIANO, C., Department of Microbiology, The Public Health Research Institute of the City of New York, Inc., New York, New York 10016

CLARK, A. J., Department of Molecular Biology, University of California, Berkeley, California 94720

COHEN, S. N., Department of Medicine, Stanford University School of Medicine, Stanford, California 94305

COSLOY, S. D., The Public Health Research Institute of the City of New York, Inc., New York, New York 10016

445

COUNCE, S. J., Departments of Anatomy and Zoology, Duke University
     Medical Center, Durham, North Carolina 27710

DAY, J. W., Biology Division, Oak Ridge National Laboratory, Oak
     Ridge, Tennessee 37830

DUBNAU, D., Department of Microbiology, The Public Health Research
     Institute of the City of New York, Inc., New York, New York
     10016

DUJON, B., Centre de Génétique Moléculaire du C.N.R.S. 91190,
     Gif-Sur-Yvette, France

ECHOLS, H., Department of Molecular Biology, University of Cali-
     fornia, Berkeley, California 94720

ESPOSITO, M. S., Erman Biology Center, Department of Biology,
     University of Chicago, Chicago, Illinois 60637

ESPOSITO, R. E., Erman Biology Center, Department of Biology,
     University of Chicago, Chicago, Illinois 60637

FINK, G. R., Department of Genetics Development and Physiology,
     Cornell University, Ithaca, New York 14850

FOGEL, S., Department of Genetics, University of California,
     Berkeley, California 94720

FOX, M. S., Department of Biology, Massachusetts Institute of
     Technology, Cambridge, Massachusetts 02139

GELBART, W. M., Genetics and Cell Biology Section, Biological
     Sciences Group, The University of Connecticut, Storrs,
     Connecticut 06268

GILLEN, J. R., Department of Molecular Biology, University of
     California, Berkeley, California 94720

GOLDMAN, S. L., Department of Biology, The University of Toledo,
     Toledo, Ohio 43606

GOODGAL, S. H., Department of Microbiology, University of Pennsyl-
     vania, Philadelphia, Pennsylvania 19104

GREEN, L., Department of Molecular Biology, University of California,
     Berkeley, California 94720

GRELL, R. F., Biology Division, Oak Ridge National Laboratory, Oak
     Ridge, Tennessee 37830

GROMKOVA, R., Department of Microbiology, University of Pennsylvania, Philadelphia, Pennsylvania 19104

GUTZ, H., Division of Biological Sciences, The University of Texas at Dallas, Dallas, Texas 75230

HENDERSON, D., Department of Molecular Biology, Vanderbilt University, Nashville, Tennessee 37203

HINTON, C. W., Department of Biology, The College of Wooster, Wooster, Ohio 44691

HOLLIDAY, R., National Institute for Medical Research, Mill Hill, London NW7 1AA, England

HOLLOMAN, W. K., National Institute for Medical Research, Mill Hill, London NW7 1AA, England

HOTCHKISS, R. D., The Rockefeller University, New York, New York 10021

IMADA, S., Department of Molecular, Cellular and Developmental Biology, University of Colorado, Boulder, Colorado 80302

KARU, A. E., Department of Biochemistry, University of California, Berkeley, California 94720

KUSHNER, S. R., Department of Biochemistry, University of Georgia, Athens, Georgia 30602

LACKS, S., Biology Department, Brookhaven National Laboratory, Upton, New York 11973

LECLERC, E., Department of Biological Chemistry, Harvard Medical School, Boston, Massachusetts 02115

LINN, S., Department of Biochemistry, University of California, Berkeley, California 94720

McCARRON, M., Genetics and Cell Biology Section, Biological Sciences Group, The University of Connecticut, Storrs, Connecticut 06268

MOENS, P. B., York University, Downsview, Ontario, Canada

MOORE, C. W., Department of Biology, University of Rochester, Rochester, New York 14627

MORTIMER, R. K., Division of Medical Physics and Donner Laboratory, University of California, Berkeley, California 94720

MOSES, M. J., Departments of Anatomy and Zoology, Duke University
    Medical Center, Durham, North Carolina 27710

MOSIG, G., Department of Molecular Biology, Vanderbilt University,
    Nashville, Tennessee 37203

NAGAISHI, H., Department of Molecular Biology, University of
    California, Berkeley, California 94720

OISHI, M., The Public Health Research Institute of the City of
    New York, Inc., New York, New York 10016

PANDEY, J., Genetics and Cell Biology Section, Biological Sciences
    Group, The University of Connecticut, Storrs, Connecticut
    06268

PLOTKIN, D. J., Erman Biology Center, Department of Biology,
    University of Chicago, Chicago, Illinois 60637

PUGH, J. E., National Institute for Medical Research, Mill Hill,
    London NW7 1AA, England

RADDING, C. M., Department of Medicine and Molecular Biophysics and
    Biochemistry, Yale University, New Haven, Connecticut 06510

SAKAKI, Y., The Mitsubishi-Kasei Institute of Life Sciences, 11
    Minamiooya, Machida-shi, Tokyo, Japan

SETLOW, J. K., Department of Biology, Brookhaven National Laboratory,
    Upton, New York 11973

SHAFER, A. J., Division of Biology, California Institute of Tech-
    nology, Pasadena, California 91109

SHEAR, C. G., Department of Biology, Emory University, Atlanta,
    Georgia 30322

SHERMAN, F., Department of Radiation Biology and Biophysics,
    University of Rochester, Rochester, New York 14642

SHINNICK, T. M., McArdle Laboratory for Cancer Research, University
    of Wisconsin, Madison, Wisconsin 53706

SINSHEIMER, R. L., Division of Biology, California Institute of
    Technology, Pasadena, California 91109

SKALKA, A., Roche Institute of Molecular Biology, Nutley, New
    Jersey 07110

SMITH, P. D., Department of Biology, Emory University, Atlanta, Georgia 30322

SOBELL, H. M., Department of Chemistry, The University of Rochester, River Campus Station, Rochester, New York 14627 and Department of Radiation Biology and Biophysics, The University of Rochester School of Medicine and Dentistry, Rochester, New York 14620

STAHL, F. W., Institute of Molecular Biology, University of Oregon, Eugene, Oregon 97403

STAHL, M. M., Institute of Molecular Biology, University of Oregon, Eugene, Oregon 97403

STERNBERG, N., Laboratory of Molecular Genetics, NICHD, NIH, Bethesda, Maryland 20014

SUEOKA, N., Department of Molecular, Cellular and Developmental Biology, University of Colorado, Boulder, Colorado 80302

SYVANEN, M., Department of Biochemistry, Stanford University School of Medicine, Stanford, California 94305

SZYBALSKI, W., McArdle Laboratory for Cancer Research, University of Wisconsin, Madison, Wisconsin 53706

TIRABY, J.-G., Laboratoire de Génétique, Université de Toulouse, 118, Route de Narbonne, 31-Toulouse, France

UNRAU, P., National Institute for Medical Research, Mill Hill, London NW7 1AA, England

WACKERNAGEL, W., Abteilung Biologie, Lehrstuhl Biologie der Mikroorganismen, Ruhr-Universität, 463 Bochum, West Germany

WEIL, J., Department of Molecular Biology, Vanderbilt University, Nashville, Tennessee 37235

WEISBERG, R. A., Laboratory of Molecular Genetics, NICHD, NIH, Bethesda, Maryland 20014

WHITE, R. L., Department of Biochemistry, Stanford University School of Medicine, Stanford, California 94304

ZINDER, N. D., The Rockefeller University, New York, New York 10021

ZUCCARELLI, A. J., Fachbereich Biologie, Universität Konstanz, D-775 Konstanz, West Germany